Cooking Light.

THE FOOD LOVER'S
HEALTHY
HABITS
COOKBOOK

ISBN-13: 978-0-8487-3476-3
ISBN-10: 0-8487-3476-9

Library of Congress Control Number: 2011941972
Printed in the United States of America
First printing 2012

Be sure to check with your health-care provider before making any changes in your diet.

Oxmoor House
Editorial Director: Leah McLaughlin
Creative Director: Felicity Keane
Brand Manager: Michelle Turner Aycock
Senior Editor: Heather Averett
Managing Editor: Rebecca Benton

Cooking Light *The Food Lover's Healthy Habits Cookbook*
Editor: Rachel Quinlivan West, RD
Art Director: Claire Cormany
Project Editor: Emily Chappell
Assistant Designer: Allison Sperando Potter
Director, Test Kitchen: Elizabeth Tyler Austin
Assistant Directors, Test Kitchen: Julie Christopher, Julie Gunter
Recipe Developers and Testers: Wendy Ball, RD; Victoria E. Cox; Tamara Goldis;
    Stefanie Maloney; Callie Nash; Karen Rankin; Leah Van Deren
Recipe Editor: Alyson Moreland Haynes
Food Stylists: Margaret Monroe Dickey, Catherine Crowell Steele
Photography Director: Jim Bathie
Senior Photographer: Hélène Dujardin
Senior Photo Stylist: Kay E. Clarke
Photo Stylist: Mindi Shapiro Levine
Assistant Photo Stylist: Mary Louise Menendez
Senior Production Manager: Greg A. Amason
Production Manager: Theresa Beste-Farley

Contributors
Author: Janet Helm, MS, RD
Writer: Hallie Levine Sklar
Designers: Hudd Byard, Carol Damsky, Emily Albright Parrish, David Terry
Cooking and Lifestyle Coach: Allison Fishman
Fitness Expert: Myatt Murphy, CSCS
Copy Editors: Julie Bosché, Dolores Hydock, Tara Trenary
Proofreader: Jacqueline Giovanelli
Indexer: Mary Ann Laurens
Recipe Developers and Testers: Martha Condra, Erica Hopper,
    Kathleen Royal Phillips
Food Stylists: Abby Gaskins, Tami Hardeman, Ana Kelly, Angie Mosier
Photographers: Iain Bagwell, Mark Manne, Mary Britton Senseney
Photo Stylist: Katherine Eckert Coyne
Interns: Erin Bishop; Morgan Bolling; Jessica Cox, RD; Laura Hoxworth;
    Susan Kemp; Alison Loughman; Anna Pollock; Emily Robinson;
    Lindsay A. Rozier; Maria Sanders; Katie Strasser

Time Home Entertainment Inc.
Publisher: Jim Childs
VP, Strategy & Business Development: Steven Sandonato
Executive Director, Marketing Services: Carol Pittard
Executive Director, Retail & Special Sales: Tom Mifsud
Director, Bookazine Development & Marketing: Laura Adam
Executive Publishing Director: Joy Butts
Associate Publishing Director: Megan Pearlman
Finance Director: Glenn Buonocore
Associate General Counsel: Helen Wan

Cooking Light
Editor: Scott Mowbray
Creative Director: Carla Frank
Executive Managing Editor: Phillip Rhodes
Executive Editor, Food: Ann Taylor Pittman
Special Publications Editor: Mary Simpson Creel, MS, RD
Senior Food Editors: Timothy Q. Cebula, Julianna Grimes
Senior Editor: Cindy Hatcher
Assistant Editor, Nutrition: Sidney Fry, MS, RD
Assistant Editors: Kimberly Holland, Phoebe Wu
Test Kitchen Director: Vanessa T. Pruett
Assistant Test Kitchen Director: Tiffany Vickers Davis
Recipe Testers and Developers: Robin Bashinsky, Adam Hickman, Deb Wise
Art Directors: Fernande Bondarenko, Shawna Kalish
Associate Art Director: Rachel Cardina Lasserre
Senior Designer: Anna Bird
Designer: Hagen Stegall
Assistant Designer: Nicole Gerrity
Photo Director: Kristen Schaefer
Assistant Photo Editor: Amy Delaune
Senior Photographer: Randy Mayor
Senior Photo Stylist: Cindy Barr
Chief Food Stylist: Kellie Gerber Kelley
Food Styling Assistant: Blakeslee Wright
Production Director: Liz Rhoades
Production Editor: Hazel R. Eddins
Assistant Production Editor: Josh Rutledge
Copy Chief: Maria Parker Hopkins
Assistant Copy Chief: Susan Roberts
Research Editor: Michelle Gibson Daniels
Administrative Coordinator: Carol D. Johnson
CookingLight.com Editor: Allison Long Lowery
CookingLight.com Nutrition Editor: Holley Johnson Grainger, MS, RD
CookingLight.com Associate Editor/Producer: Mallory Daugherty Brasseale

To order additional publications, call 1-800-765-6400 or
1-800-491-0551.

For more books to enrich your life, visit **oxmoorhouse.com**

To search, savor, and share thousands of recipes, visit **myrecipes.com**

Cooking Light

THE FOOD LOVER'S
HEALTHY HABITS
COOKBOOK

with JANET HELM, MS, RD

Oxmoor
House®

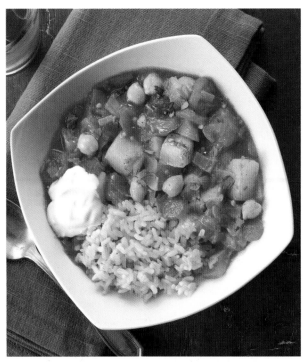

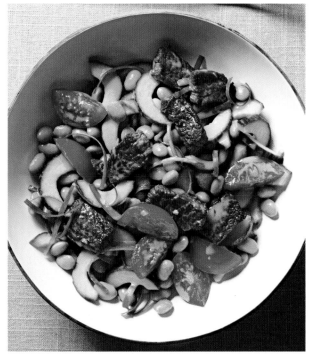

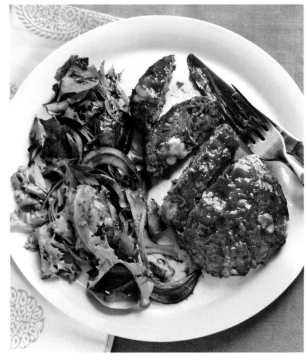

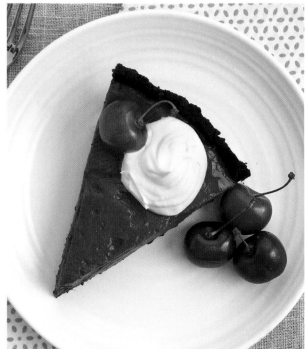

WELCOME

It's all here. This book is the culmination of the 12 Healthy Habits program that began in *Cooking Light* magazine and on CookingLight.com. Our hope is that this book will help you make changes that will have a positive effect on your health and happiness. I was especially thrilled to be a part of this project because the approach is so consistent with my own nutrition philosophy as a registered dietitian. The emphasis is on health, not weight. No foods are forbidden, and eating is revered as a source of pleasure, not guilt or regret.

Rooted in the science of habit formation, this book is a guide to making positive, lasting changes in your life. Basically, everything we do is a bunch of habits. All the choices we make every day—the foods we buy, how much we eat, and how often we exercise—may seem like well-considered decisions, but most of the time they're automatic choices.

It's tough to fully eradicate old habits; they must be replaced by new behaviors. This book will help you do that. Each chapter is an action plan for adopting a new habit. The goal is to make these behaviors your new routine. Our 6-week plan starting on page 328 will help you get started and keep you on track.

Change seems more doable when we see others succeed. That's why researchers have found that healthy behaviors can be contagious in social networks—whether that community is virtual, at work, or in your neighborhood. We saw just how influential online communities can be with the 12 Healthy Habits program. You can benefit from those inspiring personal stories and the tips and tricks that have worked for others. Now it's up to you, and we hope you enjoy the journey.

To your health and happiness,

Janet Helm, MS, RD

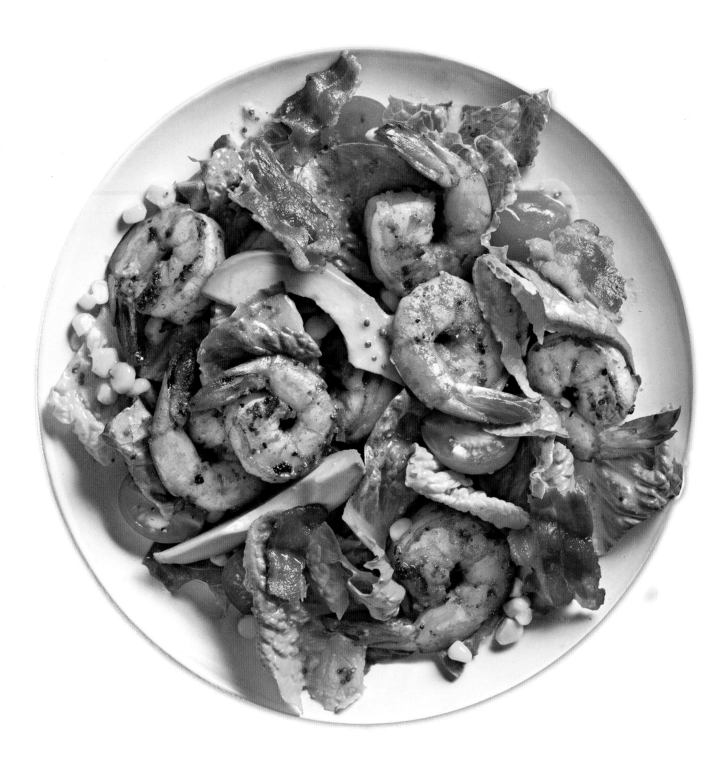

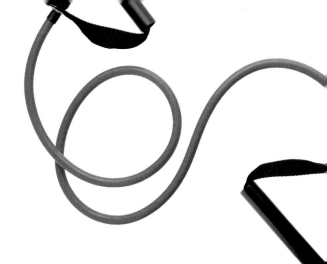

CONTENTS

Introduction 8

Get Cooking............................. 14

Eat Breakfast Daily 50

Go for Whole Grains 76

Get Moving............................. 110

Veggie Up................................ 132

Eat More Fish 168

Eat More Healthy Fats............. 202

Go Meatless One Day a Week 224

Get Stronger............................ 248

Eat Less Salt............................. 266

Be Portion-Aware...................... 286

Eat Mindfully............................ 308

6-Week Plan............................. 328

Nutritional Analysis 342

Metric Equivalents 343

References 344

Index…...347

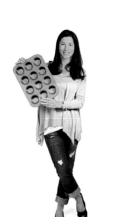
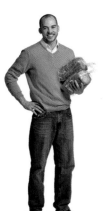
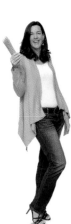
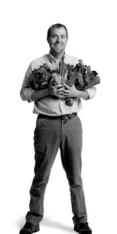
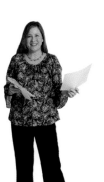
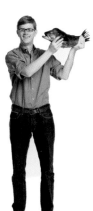

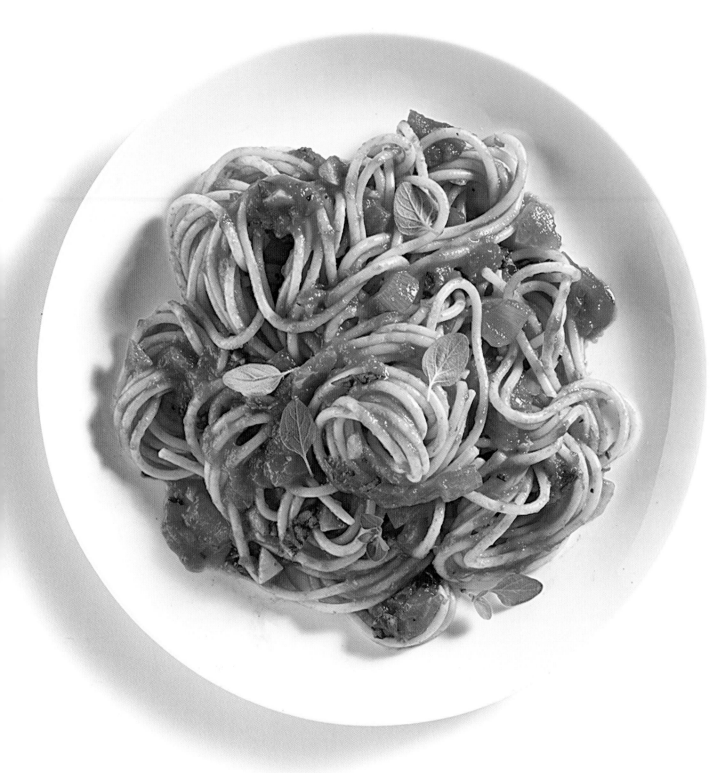

WELCOME TO THE 12 HEALTHY HABITS

Get ready to change your life, one delicious meal and one healthy habit at a time. Delicious and healthy can happily coexist, and they should. *The Food Lover's Healthy Habits Cookbook* will show you how. It's a book that helps you improve your health and encourages you to embrace the joyous pleasures of the table.

This is not a diet book. Instead of taking a quick-fix approach, this book highlights the importance of healthy habits. The focus is on changing behaviors and learning how to eat for a lifetime. After all, healthy eating should be enjoyable, easy, and gimmick-free, not bogged down by rules and restrictions.

With our approach, you'll find that nothing is off limits. In fact, nearly all the 12 healthy habits are positive changes—things to add instead of eliminate, such as vegetables, fruits, whole grains, healthy fats, seafood, and breakfast. The emphasis is on savoring flavorful whole foods, practicing moderation, being mindful, and staying active. You won't find a list of foods to avoid. Strict boundaries and extremes aren't sustainable. A healthy approach to eating includes permission to satisfy that part of the soul that craves chocolate, gooey mac and cheese, or juicy burgers. The key is balance.

HEALTHY LIFESTYLE HABITS

As much as you may want to make healthier choices, change can be hard. Even the awareness of what to do is not always enough. You've heard many times before what it means to eat healthier and why physical activity is important. The challenge is making it happen.

It all comes down to establishing a different daily routine and adopting new habits. A habit has been described as an intersection of knowledge, skill, and desire. To make something a habit, you need all three.

We're here to help you move past knowledge, giving you new skills, realistic solutions, concrete ideas, and delicious recipes to adopt a dozen healthy habits—behaviors that science tells us will have the greatest impact on our health. We also hope to inspire and motivate you by showcasing other people who are on the same journey to change their habits and live a healthier life.

Enjoy your food, but eat less.

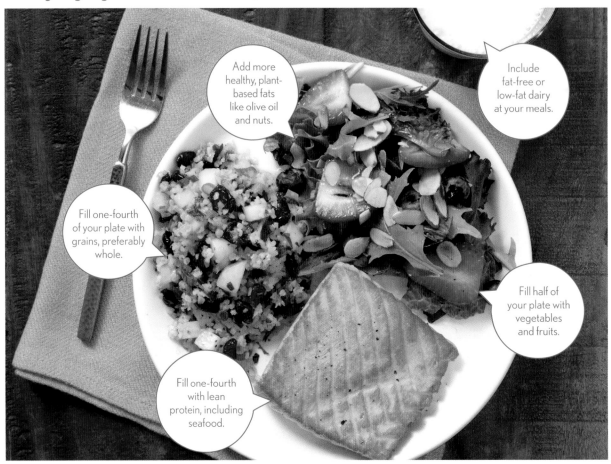

Add more healthy, plant-based fats like olive oil and nuts.

Include fat-free or low-fat dairy at your meals.

Fill one-fourth of your plate with grains, preferably whole.

Fill half of your plate with vegetables and fruits.

Fill one-fourth with lean protein, including seafood.

WHAT THIS BOOK IS ABOUT

This book is a reflection of the stories we heard, the challenges people faced, and the positive changes they've made. Think of it as your guide to a healthier lifestyle with lots of road-tested tips and tricks that have worked for others. You'll find simple moves and good food that can change your life.

Sometimes all the "shoulds" can be overwhelming. That's why we've taken the big picture of good health and broken it down into bite-sized nuggets so you can focus on one habit at a time. Each habit includes a measurable goal, along with specific steps to help you reach it. All 12 healthy habits are intended to get you closer to the latest nutrition and physical fitness guidelines. These are the daily behaviors that will help you live a long, healthy life.

YOUR 12 HEALTHY HABIT GOALS

➤ Cook at least three more meals per week.

➤ Eat a healthy breakfast every day of the week.

➤ Eat three servings of whole grains each day.

➤ Be active for 30 minutes a day, three times a week.

➤ Eat three servings of veggies each day.

➤ Make seafood the centerpiece of two meals a week.

➤ Increase healthy fats and decrease unhealthy fats every day.

➤ Go meatless one day a week for all three meals.

➤ Add strength training at least two times a week.

➤ Reduce the amount of sodium you eat every day.

➤ Find strategies to help you eat less without thinking about it.

➤ Be mindful, purposeful, and joyful each time you eat.

WHAT THIS BOOK IS NOT ABOUT

This is not a book to help you quickly lose weight or get ready for bikini season. It's not about blasting belly fat. You won't see the words "detox" or "cleanse" anywhere on these pages. Instead, this book will help you get off the diet merry-go-round and find a way to eat (and enjoy) food for the rest of your life. The answer doesn't lie in the latest fad diet. The path to better health and a trimmer waistline is through establishing new habits. It's about embracing new behaviors that you can sustain for life. Keeping pleasure in the picture will help.

HOW TO USE THIS BOOK

Try to focus on one habit at a time, and commit to it intently for one month. Pick one habit that you want to start with, and then work your way through the book. You can go in order or skip around if you'd like, although you may want to start with the first habit of cooking more at home, which will make it easier for you to adopt the other 11 habits. For instance, it will be tough for you to slash the salt if you rarely cook your own meals.

When you start a new chapter, think about your personal habit hurdles—those specific challenges that are standing in your way—and figure out how far you need to go to reach the goal that's part of each habit, such as eating three more servings of veggies a day or incorporating fish or shellfish into your meals twice a week. You need to understand your existing habits to know what changes you need to make and to discover what will work for you.

Take a look at the challenges of the real-life people we've profiled. Do you have similar barriers? If so, find out what you can glean from their stories. Whatever you do, be sure to take baby steps instead of giant leaps. Changing habits takes time, and you need a process. (On page 329, you'll find a 6-week meal plan that can help get you started.) Research tells us that long-term behavior change is the result of small victories and little daily tweaks over a long period of time. What you had to consciously decide to do at first eventually becomes automatic.

Each chapter outlines specific strategies you can use to meet your personal goals. Again, it's about starting slow and being consistent. You're in this for the long haul.

Once you feel like you're well on your way to embracing a habit, then move on to a new one. Each new healthy habit begets the next. You may discover a "keystone" habit that helps the other habits fall into place. Your aim is to incorporate all 12 of these habits in your daily life, practicing the new behaviors until they become routine. In the end, you'll be making 12 powerful changes that truly have the potential to change your life.

A COMMUNITY-BASED APPROACH

The Food Lover's Healthy Habits Cookbook was written with the help of the CookingLight.com community. It's a multi-platform book that was built with the shared wisdom and insights from the followers of the 12 Healthy Habits program. What started in the magazine and on the web as a year-long series sparked a groundswell of online conversations in which people shared their struggles and triumphs, gained inspiration and new ideas, and found solutions to change their habits. One of the most marvelous things was that people learned from each other.

We tapped into some of the best solutions and profiled members of the community who overcame challenges and adopted healthier habits. (It was easier than they thought!) People blogged, tweeted, uploaded photos, and posted on Facebook. They joined in the conversation to connect and share their stories about each of the 12 healthy habits. We had live online chats, two-way dialogue with readers, and digital coaching with chef Allison Fishman and fitness expert Myatt Murphy. The food and nutrition blogging community got involved, offering their own habit-changing advice. Many of the recipes were crowdsourced from the community to find the top dishes that made each habit easy and tasty to adopt. All helped to shape the direction of this book.

Expert Chatter:
Talking Fish

@TanyaZuckerbrot: Fish = healthy. Fried fish, smothered in cream sauce, topped with cheese, and wedged between a bun? Not so much.

@GreenEating: Did u know risk of NOT eating fish is much greater than risk of eating it, even for kids and moms-to-be?

@RMNutrition: I like canned/pouch salmon and tuna. Inexpensive, quick, ready to eat. Love them on top of salads.

@NourRD: I keep a bag of frozen fish fillets in my freezer at all times. Season and bake. Great when I can't go to the store.

@MarisaMoore: Quick, healthy, and inexpensive: Canned tuna or salmon w/white beans, tomatoes, arugula, or spinach, and an olive oil vinaigrette.

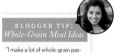

BLOGGER TIP:
Whole-Grain Meal Ideas

"I make a lot of whole-grain pastas at home. If you use the right sauce you seriously can't tell. If I have extra pasta on hand, I like to make a quick salad and throw some in. It's a great way to add healthy carbs and feel full."
—*Nisha Singh, blogger,*
Honey What's Cooking

Are you going
meatless one
day a week?

"We've made a slow transition into meatless meals, less because of a conscious choice and more because we've just found awesome recipes that work for us."
—*Alyson Lewis*

READER TIP:
The Switch-It-Up Solution

"I realized that my long stretches of absence in the gym weren't really due to a lack of time or motivation—it was boredom that kept me from coming back. In our coaching sessions, Myatt Murphy suggested I do each exercise four different ways. I now rotate between the four methods—barbell, dumbbell, machines, and resistance bands. Focusing on one side at a time allows me to concentrate on each specific muscle. I feel like I get a better workout, and I enjoy the effort it takes to maintain proper form and control. Adding some variety to my workouts has helped me stay with the program and get in better shape."
—*Gabe Chernov,*
Healthy Habits Graduate

EXPERT TIP:
A Perfect Meatless
Pasta Formula

"Our family is eating less meat these days, and I've created a simple formula for a hearty, satisfying non-meat pasta dish that's suited for any night of the week. It's a combination of pasta + frozen or fresh veggies + a spoonful of high-quality oil or oil-based sauce + a sprinkling of hard, aged cheese + 2 tablespoons of nuts. It's easy to prepare and incredibly flexible. A favorite is whole-wheat penne, chopped spinach, pesto, sharp white cheddar, and pistachios."
—*Regan Jones, RD,*
blogger, The Professional Palate

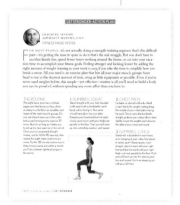

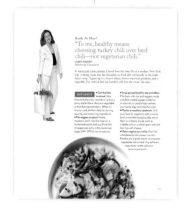

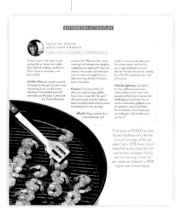

12 WAYS TO MAKE YOUR HEALTHY HABITS STICK

1. Start small. Do not completely overhaul your current routine in one day. It's easy to get over-motivated and try to tackle too much, which can backfire. Focus on taking a series of small steps, each of which is attainable, rather than attempting to change all at once.

2. Have a plan. It's been said many times: If you fail to plan, you plan to fail. Map out the specific ways you'll turn these small steps into habits. Plan out your meals and snacks. Studies show that if people devise and follow a concrete plan, they're better at acting on their intentions.

3. Write it down. Writing helps to solidify your commitment and helps you focus on the end result. Write down what you want to achieve this month. Leave reminders on your calendar or in your day planner. Scribble daily goals and motivating messages on sticky notes.

4. Be specific. Studies show that goals are easier to reach if they're action-oriented. That means being specific, such as "I'll get up 30 minutes earlier so I can walk in the morning before work" instead of "I'll get more exercise."

5. Keep track. Self-monitoring is a powerful tool to help instill new habits and achieve success. That could be writing down what you eat in a food diary, using a mobile app to calculate calories, checking off vegetable servings, logging your daily activity, or tracking the steps you take with a pedometer.

6. Find a buddy. Making changes is easier and more enjoyable when you have someone who will keep you motivated. Seek out a friend, coworker, or family member who will adopt these healthy habits with you, or join other readers in the CookingLight.com community to get support and trade tips.

7. Change your environment. Create a home that supports your healthy habits. Get rid of tempting foods, snacks, and drinks that trigger unhealthy behavior. Keep fresh fruit in bowls on the counter, and wash and cut fresh veggies ahead of time for easy snacking. Make it convenient to make healthy choices.

8. Be positive. The belief that you can make a change is a powerful force. Behavioral scientists call this self-efficacy. You're much more likely to reach a goal if you have confidence in yourself.

What we believe can significantly affect what we can achieve, so have faith in your ability to succeed.

9. Get inspired. Find someone who has succeeded in making the positive changes you want to mirror. Use these role models to keep you motivated.

10. See for yourself. Create your action plan and visualize yourself carrying it out. Researchers have found that visualization techniques—or mentally rehearsing buying, preparing, and eating healthy food—helps people actually change their eating habits.

11. Celebrate victories. Pat yourself on the back for making some new, positive changes—no matter how small. When you begin to succeed, you gain self-confidence, which leads to greater success. As behavioral experts say, "Nothing succeeds like success."

12. Give it time. Don't get impatient. It takes time to establish a new habit. One recent study found that it takes an average of 66 days before a new habit becomes automatic. So commit to 30 days, then the next month will be much easier to sustain.

YOU'RE ON YOUR WAY

Congratulations on making this commitment. These 12 healthy habits add up to something big— they're the building blocks to a healthier life. Keep in mind, however, that there are other habits that can work against your good intentions. It's also vital not to smoke, to get adequate sleep each night, and to find ways to manage stress.

Additionally, studies examining the habits of the world's longest-lived people underscore the importance of family, friends, and having a sense of purpose, as well as understanding your values, passions, and talents, and then finding ways to put your skills into action.

Now, are you ready to get started?

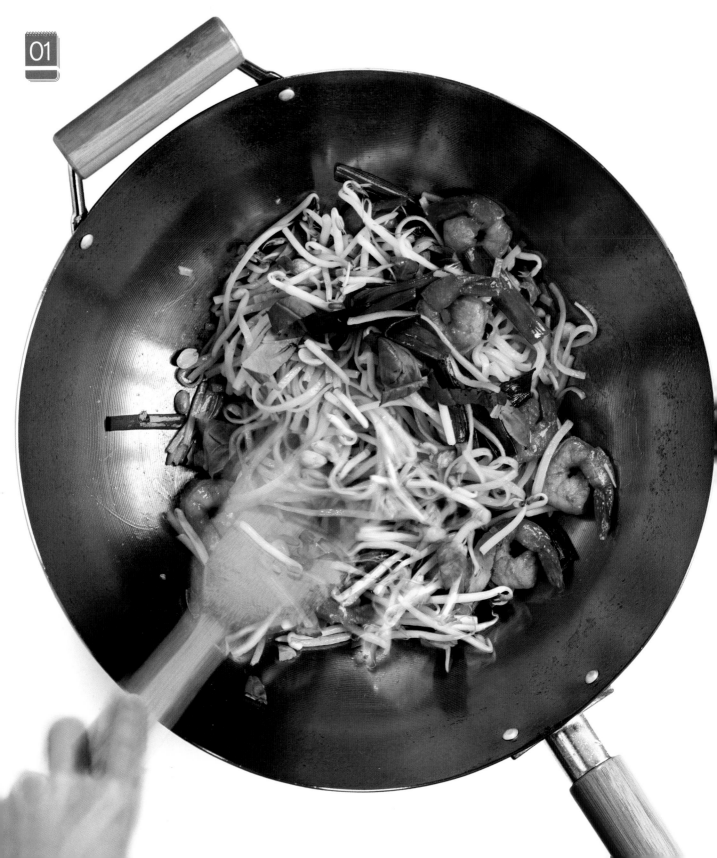

GET COOKING

THE MORE YOU COOK, THE MORE YOU MASTER.

COOKING AT HOME is the foundation of all your food-related healthy habits. And although the great American time squeeze often tempts you to opt for takeout or fast food, it's worth a little schedule shifting to implement this habit. You'll typically consume 50% more calories when eating out, and fast-food options easily pack in a day's worth of saturated fat and sodium (not to mention, you'll rarely meet up with a veggie other than fries).

Sure, prepackaged processed foods are convenient, but they're usually loaded with salt (they often contain more than one-fourth of a day's maximum recommended intake) and low on healthy ingredients like fruits, vegetables, and whole grains. Only when we cook do we really control what we eat.

Easy for you to say, you say. The time squeeze is real! True, and that's why this first chapter focuses on cooking strategies to help you solve the nightly dinner dilemma and also provides tips and recipes for make-ahead and quick meals that you can fit into your time-crunched schedule.

Since cooking can begin to feel like another of the many things on your ever-growing to-do list, even for passionate cooks, we'll also show you how to expand your cooking repertoire for fun and variety. Trust us, it is possible to get back to preparing healthy, nutritious meals for you and your family—even when your calendar is covered in ink, appointments, and reminders.

YOUR GOAL

Cook at least
three more meals
per week.

The 12 Healthy Habits

| · 01 · GET COOKING | · 02 · BREAKFAST DAILY | · 03 · WHOLE GRAINS | · 04 · GET MOVING | · 05 · VEGGIE UP | · 06 · MORE SEAFOOD | · 07 · HEALTHY FATS | · 08 · GO MEATLESS | · 09 · GET STRONGER | · 10 · LESS SALT | · 11 · BE PORTION- AWARE | · 12 · EAT MINDFULLY |

Fortify Your Kitchen

KEEP THESE 20 ALL-STAR ESSENTIAL INGREDIENTS on hand in your kitchen, and you'll never run out of inspiration for fast and flavorful meals.

IN THE PANTRY

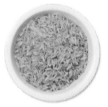 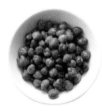 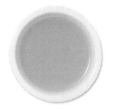 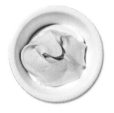 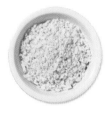

Boil-in-bag brown rice
It's one of the quickest ways to get more whole grains in your diet.
Use for: Rice pilaf, rice salad, soups, and stews

Capers
They deliver bright, briny flavor in a flash.
Use for: Pasta dishes, roasted vegetables, and sauces for chicken and fish

Fat-free, lower-sodium chicken broth
It's indispensable for fast cooking.
Use for: Poaching liquid, sauces, braising and stewing liquid

Canola mayonnaise
It has less saturated fat than conventional store-bought mayo.
Use for: Marinades, flavored sandwich spreads, and dips

Panko (Japanese breadcrumbs)
They're every bit as convenient but taste better than bland, dry breadcrumbs. Panko also gives foods a supercrisp crust.
Use for: Filler for crab cakes and meatballs, breading for oven-fried shrimp or fish fillets, and casserole toppings

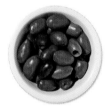 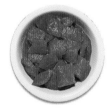 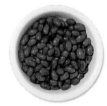 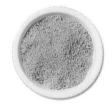

Pitted kalamata olives
They add a rich and unique flavor to any dish they grace.
Use for: Tapenade, pasta dishes, and roasting along with chicken or vegetables

Canned no-salt-added diced tomatoes
They save you the time and effort of seeding, chopping, and peeling fresh tomatoes.
Use for: Marinara sauce, bruschetta, salsa, and soups

Canned organic black beans
These offer options for main dishes and sides, and going with organic ensures there's minimal added salt.
Use for: Black bean cakes, filling for tacos or burritos, and salsa

Whole-wheat couscous
It's one of the easiest and most versatile starches you can find.
Use for: Salads, stuffing roasted veggies like zucchini, and serving with Moroccan tagines and other stews

IN THE FRIDGE

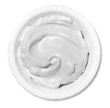

Greek yogurt
The fat-free or 2% reduced-fat is luscious, smooth, and rich, not chalky like traditional plain yogurt.
Use for: Dips, sauces, and marinades

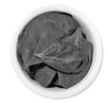

Bagged baby spinach
It saves you time and the trouble of removing stems.
Use for: Pizza topping, pasta dishes, and a tasty side dish or salad

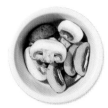

Presliced fresh cremini mushrooms
They allow you to simply dump and stir.
Use for: Sauces, casseroles, stuffings, and fillings

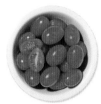

Grape tomatoes
They add a quick splash of color and flavor.
Use for: Pasta tosses, salads, and garnishes

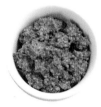

Pesto spread
Commercial pesto is convenient and high-flavor. Even though pesto is made with high-calorie ingredients (nuts, olive oil, and cheese), it's still a good-for-you spread filled with healthy fats.
Use for: Pizza, pasta dishes, and sandwiches

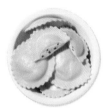

Fresh pasta
It cooks in half the time as dried. Look for whole-wheat ravioli and fettuccine in the refrigerated case of your grocery store.
Use for: Soups, baked casseroles, and appetizers

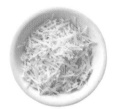

Parmigiano-Reggiano cheese
It adds an incomparable flavor, texture, and richness to foods.
Use for: Grating over pasta dishes, salads, and roasted veggies, and stirring into soups and risottos

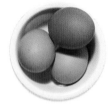

Eggs
They're a quick protein and amazingly versatile.
Use for: Binders in patties and meatballs, salad toppers, thickening and enriching sauces and salad dressings, and bulking up fried rice

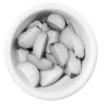

Red potato wedges
They're ready to cook straight out of the bag.
Use for: Potato salad, roasted potato sides, and soup

IN THE FREEZER

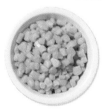

Corn kernels
They save you the time spent shucking and cutting kernels from the cob.
Use for: Cream-style corn, salsa, salads, and corn bread

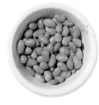

Shelled edamame (green soybeans)
They're a super convenient way to add color, texture, and protein to most any dish.
Use for: Salads, pastas, and pureed dips or spreads

Jump-Start Meal Prep

THE MOROCCAN CHICKPEA STEW PICTURED BELOW may seem like a daunting recipe for a weeknight, but with a little advance prep work it becomes an easy dinner that you can get on the table in under 30 minutes. The following tips offer advice that you can use for preparing a variety of dishes.

Precook some items. The next time you're cooking rice, make a large batch so you can freeze the extra. Simply reheat in the microwave.

Make and freeze. When you cook the stew, freeze individual portions to create a frozen meal to take to work for lunch or to reheat for dinner later in the week.

Plan for leftovers. Soups and stews have good fridge shelf lives since they're packed in moisture. Later in the week, prep some quick sides and serve, or you can even roast a piece of fish and pour the stew on top as a sauce.

Jump-start your ingredient prep. In the morning or the night before, wash and chop the vegetables so all you have to do is throw the ingredients into the pan when you get home.

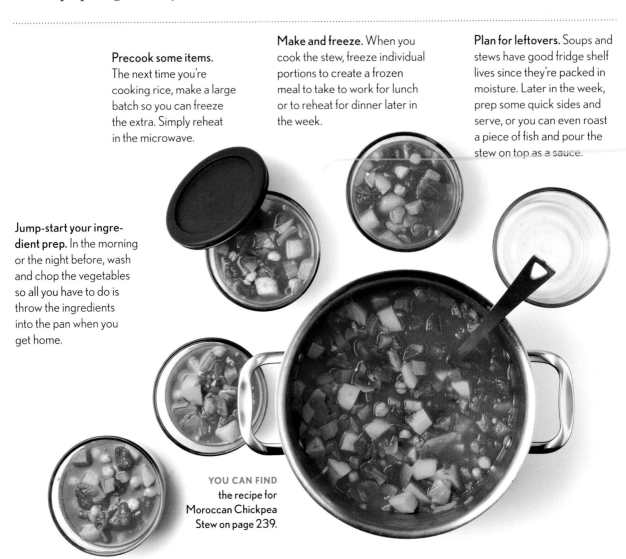

YOU CAN FIND
the recipe for
Moroccan Chickpea
Stew on page 239.

The Lapsed Solo Cook

"I need to get reacquainted with my kitchen."

CAROL "C.J." JOHNSON
Cooking Light *Administrative Coordinator*

➤ **HER CHALLENGE:** For the last year, C.J. has been time crunched and energy depleted. When mealtime came, "It was just way too easy to go through somebody's drive-through," she says. Although she loves to cook, the idea of shopping and cooking for one was too tiring to even think about. The result: an upsurge in restaurant food spending and an increase in pounds.

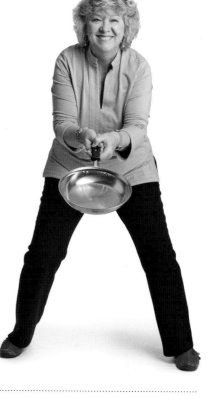

OUR ADVICE ▪ **Cook and freeze.** On the weekend, if you're cooking a lasagna, enchiladas, or a casserole like mac and cheese, make double portions and freeze one. That way, you've cooked once, but you get at least two home-cooked meals.

▪ **A healthy breakfast is just a muffin tin away.** Bake and freeze muffins or individual frittatas (baked in muffin tins) for pre-portioned, grab-and-go breakfasts.

▪ **Make a batch of pasta salad for the week.** Try penne with diced red bell pepper and red onion plus purchased or homemade vinaigrette.

Add something new each day so you don't get sick of it—toasted nuts and feta cheese, sliced grilled chicken breast, or olives and canned tuna.

▪ **Learn to cook *en papillote*.** It's a smart option for those cooking for one—a great one-dish meal with almost no cleanup. (See page 197 for tips.)

▪ **Cook with friends.** Open a bottle of wine, and have a friend or two over. You might be more willing to tackle a new technique together, and you'll learn from each other—a new ingredient, a cool tip, or a time-saving option.

You can find some muffin options on page 66.

Frequent home cooking may even help you live longer, suggests a 10-year study published in *Public Health Nutrition.*

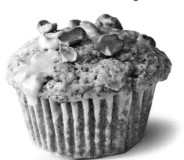

Simplify Your Meals

MAKING DINNER DOESN'T HAVE TO TAKE AN HOUR. There are great time-cutting products out there to make even the freshest cooking easier and faster. Here are five healthy off-the-shelf convenience foods to help simplify dinner prep.

PREMADE PIZZA DOUGH

In as little as 30 minutes, you can make a fantastic pie with a crispy-chewy, deliciously brown crust warm from the oven. Load it with fresh veggies for a wonderfully healthy salad pizza.

PASTA SAUCE

A good basic bottled marinara sauce can make quick work of so many dinners—from spaghetti and meatballs to lasagna. Plus it's great as a quick pizza or dipping sauce.

HUMMUS

It's a tasty base for a wide range of easy, veggie-packed sandwiches made special with the robust flavors of garlic and nutty tahini. And hummus is loaded with protein and fiber.

PRECOOKED BROWN RICE

We all need to eat more whole grains, but they're not always an easy choice for the fast cook—some can take an hour to prepare. Instead, say hello to precooked brown rice, which is cooked and then put in a shelf-stable pouch.

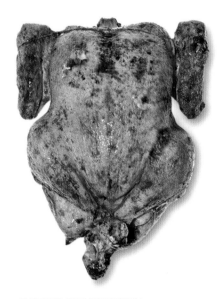

ROTISSERIE CHICKEN

Rotisserie chicken is a convenient and healthy choice. Always remove the skin before chopping or shredding the meat. Here are 10 things to do with rotisserie chicken:

1. Stir chopped or shredded breast meat into chilis, stews, and soups.
2. Turn a variety of salads into main dishes by using chicken as the protein.
3. Add shredded chicken to any number of casseroles, from green bean to stratas. Use the dark meat; it can stand up to the extra cooking time without drying out.
4. Make a simple chicken salad by adding canola mayonnaise, prechopped celery and onion, chopped walnuts, and halved red grapes.
5. Toss chicken chunks with jarred salsa verde and preshredded Mexican blend cheese as a quick-and-easy filling for enchiladas, quesadillas, or tacos.
6. Combine shredded chicken with a mix of bottled barbecue sauce and light ranch dressing for a deliciously different potato topper. Stir in chopped green onions for flavor and color.
7. Tuck breast meat slices into sandwiches for an easy, lower-sodium alternative to cold cuts.
8. Mix chopped chicken into potato hash in place of corned beef or pork.
9. Make fried rice a full meal by adding shredded breast and thigh meat.
10. To save cooking time, use rotisserie chicken whenever a recipe calls for cooked chicken.

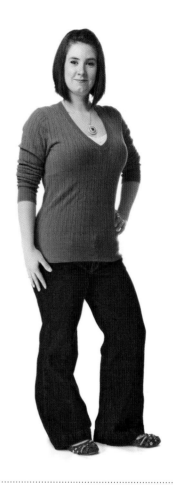

Healthy Habits Success Story

"Cooking gives me good food and quality time with my family."

HEATHER WALKER
Stay-at-Home Mom

➤ **HEALTHY HABITS GRADUATE:** This new mom lost almost 72 pounds in a year simply by cutting back on calorie-laden takeout and cooking at home more. Here, her top five strategies for keeping it simple:

HEATHER'S STRATEGIES

■ **Get a game plan.** "I sit down on Monday evenings after my daughter has gone to bed, and I make a meal plan for the week that focuses primarily on dinner. I try to cook meals that will have a lot of leftovers that save well to use as lunches throughout the week."

■ **Embrace the slow cooker.** "I use it probably twice a week. It works well for me because it frees up my days and allows me time to get out of the house, run errands, or visit family. One of our family favorites is carnitas (pulled pork) that you can cook for seven to eight hours on low." Vegetarian chili, chicken stew, or braised collard greens are also great options (see our recipes starting on page 42).

■ **Invest in a few good tools.** "Buy a good set of knives. I also have a huge Calphalon sauté pan that I use almost every day—sometimes twice a day. Just having good utensils makes food prep and cooking a lot easier."

■ **Gather your favorite go-to recipes.** "Any time I find a recipe I really like, I put it in a special folder. That way, if I'm feeling sluggish one week, I can make one of those."

■ **Tackle meal prep as a team.** "I marinate meat first thing in the morning and put it in the fridge. When my husband gets home from work, he puts it on the grill while I prep salads and chop veggies. We're ready to eat in 15 minutes, no muss, no fuss!"

Have a pot of slow-cooker Provençal Beef Daube (page 43) ready when you get home.

A slow cooker was the #1 favorite kitchen helper identified by the *Cooking Light* community; it won hands down at 46%.

Avoid the Most Common Cooking Mistakes

EVERY COOK, BEING HUMAN, ERRS, bungles, botches, and screws up in the kitchen once in a while. Here, some of the most common, avoidable culinary boo-boos, and ways to prevent them:

OOPS! You don't read the entire recipe before you start cooking.
Result: Flavors are dull, entire steps or ingredients get left out.
What to do: A wise cook approaches each recipe with a critical eye and reads the recipe well before it's time to cook. Follow the pros' habit of creating your *mise en place*—that is, having all the ingredients gathered, prepped, and ready to go before you turn on the heat.

OOPS! You don't taste as you go.
Result: The flavors or textures of an otherwise excellent dish are out of balance or unappealing.
What to do: Your palate is the control factor, so taste every two to three steps. Recipes don't always call for the "right" amount of seasoning, cooking times are estimates, and results vary depending on your ingredients, your stove, altitude...and a million other factors.

OOPS! You overcrowd the pan.
Result: Soggy food that doesn't brown
What to do: It's easy to overcrowd a pan when you're in a hurry, but the brown, crusty bits are critical for flavor. Leave breathing room in the pan, and you'll get much better results. If you need to speed things up, use two pans at once.

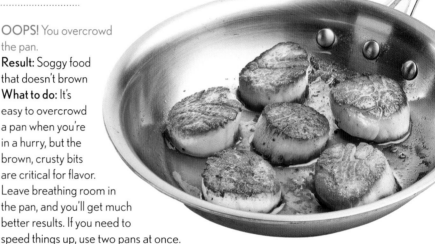

EXPERT TIP: *Avoiding "Oops" in the Kitchen*

"Organize and prepare are the two critical acts in a kitchen. Begin any task with these two acts, and you're on your way. Ignore them, and you've put yourself at risk even before you begin. Ninety-five percent of kitchen failures can be traced back to a failure to organize and prepare at the outset."

—*Michael Ruhlman, author of* Ruhlman's Twenty: 20 Techniques, 100 Recipes, A Cook's Manifesto

OOPS! You don't use a meat thermometer.

Result: Your roast chicken, leg of lamb, or beef tenderloin turns out over- or undercooked.

What to do: Invest in a small, inexpensive meat thermometer. Using one is the surefire way to achieve a perfect roast chicken or beautiful medium-rare lamb roast, because temperatures don't lie and appearances can deceive. We love digital probe thermometers, which allow you to set the device to the desired temperature.

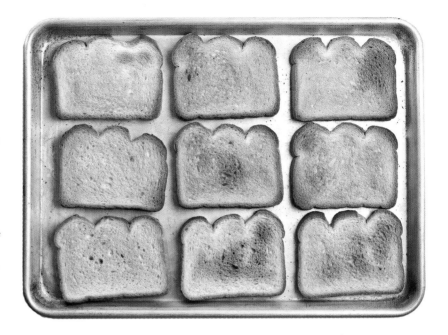

OOPS! You turn the food too often.

Result: You interfere with the sear, food sticks, or you lose the breading.

What to do: Learning to leave food alone is one of the hardest lessons in cooking; it's so tempting to turn, poke, flip. But your breaded chicken or steak won't develop a nice crust unless you allow it to cook, undisturbed, for the specified time. One sign that it's too early to turn: You can't slide a spatula cleanly under the crust.

OOPS! You don't know your oven's quirks and idiosyncrasies.

Result: Food cooks too fast, too slowly, or unevenly.

What to do: Ideally, every oven set to 350° would heat to 350°. But many ovens don't, including expensive ones, and some change as they age. Always use an oven thermometer. Next, be aware of hot spots. If you've produced cake layers with wavy rather than flat tops, hot spots are the problem. One way to check is the "bread test."

Arrange bread slices on a large jelly-roll pan or baking sheet, and place on the middle rack. Bake at 350° for a few minutes, and see which slices get singed—their location marks your oven's hot spots. If you know you have a hot spot in, say, that back left corner, avoid putting pans in that location or rotate accordingly.

OOPS! You don't get the pan hot enough before you add the food.

Result: Food that sticks, scallops with no sear, pale meats

What to do: A hot pan is essential for sautéing veggies or creating a great crust on meat, fish, and poultry. It also helps prevent food from sticking. Senior Food Editor Tim Cebula was once advised: "If you think your pan is hot enough, step back and heat

it a couple more minutes. When you're about ready to call the fire department, then add oil and proceed to cook the food."

OOPS! You pop meat straight from the fridge into the oven or on the grill.

Result: Food cooks unevenly: The outside is overdone, the inside rare or raw.

What to do: Meats will cook much more evenly if you allow them to stand at room temperature for 15 to 30 minutes (depending on the size of the cut) to take the chill off.

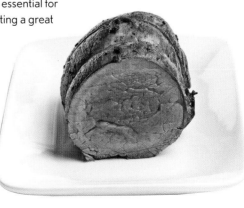

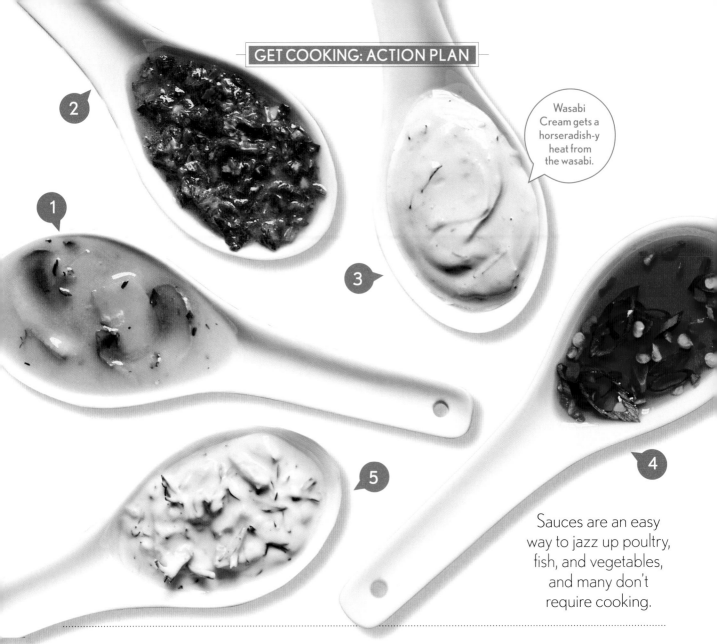

Wasabi Cream gets a horseradish-y heat from the wasabi.

Sauces are an easy way to jazz up poultry, fish, and vegetables, and many don't require cooking.

Try New Flavor Combinations

7 DIFFERENT PROTEINS + 5 DIFFERENT SAUCES = a variety of delicious dinner options that help beat boredom. Here, supersimple ways to jazz up mainstays like chicken or beef and get dinner on the table in 15 minutes or less:

PICK YOUR PROTEIN

- Fish fillets
- Skinless, boneless chicken breast halves
- Boneless center-cut pork chops
- Beef tenderloin steaks
- Shrimp, peeled and deveined
- Scallops
- Lean ground beef

PICK YOUR SAUCE

1. Mushroom Sauce

Goes with: Steak, roasted or grilled chicken or pork

Pair with: Creamed spinach and mashed potatoes

To prepare: Heat a large skillet over medium-high heat. Coat pan with cooking spray. Add 1 (8-ounce) package presliced mushrooms; sauté 4 minutes or until lightly browned. Stir in ½ cup fat-free, lower-sodium chicken broth; ¼ cup white wine; 2 teaspoons cornstarch; ⅛ teaspoon salt, and ⅛ teaspoon black pepper. Cook 2 minutes or until sauce is slightly thick. Remove from heat; add 2 tablespoons butter, stirring until butter melts. Serves 8 (serving size: about 3 tablespoons).

CALORIES 37; FAT 2.9g (sat 1.8g, mono 0.8g, poly 0.1g); PROTEIN 0.8g; CARB 1.9g; FIBER 0.2g; CHOL 8mg; IRON 0.2mg; SODIUM 87mg; CALC 7mg

2. Chimichurri

Goes with: Steak, chicken, or fish

Pair with: Roasted red potatoes and steamed asparagus

To prepare: Place 1 cup fresh flat-leaf parsley leaves, 1 cup fresh cilantro, ¼ cup fresh oregano, and 2 garlic cloves in a food processor; process until finely chopped. Add ½ teaspoon grated lime rind, 2 tablespoons fresh lime juice, 2 tablespoons extra-virgin olive oil, ¼ teaspoon salt, and ¼ teaspoon crushed red pepper; process until mixture is well combined. Serves 4 (serving size: 2 tablespoons).

CALORIES 79; FAT 7.2g (sat 1g, mono 5g, poly 0.9g); PROTEIN 0.9g; CARB 4.2g; FIBER 1.9g; CHOL 0mg; IRON 2.4mg; SODIUM 155mg; CALC 73mg

3. Wasabi Cream

Goes with: Grilled or roasted beef, chicken, or pork; burgers; sautéed or grilled shrimp or scallops

Pair with: Baked potato and cabbage slaw

To prepare: Combine 1 cup reduced-fat sour cream, 2 tablespoons chopped fresh cilantro, 2 tablespoons fresh lime juice, and 2 teaspoons wasabi paste. Serves 8 (serving size: 2 tablespoons).

CALORIES 57; FAT 3.9g (sat 2.4g, mono 1g, poly 0.2g); PROTEIN 1.4g; CARB 3.1g; FIBER 0.1g; CHOL 16mg; IRON 0mg; SODIUM 43mg; CALC 50mg

4. Ponzu

Goes with: Beef, chicken, shrimp, or scallops

Pair with: Brown rice and sautéed snow peas

To prepare: Combine 1 tablespoon chopped green onions, 3 tablespoons

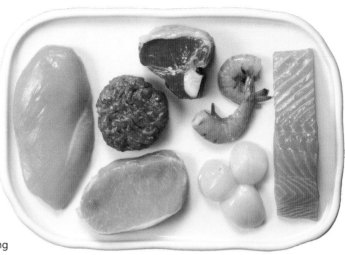

fresh lemon juice, 2 tablespoons mirin (sweet rice wine), 2 tablespoons lower-sodium soy sauce, 1 teaspoon brown sugar, ¼ teaspoon crushed red pepper, and ¼ teaspoon fish sauce. Serves 4 (serving size: 2 tablespoons).

CALORIES 30; FAT 0g (sat 0g, mono 0g, poly 0g); PROTEIN 0.6g; CARB 5.2g; FIBER 0.1g; CHOL 0mg; IRON 0.1mg; SODIUM 225mg; CALC 5mg

5. Tzatziki

Goes with: Beef, lamb, or chicken kebabs; pita sandwiches or burgers

Pair with: Avocado salad and pita bread

To prepare: Combine ¾ cup plain low-fat Greek yogurt, ¼ cup grated peeled English cucumber, 1 tablespoon chopped fresh dill, 2 teaspoons red wine vinegar, ¼ teaspoon salt, ⅛ teaspoon black pepper, and 2 minced garlic cloves. Serves 4 (serving size: 3 tablespoons).

CALORIES 36; FAT 1g (sat 0.8g, mono 0g, poly 0g); PROTEIN 4.4g; CARB 2.7g; FIBER 0.1g; CHOL 3mg; IRON 0.1mg; SODIUM 162mg; CALC 50mg

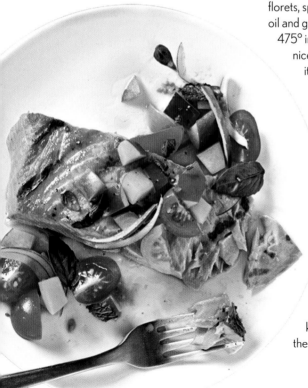

COACHING SESSION
with ANN PITTMAN

SIMPLE DINNER SOLUTIONS: "WHAT I MADE THIS WEEK"

Cooking Light Executive Editor Ann Pittman works full time, and when she's not testing recipes for the magazine she's mothering 6-year-old twin boys. But despite her schedule, she still manages to put nutritious meals on her table every night, even when her larder is running low. Here's how she does it:

■ **Monday:** The pantry and fridge were starting to look bare (Wednesday is grocery shopping day), so I threw together what I had on hand and made a roasted cauliflower pasta. Fortunately, I had some campanelle—that beautiful pasta shaped like small flowers—which my 6-year-old twins always think is really fun. It took less than 20 minutes to make: I cut the cauliflower into florets, sprinkled them with some olive oil and garlic, and roasted them at 475° in the oven until they were nice and toasty brown. I topped it with shaved Parmesan cheese and capers for some salty flavor.

■ **Tuesday:** It was a crazy day at work and I didn't feel much like cooking, so I stopped at Whole Foods to buy pizza dough, fresh mozzarella, and a lower-sodium marinara pasta sauce. Cheese pizza probably isn't the most nutritious stand-alone meal, but at least I knew it was healthier than the delivery version.

■ **Wednesday:** Grocery day! Among the items on my shopping list: Bone-in, thin-cut pork chops; brown rice; and fresh broccoli. The pork chops were simple but delicious: I sautéed them with salt and pepper and drizzled some lemon juice on at the end. I cheated and used Uncle Ben's boil-in-bag brown rice: I love the texture and how fluffy it looks at the end. I tossed it with a tablespoon of browned butter and toasted pecans to give it more flavor. I steamed the broccoli. Supereasy!

■ **Thursday:** Taco night! I chopped up some flank steak, seared it off in my go-to cast-iron pan, sprinkled on a little bit of salt, pepper, and smoked paprika, and served it on corn tortillas. My husband and I topped ours off with some spicy store-bought salsa for an extra serving of veggies; the kids had grape tomatoes on theirs. As a side dish, I sautéed some chopped zucchini and frozen corn with a little bit of olive oil and a whole lot of garlic.

■ **Friday:** My husband and I are always exhausted from the week, so Fridays are traditionally takeout and family movie night. I picked up some brown rice sushi and frozen edamame at Whole Foods on my way home. Everyone in my household loves sushi, and the brown rice is a great way to get in an extra helping of healthy whole grains.

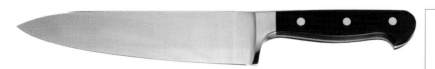

■ Saturday: Saturday was our fun fish dinner—my kids love seafood! I sautéed some salmon (I left the skin on, to keep it crisp and crunchy for my boys) and served it with couscous tossed with grape tomatoes and a salad topped with a supereasy homemade Dijon vinaigrette (see the recipe on page 222 for tips on making your own).

■ Sunday: Sundays are traditionally my big cooking day—I try to make something pretty substantial that we can have for leftovers later in the week. Today's project was a pork roast. I trimmed all the fat from the outside, coated it with salt and pepper, browned it for a bit on the stovetop, and then popped it in the oven with 8 cups of water and a pound of dried white beans. I let it cook in the oven at 300° for four hours while my boys and I played outside. I served it with steamed green beans. Best of all, there were plenty of leftovers to make pork tacos and nachos later in the week.

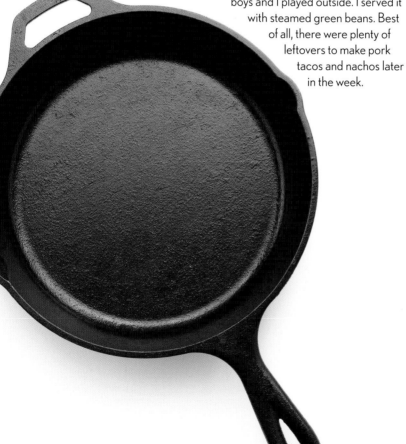

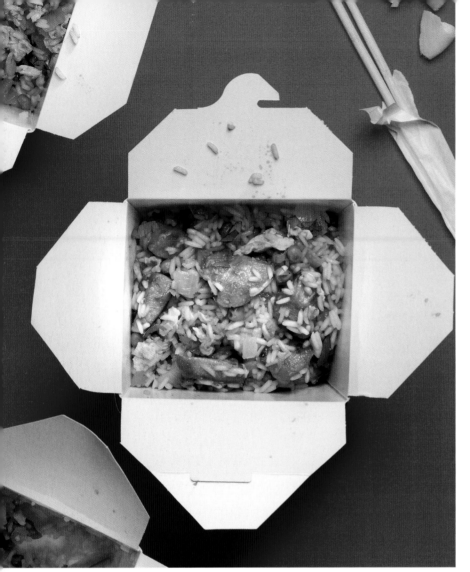

Chicken Fried Rice

Fried rice is one of those comforting Chinese-American hybrids that populates nearly every Chinese takeout menu in the country. This version scales down the salty, greasy part by using a lower-sodium soy sauce with sweet-salty hoisin sauce and fiery chile paste. The sodium savings is about 60% compared to typical takeout.

2 (3½-ounce) bags boil-in-bag rice
7 teaspoons lower-sodium soy
    sauce, divided
1 teaspoon cornstarch
12 ounces skinless, boneless chicken
    breast halves, cut into ½-inch
    pieces
2 tablespoons hoisin sauce
2 tablespoons rice wine vinegar
2 tablespoons fresh lime juice
1 teaspoon chile paste with garlic
2 tablespoons canola oil, divided
2 large eggs, lightly beaten
1 cup chopped white onion
1 teaspoon grated peeled fresh ginger
3 garlic cloves, minced
1 cup frozen green peas, thawed
½ cup chopped green onions

Trim Your Takeout

W E EAT OUT MORE THAN EVER BEFORE—in fact, it provides about one-third of the calories in American diets. Studies link frequent dining out to obesity, and no wonder: An order of chicken fried rice at your favorite Chinese restaurant can set you back 1,000 calories or more. But it's not difficult to duplicate the food on your Chinese and Thai takeout menus. Keep a variety of rices and noodles in your pantry and Asian staples like hoisin sauce, chile paste with garlic, and lower-sodium soy sauce in your fridge so you're ready when the urge strikes. Your waistline—and wallet—will thank you.

1. Cook rice according to package directions, omitting salt and fat.
2. Combine 1 tablespoon soy sauce, cornstarch, and chicken in a bowl; toss well. Combine remaining 4 teaspoons soy sauce, hoisin sauce, and next 3 ingredients in a small bowl.
3. Heat a wok or large nonstick skillet over medium-high heat. Add 1 tablespoon oil to pan; swirl to coat. Add chicken mixture; stir-fry 4 minutes or until lightly browned. Push chicken to 1 side of pan; add eggs to open side of pan. Cook 45 seconds, stirring constantly; stir eggs and chicken mixture together.

Remove chicken mixture from pan; keep warm. Add remaining 1 tablespoon oil to pan; swirl to coat. Add white onion, ginger, and garlic; cook 2 minutes or until fragrant. Add rice; cook 1 minute. Add peas; cook 1 minute. Add chicken mixture and soy sauce mixture; cook 2 minutes or until thoroughly heated. Remove pan from heat; stir in green onions. Serves 4 (serving size: about 1½ cups).

CALORIES 477; FAT 11.7g (sat 1.7g, mono 5.7g, poly 2.7g); PROTEIN 30.2g; CARB 58.3g; FIBER 3.5g; CHOL 139mg; IRON 3.5mg; SODIUM 488mg; CALC 58mg

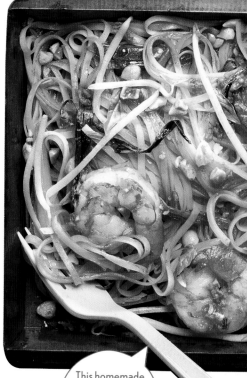

This homemade version of Pad Thai has about 30% less sodium than the restaurant version.

Shrimp Pad Thai

8 ounces uncooked flat rice noodles
2 tablespoons dark brown sugar
2 tablespoons lower-sodium soy sauce
1½ tablespoons fresh lime juice
1 tablespoon fish sauce
1 tablespoon Sriracha (hot chile sauce) or chili garlic sauce
3 tablespoons canola oil
1 cup (2-inch) green onion pieces
8 ounces peeled and deveined large shrimp
5 garlic cloves, minced
1 cup fresh bean sprouts
¼ cup chopped unsalted, dry-roasted peanuts
3 tablespoons thinly sliced fresh basil

1. Cook noodles according to package directions; drain.
2. While water comes to a boil, combine sugar and next 4 ingredients in a small bowl.
3. Heat a large skillet or wok over medium-high heat. Add oil to pan;

swirl to coat. Add onion pieces, shrimp, and garlic; stir-fry 2 minutes or until shrimp is almost done. Add cooked noodles; toss to combine. Stir in sauce; cook 1 minute, stirring constantly. Arrange about 1 cup noodle mixture on each of 4 plates; top each serving with ¼ cup bean sprouts, 1 tablespoon peanuts, and 2 teaspoons basil. Serves 4.

CALORIES 462; FAT 16.1g (sat 1.6g, mono 9.1g, poly 4.8g); PROTEIN 15.8g; CARB 64.3g; FIBER 2.6g; CHOL 86mg; IRON 3.7mg; SODIUM 637mg; CALC 90mg

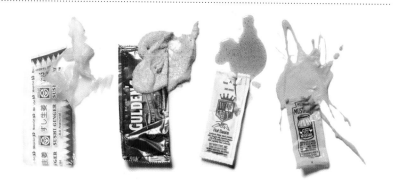

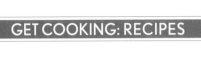
Enjoy Pizza Night

TOO WIPED OUT TO COOK? NO PROBLEM. On your way home, swing by your supermarket or local pizza shop to buy fresh dough. In the time it takes to call for delivery, you can roll a 1-pound ball of fresh dough into a 14-inch base, top it with one of these tasty topping combinations, bake, and divide by 8. Each slice clocks in at under 200 calories. Buon appetito!

THE BAGEL-AND-LOX TREATMENT

Base: 1 tablespoon fresh lemon juice + 1/2 cup 1/3-less-fat cream cheese

Toppers: 4 ounces sliced smoked salmon + 1/3 cup thinly sliced red onion + 1 tablespoon chopped fresh dill

THE CHICKEN PESTO PARTY

Base: 1/4 cup prepared pesto

Toppers: 3/4 cup shredded roasted chicken breast + 1/2 cup sliced red bell pepper + 1/3 cup shaved fresh Parmigiano-Reggiano cheese

THE CAN'T-BEET-THIS COMBO

Base: 1 1/2 tablespoons olive oil

Toppers: 8 ounces sliced roasted beets + 1/3 cup toasted walnut halves + 1/3 cup crumbled goat cheese + 2 tablespoons chopped fresh flat-leaf parsley

THE HAPPY HAWAIIAN

Base: 1/2 cup lower-sodium marinara sauce

Toppers: 4 ounces turkey pepperoni slices + 1 cup pineapple chunks (fresh or canned) + 1/2 cup shredded part-skim mozzarella cheese

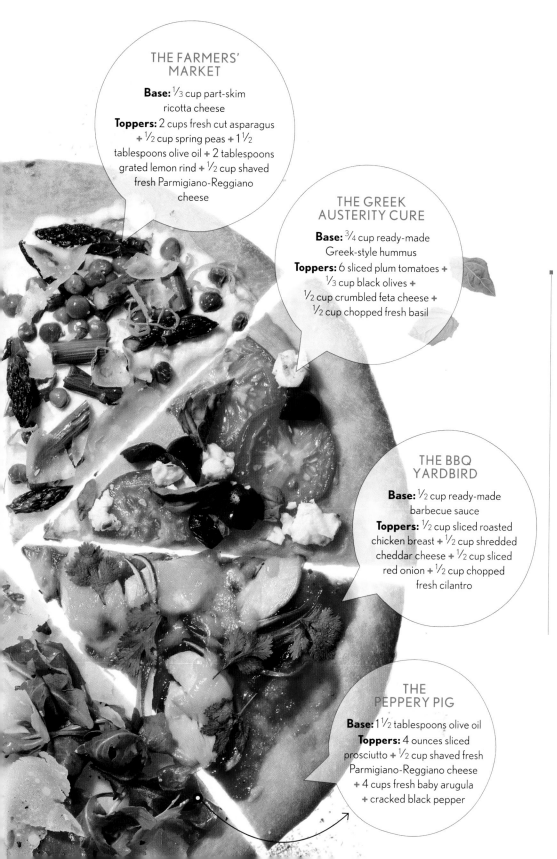

THE FARMERS' MARKET

Base: 1/3 cup part-skim ricotta cheese

Toppers: 2 cups fresh cut asparagus + 1/2 cup spring peas + 1 1/2 tablespoons olive oil + 2 tablespoons grated lemon rind + 1/2 cup shaved fresh Parmigiano-Reggiano cheese

THE GREEK AUSTERITY CURE

Base: 3/4 cup ready-made Greek-style hummus

Toppers: 6 sliced plum tomatoes + 1/3 cup black olives + 1/2 cup crumbled feta cheese + 1/2 cup chopped fresh basil

THE BBQ YARDBIRD

Base: 1/2 cup ready-made barbecue sauce

Toppers: 1/2 cup sliced roasted chicken breast + 1/2 cup shredded cheddar cheese + 1/2 cup sliced red onion + 1/2 cup chopped fresh cilantro

THE PEPPERY PIG

Base: 1 1/2 tablespoons olive oil

Toppers: 4 ounces sliced prosciutto + 1/2 cup shaved fresh Parmigiano-Reggiano cheese + 4 cups fresh baby arugula + cracked black pepper

HOW THE DELIVERY STACKS UP

All that cheesy cheesiness promoted in TV ads adds calories to single plain slices of hand-tossed pizza—mostly from cheese.

Little Caesars
250 calories

Domino's
290 calories

Papa John's
290 calories

Godfather's
313 calories

Pizza Hut
320 calories

Make Your Own Mexican Meal

GIVE YOUR WEEKNIGHT DINNER a south-of-the-border theme by topping a six-inch corn tortilla with your choice of tasty fillings for tacos that each clock in at 200 calories or less.

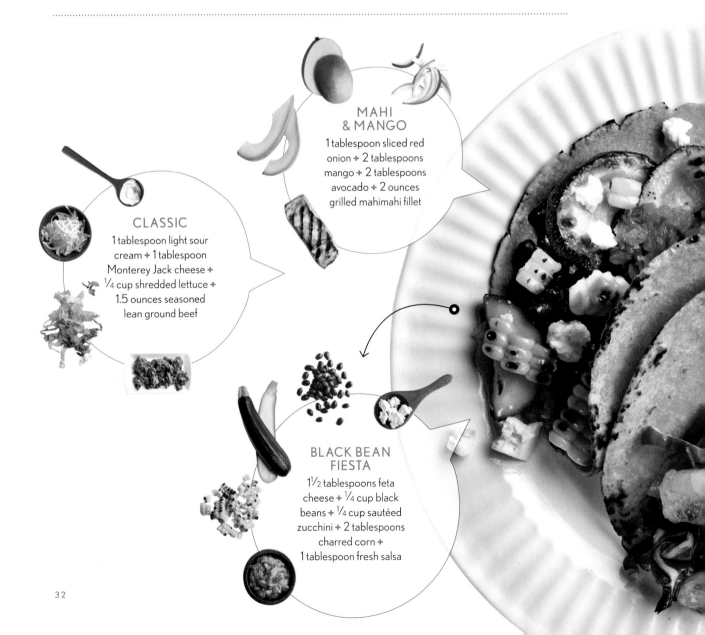

MAHI & MANGO

1 tablespoon sliced red onion + 2 tablespoons mango + 2 tablespoons avocado + 2 ounces grilled mahimahi fillet

CLASSIC

1 tablespoon light sour cream + 1 tablespoon Monterey Jack cheese + ¼ cup shredded lettuce + 1.5 ounces seasoned lean ground beef

BLACK BEAN FIESTA

1½ tablespoons feta cheese + ¼ cup black beans + ¼ cup sautéed zucchini + 2 tablespoons charred corn + 1 tablespoon fresh salsa

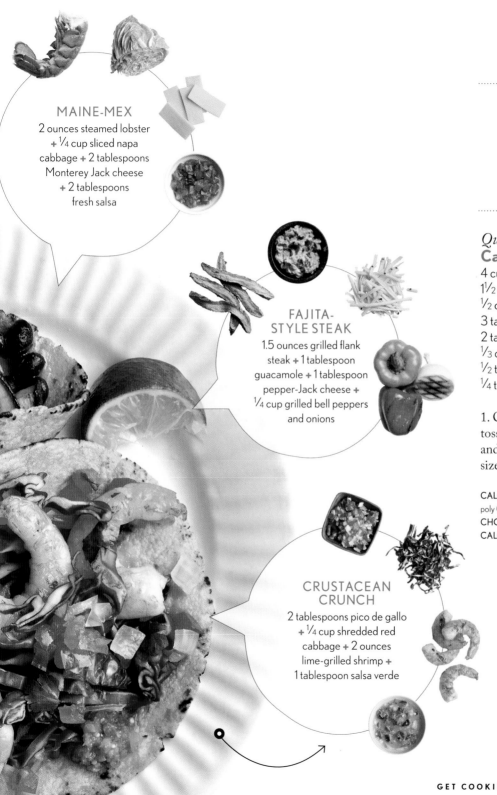

MAINE-MEX
2 ounces steamed lobster + ¼ cup sliced napa cabbage + 2 tablespoons Monterey Jack cheese + 2 tablespoons fresh salsa

FAJITA-STYLE STEAK
1.5 ounces grilled flank steak + 1 tablespoon guacamole + 1 tablespoon pepper-Jack cheese + ¼ cup grilled bell peppers and onions

CRUSTACEAN CRUNCH
2 tablespoons pico de gallo + ¼ cup shredded red cabbage + 2 ounces lime-grilled shrimp + 1 tablespoon salsa verde

Our Cabbage Slaw adds just the right amount of fresh crunch to any of these taco options.

Quick Side
Cabbage Slaw
4 cups shredded cabbage
1½ cups thinly sliced radishes
½ cup diagonally cut green onions
3 tablespoons olive oil
2 tablespoons fresh lemon juice
⅓ cup chopped fresh mint
½ teaspoon salt
¼ teaspoon ground red pepper

1. Combine first 5 ingredients; toss. Sprinkle with mint, salt, and pepper. Serves 6 (serving size: ½ cup).

CALORIES 81; FAT 6.9g (sat 1g, mono 4.9g, poly 0.8g); PROTEIN 1g; CARB 5g; FIBER 2g; CHOL 0mg; IRON 0.6mg; SODIUM 218mg; CALC 36mg

Mix It Up with Middle Eastern Food

GRABBING A FALAFEL or pita sandwich may be a better alternative to fast food, but you can easily make your own Middle Eastern favorites at home. Keep a few ingredients on hand—like tahini and bulgur—and enjoy healthy exotic fare without much fuss.

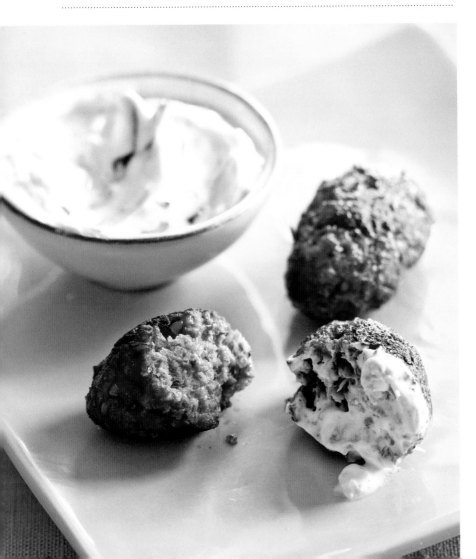

Kibbeh Meatballs with Spiced Yogurt Sauce

Considered the national dish of Lebanon, kibbeh is made of minced meat with bulgur and spices. You'll find it in many forms, including a raw version that's similar to steak tartare. Our style of kibbeh is formed into football-shaped meatballs and cooked until brown.

1½ cups plain fat-free Greek yogurt
1 cup shredded seeded cucumber
½ teaspoon ground cumin
½ teaspoon minced garlic
⅛ teaspoon salt
⅛ teaspoon black pepper
¾ cup uncooked bulgur
2 cups cold water
1 pound lean ground lamb
¼ cup minced shallots
¼ cup minced fresh parsley
¾ teaspoon salt
½ teaspoon ground cumin
½ teaspoon ground allspice
½ teaspoon ground cinnamon
¼ teaspoon ground red pepper
1 tablespoon olive oil

1. Combine first 6 ingredients; chill.
2. Combine bulgur and 2 cups water in a medium bowl. Let stand 30 minutes; drain bulgur through a fine sieve, pressing out excess liquid. Place bulgur, lamb, and next 7 ingredients in a food processor; process just until smooth. Cover and chill 30 minutes. Form lamb mixture into 20 (2½-inch) football-shaped meatballs.

3. Heat a nonstick skillet over medium-high heat. Add oil to pan; swirl to coat. Add meatballs to pan; cook 12 minutes, browning on all sides. Serve with sauce. Serves 10 (serving size: 2 meatballs and 3 tablespoons sauce).

CALORIES 161; FAT 7.7g (sat 2.7g, mono 3.6g, poly 0.6g); PROTEIN 12.2g; CARB 10.8g; FIBER 2.3g; CHOL 30mg; IRON 1.1mg; SODIUM 248mg; CALC 43mg

Spicy Chicken Shawarma

Shawarma is traditionally made by layering strips of meat on a large rotating cone and roasting over an open flame. The chicken or lamb is then shaved off with a large knife to roll into pita or flatbread for sandwiches. Here's a much easier way for you to enjoy this dish.

2 tablespoons finely chopped
  fresh parsley
1/2 teaspoon salt
1/2 teaspoon crushed red pepper
1/4 teaspoon ground ginger
1/4 teaspoon ground cumin
1/8 teaspoon ground coriander
5 tablespoons plain 2% reduced-fat
  Greek yogurt, divided
2 tablespoons fresh lemon juice,
  divided
3 garlic cloves, minced and divided
1 pound skinless, boneless chicken
  breast halves, thinly sliced
2 tablespoons extra-virgin olive oil
1 tablespoon tahini
4 (6-inch) pitas, cut in half
1/2 cup chopped cucumber
1/2 cup chopped plum tomato
1/4 cup prechopped red onion

1. Combine first 6 ingredients in a large bowl; stir in 1 tablespoon yogurt, 1 tablespoon juice, and 2 garlic cloves. Add chicken; toss to coat. Heat a large nonstick skillet over medium-high heat. Add oil to pan; swirl to coat. Add chicken mixture to pan; sauté 6 minutes or until browned, stirring frequently.
2. While chicken cooks, combine remaining 1/4 cup yogurt, remaining 1 tablespoon lemon juice, remaining 1 garlic clove, and tahini, stirring well. Spread 1 1/2 teaspoons tahini mixture inside each pita half; divide

Instead of the tahini sauce, try the sandwich with homemade hummus. Check out page 162 for recipes.

chicken evenly among pita halves. Fill each pita half with 1 tablespoon cucumber, 1 tablespoon tomato, and 1 1/2 teaspoons onion. Serves 4 (serving size: 2 stuffed pita halves).

CALORIES 402; FAT 10.7g (sat 1.9g, mono 6g, poly 2g); PROTEIN 36.4g; CARB 40g; FIBER 2.1g; CHOL 67mg; IRON 4.1mg; SODIUM 541mg; CALC 93mg

Bone Up On a Classic

A WHOLE ROAST CHICKEN is a surprisingly simple but elegant dinner option that provides plenty of leftovers for the rest of the week. Our version calls for baking the bird and then cranking up the heat at the end. Be prepared to turn on the oven vent, since the high finish heat may generate smoke.

HOW TO ROAST A WHOLE CHICKEN

1. Truss. Simply cross the legs and tie them together with kitchen twine. Next, lift the wing tips up, and tuck them under the bird. Once cooked, discard the twine, and the chicken will hold this tidy shape.

2. Season and roast. Season the flesh, leaving the skin intact. (Season the skin, too, for a nice presentation.) Then place the chicken on a rack in a roasting pan. Elevating the bird allows air to circulate and promotes even browning.

3. Check the temperature. Cooking to the proper temperature is the most critical step. Insert a thermometer into a meaty part of the leg (avoiding the bone). When the temperature reaches 165°, pull the bird from the oven. Let it rest 10 minutes.

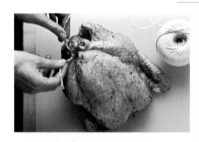

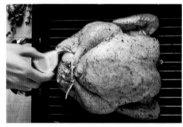

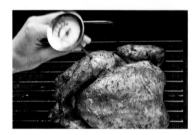

Classic Roast Chicken

"This was the best chicken I've ever roasted," said Cat111719 on CookingLight.com. "So juicy and flavorful, and the skin is perfectly crispy. You can adjust the flavor by changing up the herbs, but really, it was perfect, so why mess with it? I have already made it twice and plan to make it weekly just to have such great chicken meat on hand."

1 (4-pound) roasting chicken
2 teaspoons unsalted butter, softened
1½ teaspoons minced fresh thyme
1 teaspoon paprika
1 teaspoon ground coriander
2 teaspoons extra-virgin olive oil
¾ teaspoon salt
¼ teaspoon freshly ground black pepper
2 garlic cloves, minced
3 shallots, peeled and halved
3 thyme sprigs
1 lemon, quartered
Thyme sprigs (optional)

1. Preheat oven to 350°.
2. Discard giblets and neck from chicken. Starting at neck cavity, loosen skin from breasts and drumsticks by inserting fingers, gently pushing between skin and meat.

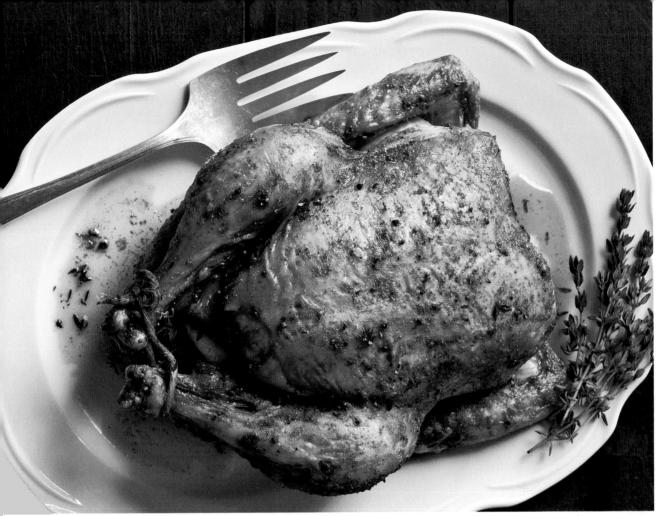

3. Combine butter and next 7 ingredients in a small bowl. Rub mixture under loosened skin, over flesh; rub over top of skin. Tie ends of legs together with twine. Lift wing tips up and over back; tuck under chicken. Place chicken, breast side up, on a rack; place rack in roasting pan. Place shallots, thyme sprigs, and lemon in cavity of chicken.

4. Bake at 350° for 45 minutes. Increase oven temperature to 450° (do not remove chicken); bake at 450° for 15 minutes or until a thermometer inserted in meaty part of leg registers 165°. Remove chicken from pan; let stand 10 minutes. Discard skin. Garnish with thyme sprigs, if desired. Serves 4 (serving size: 1 breast half or 1 leg quarter).

CALORIES 278; **FAT** 13.6g (sat 4.1g, mono 5.7g, poly 2.5g); **PROTEIN** 35.7g; **CARB** 0.9g; **FIBER** 0.3g; **CHOL** 111mg; **IRON** 1.9mg; **SODIUM** 563mg; **CALC** 23mg

READER TIP:
Count on Leftovers

"I make sure that one meal will provide leftovers for another night or the base of another meal. Extra chicken can be used later in a soup, salad, or panini. I also try to bring my lunch to work every day, so I grill extra chicken and veggies on Sunday to use in wraps for lunch during the week."

—*Christina Corieri*

Go Beyond Chicken Basics

SKINLESS, BONELESS CHICKEN BREASTS ARE LEAN and cook in a flash, but they can get boring if you don't mix it up with various techniques and flavors. Here, two ways to diversify your weeknight chicken dinners:

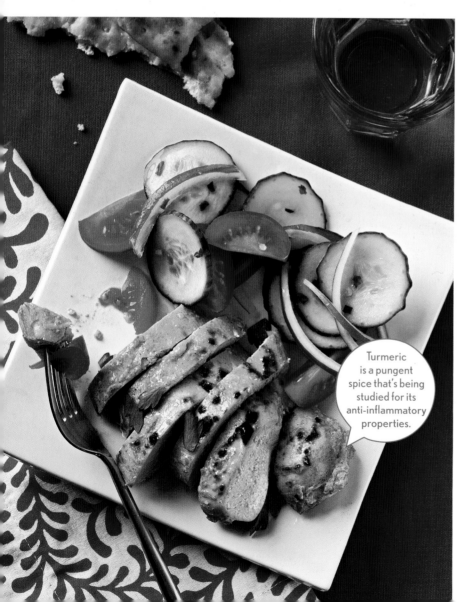

Turmeric is a pungent spice that's being studied for its anti-inflammatory properties.

Tandoori-Spiced Chicken

The yogurt-based marinade helps keep the chicken juicy and tender while adding plenty of flavor.

$1\frac{1}{2}$ cups plain 2% reduced-fat Greek yogurt
2 tablespoons grated onion
1 tablespoon grated peeled fresh ginger
1 tablespoon canola oil
1 teaspoon ground cumin
$\frac{1}{2}$ teaspoon ground red pepper
$\frac{1}{4}$ teaspoon ground turmeric
3 garlic cloves, minced
4 (6-ounce) skinless, boneless chicken breast halves
$\frac{1}{2}$ teaspoon salt
Cooking spray

1. Combine first 8 ingredients in a heavy-duty zip-top plastic bag. Add chicken to bag; seal. Marinate in refrigerator 2 hours, turning occasionally.
2. Place a small roasting pan in oven. Preheat broiler to high. Remove chicken from bag; discard marinade. Sprinkle both sides of chicken evenly with salt. Place chicken on preheated pan coated with cooking

spray. Broil in lower third of oven 15 minutes or until done, turning after 7 minutes. Serves 4 (serving size: 1 breast half).

CALORIES 230; FAT 4.4g (sat 1.3g, mono 1.4g, poly 0.9g); PROTEIN 42.8g; CARB 2.4g; FIBER 0.2g; CHOL 101mg; IRON 1.4mg; SODIUM 415mg; CALC 59mg

Meyer Lemon Chicken Piccata

The tangy-sweet Meyer lemon transforms a simple chicken breast into something special.

2 (8-ounce) skinless, boneless chicken breast halves
½ teaspoon kosher salt
¼ teaspoon freshly ground black pepper
¼ cup all-purpose flour
2 tablespoons unsalted butter, divided
⅓ cup sauvignon blanc or other crisp, tart white wine
½ cup fat-free, lower-sodium chicken broth
⅓ cup fresh Meyer lemon juice (about 3 lemons)
2 tablespoons capers, rinsed and drained
¼ cup chopped fresh flat-leaf parsley

1. Split chicken breast halves in half horizontally to form 4 cutlets. Place each cutlet between 2 sheets of heavy-duty plastic wrap; pound each cutlet to ¼-inch thickness using a meat mallet or small heavy skillet. Sprinkle cutlets evenly with salt and pepper. Place flour in a shallow dish; dredge cutlets in flour.

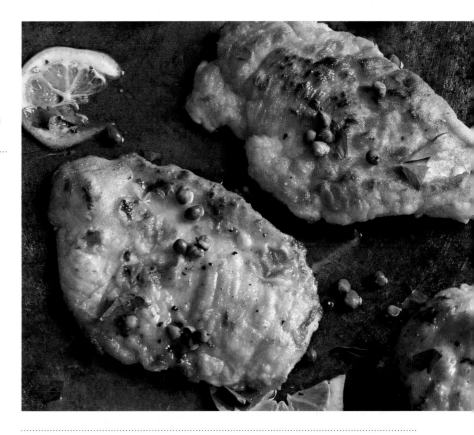

2. Melt 1 tablespoon butter in a large skillet over medium-high heat. Add 2 cutlets to pan; sauté 2 minutes. Turn cutlets over; sauté 1 minute. Remove cutlets from pan. Repeat procedure with remaining 1 tablespoon butter and 2 cutlets.
3. Add wine to pan; bring to a boil, scraping pan to loosen browned bits. Cook 1 minute or until liquid almost evaporates. Stir in broth; bring to a boil. Cook until broth mixture is reduced to 2 tablespoons (about 4 minutes). Stir in juice and capers. Serve over chicken. Sprinkle with parsley. Serves 4 (serving size:

1 cutlet, 2 tablespoons sauce, and 1 tablespoon parsley).

CALORIES 214; FAT 7.3g (sat 4.1g, mono 1.9g, poly 0.6g); PROTEIN 27.5g; CARB 8.5g; FIBER 0.6 g; CHOL 81mg; IRON 1.6mg; SODIUM 502mg; CALC 26mg

HOW TO PAN-FRY CHICKEN

Dip chicken in a marinade (or try buttermilk to add tangy flavor), coat it with flour and nuts or other tasty breading ingredients, then pan-fry it in a sensible amount of heart-healthy oil to create a crisp exterior.

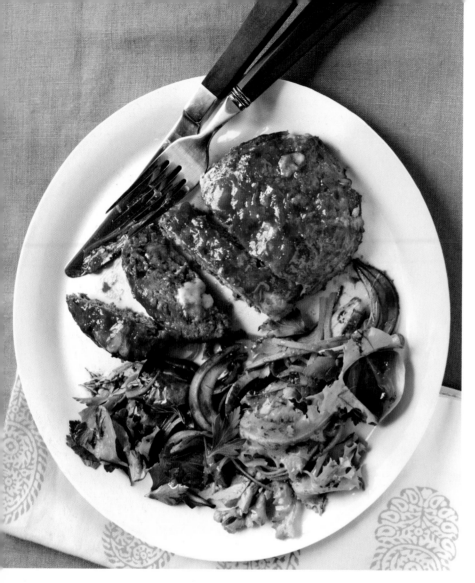

Cheesy Meat Loaf Minis

½ cup fresh breadcrumbs
   (about 1 ounce)
Cooking spray
1 cup chopped onion
2 garlic cloves, chopped
½ cup ketchup, divided
3 ounces white cheddar cheese, diced
¼ cup chopped fresh parsley
2 tablespoons grated fresh Parmesan
   cheese
1 tablespoon prepared horseradish
1 tablespoon Dijon mustard
¾ teaspoon dried oregano
¼ teaspoon freshly ground black
   pepper
⅛ teaspoon salt
1½ pounds ground sirloin
1 large egg, lightly beaten

1. Preheat oven to 425°.
2. Heat a skillet over medium-high heat. Add breadcrumbs; cook 3 minutes or until toasted, stirring frequently.
3. While breadcrumbs cook, heat a large skillet over medium-high heat. Coat pan with cooking spray. Add onion and garlic; sauté 3 minutes. Combine onion mixture, breadcrumbs, ¼ cup ketchup, and next 10 ingredients. Shape into 6 (4 x 2–inch) loaves on a broiler pan coated with cooking spray; spread 2 teaspoons ketchup over each. Bake at 425° for 25 minutes or until done. Serves 6 (serving size: 1 meat loaf).

CALORIES 256; FAT 11.6g (sat 5.7g, mono 3.9g, poly 0.9g); PROTEIN 28.5g; CARB 11.2g; FIBER 0.9g; CHOL 112mg; IRON 2.6mg; SODIUM 573mg; CALC 159mg

Find New Kid-Friendly Favorites

G ET YOUR KIDS INVOLVED in meal prep—there's a variety of tasks children of all ages can help with. Plus, they'll be more likely to try something new if they've had a hand in preparing it.

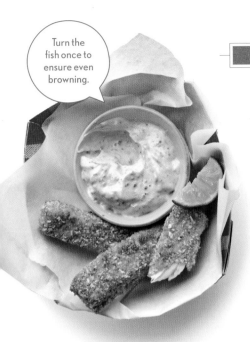

Turn the fish once to ensure even browning.

Fancy Fish Sticks

¼ cup reduced-fat mayonnaise
¼ cup fat-free sour cream
1 tablespoon Creole mustard
2 teaspoons fresh lime juice
½ teaspoon Cajun seasoning
Cooking spray
1 tablespoon canola oil
½ cup all-purpose flour
¼ teaspoon freshly ground
   black pepper
½ cup lager-style beer
1½ tablespoons creamy mustard blend
1 tablespoon fresh lime juice
2 large egg whites
1 large egg
⅔ cup panko (Japanese breadcrumbs)
⅓ cup unsalted pumpkinseed
   kernels, toasted
1 teaspoon ground cumin
½ teaspoon ground chipotle
   chile pepper
1 pound halibut or other lean white fish
   fillets (such as cod or pollock), cut into
   4 x 1-inch pieces (about 12 pieces)
¼ teaspoon kosher salt
4 lime wedges

1. Combine first 5 ingredients in a small bowl, stirring with a whisk. Cover and chill.
2. Preheat oven to 425°. Coat a baking sheet with cooking spray; spread evenly with oil. Heat in oven 12 minutes.
3. Combine flour and black pepper in a shallow dish. Combine beer and next 4 ingredients in another shallow dish; stir with a whisk until foamy. Place panko, pumpkinseeds, cumin, and chile pepper in a food processor; pulse 20 times or until coarse crumbs form. Place panko mixture in a shallow dish.
4. Sprinkle fish evenly with salt. Working with 1 piece at a time, dredge fish in flour mixture. Dip in egg mixture, and dredge in panko mixture until completely covered.
5. Remove preheated baking sheet from oven; place fish on pan, and return to oven. Bake at 425° for 15 minutes or until fish flakes easily with a fork, turning once. Serve immediately with sauce and lime wedges. Serves 4 (serving size: about 3 fish sticks, 2 tablespoons sauce, and 1 lime wedge).

CALORIES 425; FAT 17g (sat 2.5g, mono 6g, poly 6.2g); PROTEIN 36.9g; CARB 29.5g; FIBER 1.8g; CHOL 91mg; IRON 5mg; SODIUM 597mg; CALC 98mg

Turkey Tenders

1 (1-pound) turkey tenderloin
¼ cup all-purpose flour
⅓ cup egg substitute
¾ cup panko (Japanese breadcrumbs)
2 tablespoons grated fresh Parmesan
   cheese
¼ teaspoon garlic salt
¼ teaspoon black pepper
1 tablespoon canola oil

1. Preheat oven to 425°.
2. Cut tenderloin in half lengthwise; cut into 20 (2-inch) pieces.
3. Place flour in a shallow dish. Place egg substitute in another shallow dish. Combine panko, cheese, garlic salt, and pepper in another dish. Dredge turkey in flour; dip in egg substitute, and dredge in breadcrumb mixture. Heat a nonstick skillet over medium-high heat. Add oil; swirl to coat. Add turkey pieces to pan; cook 2 minutes on each side. Place pieces on a broiler pan. Bake at 425° for 5 minutes. Turn pieces over; bake an additional 5 minutes or until golden. Serves 4 (serving size: 5 pieces).

CALORIES 227; FAT 6.1g (sat 1.2g, mono 2.7g, poly 1.3g); PROTEIN 32.9g; CARB 11g; FIBER 0.5g; CHOL 47mg; IRON 2mg; SODIUM 237mg; CALC 36mg

---

EXPERT TIP: *Put Kids in Charge*

"Consider assigning each child in your family one night a week when they're in charge of dinner. Encourage them to look through cookbooks, food magazines, and online recipe sites, and then help them create a shopping list based on the recipes they select. When they see how much work goes into their meal, they'll appreciate what's on the table and be more likely to take that first bite."

—*Liz Weiss, MS, RD, and Janice Bissex, MS, RD, bloggers, Meal Makeover Moms' Kitchen*

Take Advantage of Your Slow Cooker

YOU CAN'T BEAT A SLOW COOKER for make-ahead meals. Just combine the ingredients in the removable pot up to 24 hours in advance, and store it in the refrigerator overnight. The next day, put the pot into the heating unit, and set the temperature. A pot you don't have to watch during cooking and that's easy to clean afterward? What could be better for busy days?

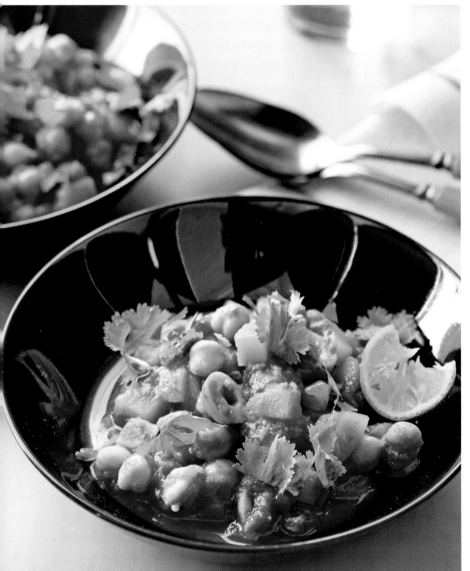

Chickpea Chili

If you use dried chickpeas, be sure to build in an hour for soaking. Or you can substitute drained canned chickpeas if you want to skip that step.

1 cup dried chickpeas
2 quarts boiling water
2 tablespoons olive oil, divided
1½ cups chopped onion
5 garlic cloves, minced
1 tablespoon tomato paste
1½ teaspoons ground cumin
½ teaspoon ground red pepper
½ teaspoon ground cinnamon
¼ teaspoon ground turmeric
¼ teaspoon kosher salt
2½ cups fat-free, lower-sodium
   chicken broth
⅔ cup sliced pimiento-stuffed olives
½ cup water
½ cup golden raisins
1 (28-ounce) can whole tomatoes,
   undrained and crushed
4 cups chopped peeled butternut
   squash
1 cup frozen green peas, thawed
¼ cup chopped fresh cilantro
6 cups hot cooked whole-wheat
   couscous
8 lime wedges

1. Place chickpeas in a saucepan; add 2 quarts boiling water. Cover and let stand 1 hour; drain. Place beans in a 6-quart electric slow cooker.
2. Heat a large skillet over medium-high heat. Add 1 tablespoon oil to pan; swirl to coat. Add onion; sauté 4 minutes, stirring occasionally. Add garlic; sauté 1 minute, stirring constantly. Stir in tomato paste and next 5 ingredients; sauté 30 seconds, stirring constantly. Add onion mixture to cooker. Add broth and next 4 ingredients to cooker; cover and cook on HIGH 8 hours.
3. Heat pan over medium-high heat. Add remaining 1 tablespoon oil to pan; swirl to coat. Add squash; sauté 5 minutes. Add squash to slow cooker. Cover and cook on HIGH 1 hour; stir in peas. Sprinkle with cilantro. Serve over couscous with lime wedges. Serves 8 (serving size: 1 cup chili and ¾ cup couscous).

CALORIES 382; FAT 7.6g (sat 0.9g, mono 4.1g, poly 0.8g); PROTEIN 12.9g; CARB 69.4g; FIBER 8.6g; CHOL 0mg; IRON 4mg; SODIUM 610mg; CALC 133mg

EXPERT TIP:
Go Slow Once a Week

"Make your life a whole lot easier and vow to use your slow cooker for at least one meal a week. Go on, find your slow cooker, dust it off, and give it a kiss. It will be your very best friend, I promise!"
—*Robin Plotkin, RD, blogger, Robinsbite*

Provençal Beef Daube

1 (2-pound) boneless chuck roast, trimmed and cut into chunks
1 tablespoon extra-virgin olive oil
6 garlic cloves, minced
½ cup boiling water
½ ounce dried porcini mushrooms
Cooking spray
¾ teaspoon salt, divided
½ cup red wine
¼ cup fat-free, lower-sodium beef broth
⅓ cup pitted niçoise olives
½ teaspoon freshly ground black pepper
2 large carrots, peeled and thinly sliced
1 large onion, peeled and chopped
1 celery stalk, thinly sliced
1 (15-ounce) can whole tomatoes, drained and crushed
1 teaspoon whole black peppercorns
3 flat-leaf parsley sprigs
2 thyme sprigs
1 bay leaf
1 (1-inch) strip orange rind
1 tablespoon water
1 teaspoon cornstarch
1½ tablespoons chopped fresh flat-leaf parsley
1½ teaspoons chopped fresh thyme

1. Combine first 3 ingredients in a large zip-top plastic bag. Seal and marinate at room temperature 30 minutes, turning bag occasionally.
2. Combine ½ cup boiling water and mushrooms; cover and let stand 30 minutes. Drain through a sieve over a bowl, reserving mushrooms and ¼ cup soaking liquid. Chop mushrooms.
3. Heat a large skillet over medium-high heat. Coat pan with cooking spray. Sprinkle beef mixture with ¼ teaspoon salt. Add half of beef mixture to pan; sauté 5 minutes, turning to brown on all sides. Place browned beef mixture in a 6-quart electric slow cooker. Repeat procedure with cooking spray and remaining beef mixture. Add wine and broth to pan; bring to a boil, scraping pan to loosen browned bits. Pour wine mixture into cooker. Add mushrooms, reserved ¼ cup soaking liquid, remaining ½ teaspoon salt, olives, and next 5 ingredients. Place peppercorns and next 4 ingredients on a double layer of cheesecloth. Gather edges of cheesecloth together; secure with twine. Add bundle to cooker. Cover and cook on LOW 6 hours or until beef and vegetables are tender. Discard bundle.
4. Combine 1 tablespoon water and cornstarch in a small bowl, stirring until smooth. Add cornstarch mixture to cooker; cook 20 minutes or until slightly thick, stirring occasionally. Sprinkle with chopped parsley and chopped thyme. Serves 8 (serving size: about ¾ cup).

CALORIES 360; FAT 22.5g (sat 8g, mono 10.6g, poly 1.1g); PROTEIN 30.2g; CARB 7.8g; FIBER 2.2g; CHOL 94mg; IRON 3.5mg; SODIUM 516mg; CALC 53mg

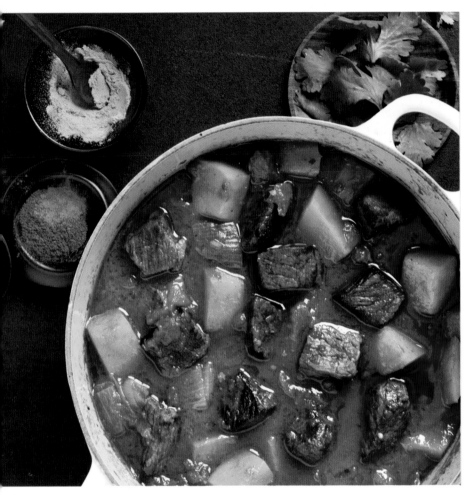

A 3½-ounce serving of beef provides 27g to 30g of protein.

Beef Tagine with Butternut Squash

Take your basic beef stew to the next level by making this simple, fragrant tagine featuring butternut squash. "Excellent!" said Stormydogblue on CookingLight.com. "I made this exactly as in the recipe, including the couscous. It was very good, and the smell was incredible. Don't skip the cilantro. It was perfect sprinkled on top. Bags of peeled and cubed squash at my local grocery store made this very simple."

2 teaspoons paprika
1 teaspoon ground cinnamon
¾ teaspoon salt
½ teaspoon ground ginger
½ teaspoon crushed red pepper
¼ teaspoon freshly ground black pepper
1 (1-pound) beef shoulder roast or petite tender roast, trimmed and cut into 1-inch cubes
1 tablespoon olive oil
4 shallots, quartered
4 garlic cloves, chopped
½ cup fat-free, lower-sodium chicken broth
1 (14.5-ounce) can no-salt-added diced tomatoes, undrained
3 cups (1-inch) cubed peeled butternut squash (about 1 pound)
¼ cup chopped fresh cilantro

Beef Up Your Beef Intake

THERE'S NO NEED TO BYPASS BEEF in your weekly meal planning—it can be a healthy choice as long as you choose lean cuts with "loin" or "round" in the name. Tenderloin is among the leanest but has a higher price tag. Less-expensive lean cuts benefit from marinating and braising to make them more tender.

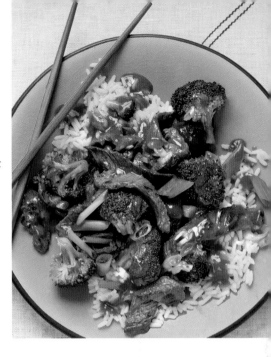

1. Combine first 6 ingredients in a medium bowl. Add beef; toss well to coat.

2. Heat a Dutch oven over medium-high heat. Add oil to pan; swirl to coat. Add beef and shallots; cook 4 minutes or until browned, stirring occasionally. Add garlic; cook 1 minute, stirring frequently. Stir in broth and tomatoes; bring to a boil. Cook 5 minutes. Add squash; cover, reduce heat, and simmer 15 minutes or until squash is tender. Sprinkle with cilantro. Serves 4 (serving size: 1½ cups).

CALORIES 283; FAT 9.5g (sat 2g, mono 4.8g, poly 0.5g); PROTEIN 25.6g; CARB 25.7g; FIBER 4.8g; CHOL 67mg; IRON 4.6mg; SODIUM 617mg; CALC 103mg

Quick Side
Scallion Couscous

Bring ¾ cup fat-free, lower-sodium chicken broth and ½ cup water to a boil in a medium saucepan. Gradually stir in 1 cup uncooked couscous. Remove from heat; cover and let stand 5 minutes. Fluff couscous with a fork. Stir in ⅓ cup chopped green onions. Serves 4.

CALORIES 169; FAT 0.3g (sat 0.1g, mono 0.1g, poly 0.1g); PROTEIN 6g; CARB 34.3g; FIBER 2.7g; CHOL 0mg; IRON 0.7mg; SODIUM 80mg; CALC 20mg

Beef-Broccoli Stir-Fry

"We loved this!" said Kellyyy624 on CookingLight.com. "This tasted just like something you would get from takeout except so much fresher! Next time, I think I will add some more veggies, perhaps carrots, snow peas, or even bean sprouts or baby corn. This is definitely a keeper!"

2 (3½-ounce) bags boil-in-bag long-grain white or brown rice
2 tablespoons dry sherry, divided
2 tablespoons lower-sodium soy sauce, divided
1 teaspoon sugar
1 (1-pound) boneless sirloin steak, cut diagonally across grain into thin slices
½ cup lower-sodium beef broth
1 tablespoon cornstarch
1 tablespoon hoisin sauce
1 teaspoon Sriracha (hot chile sauce) or ½ teaspoon crushed red pepper
2 tablespoons canola oil, divided
1 tablespoon bottled ground fresh ginger
2 teaspoons minced garlic
4 cups prechopped broccoli florets
¼ cup water
⅓ cup sliced green onions

1. Cook rice according to package directions.

2. While rice cooks, combine 1 tablespoon sherry, 1 tablespoon soy sauce, sugar, and beef in a bowl. Combine remaining 1 tablespoon sherry, remaining 1 tablespoon soy sauce, broth, cornstarch, hoisin, and Sriracha in another bowl.

3. Heat a large skillet over medium-high heat. Add 1 tablespoon oil to pan; swirl to coat. Add beef mixture; sauté 3 minutes or until browned. Remove beef from pan. Add remaining 1 tablespoon oil to pan; swirl to coat. Add ginger and garlic; cook 30 seconds, stirring constantly. Add broccoli and ¼ cup water; cook 1 minute. Add onions; cook 1 minute, stirring constantly. Add broth mixture and beef mixture; cook 2 minutes or until sauce is slightly thick. Serve beef mixture over rice. Serves 4 (serving size: about 1⅓ cups beef mixture and ½ cup rice).

CALORIES 476; FAT 12.9g (sat 2.4g, mono 6.3g, poly 2.3g); PROTEIN 32.1g; CARB 52g; FIBER 2.5g; CHOL 48mg; IRON 4.2mg; SODIUM 523mg; CALC 71mg

HOW TO EASILY SLICE BEEF INTO STRIPS

Partially freezing meat can make slicing cuts like sirloin or flank steak into thin, bite-sized pieces easier. For cuts that are 1 inch thick, cover the meat with plastic wrap and place it in the freezer for 45 to 60 minutes. You want the meat to be firm so it will remain rigid while slicing but not so hard that it can't be cut.

Keep It Lean with Pork

PORK TRULY IS the "other white meat" as many cuts are just as lean as chicken—or even leaner if you leave the skin on the chicken. Two of the leanest choices include pork tenderloin, which is incredibly versatile, and boneless center-cut loin pork chops.

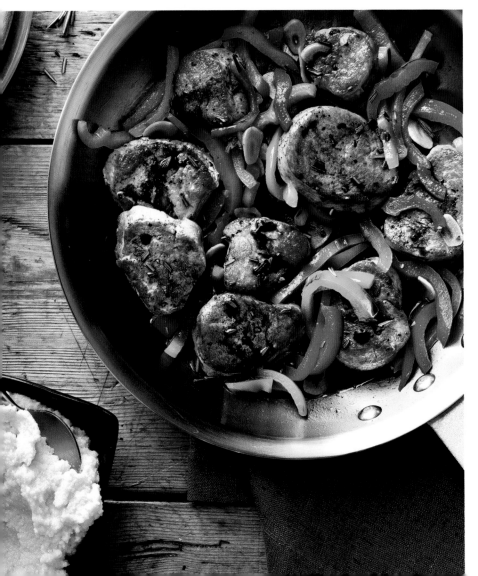

Pork Tenderloin with Red and Yellow Peppers

1 (1-pound) pork tenderloin, trimmed and cut crosswise into 1-inch-thick slices
½ teaspoon kosher salt
½ teaspoon freshly ground black pepper
1 tablespoon extra-virgin olive oil
1½ teaspoons chopped fresh rosemary, divided
4 canned anchovy fillets, drained and mashed
3 garlic cloves, thinly sliced
1 red bell pepper, cut into 1½-inch strips
1 yellow bell pepper, cut into 1½-inch strips
2 teaspoons balsamic vinegar

1. Heat a large skillet over medium-high heat. Sprinkle pork with salt and pepper. Add oil to pan; swirl to coat. Add pork to pan; cook 5 minutes. Reduce heat to medium; turn pork over. Add 1 teaspoon rosemary, anchovies, garlic, and bell peppers; cook 7 minutes or until peppers are tender and pork is done. Drizzle with vinegar. Top with remaining ½ teaspoon rosemary. Serves 4 (serving size: 3 ounces pork and about ½ cup bell pepper mixture).

CALORIES 215; FAT 10.1g (sat 2.7g, mono 5.4g, poly 1.2g); PROTEIN 25.2g; CARB 5g; FIBER 1.4g; CHOL 78mg; IRON 2mg; SODIUM 441mg; CALC 26mg

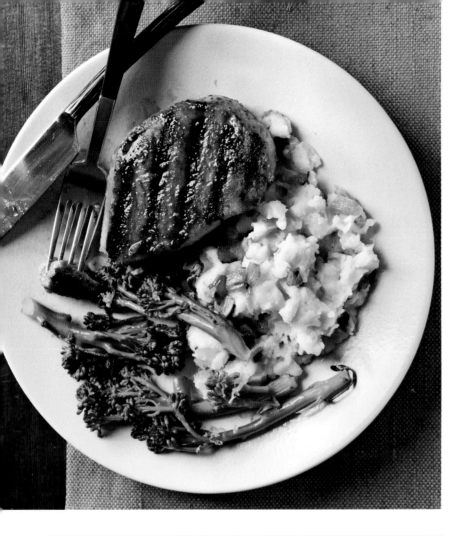

Pork chops, roasts, and tenderloins can be safely cooked to 145° (medium-rare), according to the U.S. Department of Agriculture. Because overcooking pork can make it tough, use a meat thermometer to make sure you hit the right temperature.

Expert Chatter on Cooking More at Home

@Nutritionbabes: Keep it simple. A few whole ingredients can transform into a beautiful meal in minutes.

@NutritionJill: Identify the payoff: budget, family time, health, control over choices, etc.

@ReganJonesRD: I think people hear plan ahead and think whole meal planned ahead = too much. I recommend prepping ingredients ahead so assembling is a snap later.

@AlexOppRD: I find having frozen vegetables helps me be able to make more meals because I have more ingredients on hand and ready to go.

Smoky Pan-Grilled Pork Chops

1 tablespoon cumin seeds
1 tablespoon brown sugar
½ teaspoon hot smoked paprika
¼ teaspoon salt
¼ teaspoon freshly ground black pepper
4 (4-ounce) boneless center-cut loin pork chops
Cooking spray

1. Cook cumin seeds in a small skillet over medium heat 1 minute or until fragrant, stirring frequently. Place in a clean coffee grinder or blender; process until ground. Combine ground cumin and next 4 ingredients; rub evenly over pork.
2. Heat a grill pan over medium-high heat. Coat pan with cooking spray. Add pork to pan; cook 5 minutes on each side or until done. Serves 4 (serving size: 1 chop).

CALORIES 224; FAT 11.5g (sat 4.1g, mono 5.2g, poly 0.9g); PROTEIN 24.8g; CARB 4.3g; FIBER 0.3g; CHOL 70mg; IRON 1.9mg; SODIUM 201mg; CALC 47mg

Keep It Simple with Sandwiches

THIS QUINTESSENTIAL LUNCHBOX STAPLE can carry over to dinner. Pair your sandwich with soup or salad, and use quality ingredients like bakery-fresh bread and flavorful sauces to make it more of a nighttime affair. Pile on the veggies while you're at it.

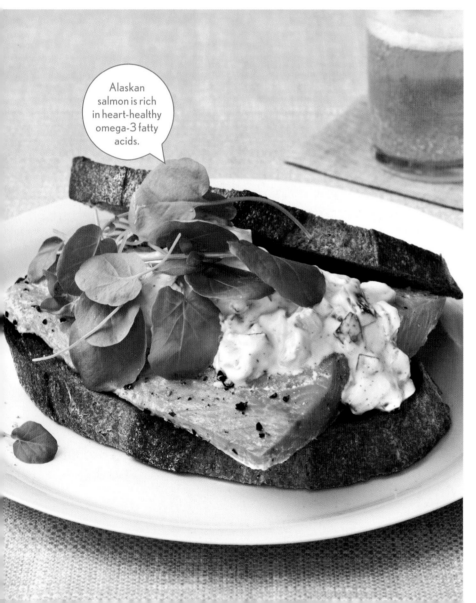

Alaskan salmon is rich in heart-healthy omega-3 fatty acids.

Salmon Sandwiches

4 (6-ounce) skinless wild Alaskan
   salmon fillets (about 1 inch thick)
Cooking spray
1 teaspoon olive oil
1/4 teaspoon salt, divided
1/8 teaspoon black pepper
1/2 cup chopped peeled cucumber
1/2 cup plain fat-free Greek yogurt
1 tablespoon minced fresh mint
2 teaspoons fresh lemon juice
1/8 teaspoon ground red pepper
8 (1-ounce) slices 100% whole-wheat
   bread, toasted
1/2 cup trimmed watercress

1. Preheat oven to 450°.
2. Place fish in a 13 x 9–inch glass or ceramic baking dish coated with cooking spray. Drizzle with olive oil; sprinkle with 1/8 teaspoon salt and black pepper. Bake at 450° for 8 minutes or until desired degree of doneness.
3. Combine remaining 1/8 teaspoon salt, cucumber, and next 4 ingredients. Place 1 fillet on each of 4 bread slices; top with 1/4 cup sauce, 2 tablespoons watercress, and 1 bread slice. Serves 4.

CALORIES 385; FAT 9.5g (sat 1.6g, mono 3.5g, poly 3g); PROTEIN 47g; CARB 25.3g; FIBER 4.1g; CHOL 97mg; IRON 2.9mg; SODIUM 550mg; CALC 113mg

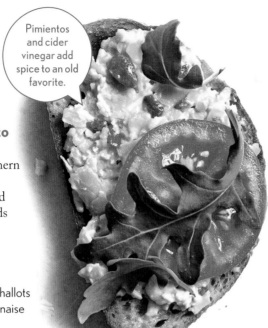

Pimientos and cider vinegar add spice to an old favorite.

Open-Faced Pimiento Cheese BLTs

Pimiento cheese is a Southern tradition. Stirring a little Parmesan into the standard cheddar-mayo mixture adds extra savory depth.

2 tablespoons bottled diced pimientos, drained
1 tablespoon grated peeled shallots
2 tablespoons canola mayonnaise
1 teaspoon cider vinegar
¼ teaspoon freshly ground black pepper
4 ounces reduced-fat shredded sharp cheddar cheese (about 1 cup)
1¼ ounces grated fresh Parmesan cheese (about ⅓ cup)
4 (1-ounce) slices sourdough bread, toasted
12 tomato slices
¼ teaspoon kosher salt
4 center-cut bacon slices, cooked and halved
1 cup baby arugula leaves

1. Combine first 7 ingredients in a large bowl. Spread 3 tablespoons cheese mixture on each bread slice; top each with 3 tomato slices. Sprinkle tomato slices evenly with salt. Top each sandwich with 2 bacon halves and ¼ cup arugula. Serves 4 (serving size: 1 sandwich).

CALORIES 266; FAT 14.9g (sat 5.5g, mono 6.1g, poly 2.2g); PROTEIN 16.4g; CARB 19.3g; FIBER 2.2g; CHOL 31mg; IRON 1.7mg; SODIUM 743mg; CALC 139mg

Grilled Eggplant Pita Sandwiches with Yogurt-Garlic Spread

2 (1-pound) eggplants, cut crosswise into ½-inch-thick slices
1 tablespoon plus ½ teaspoon kosher salt, divided
½ cup plain 2% reduced-fat Greek yogurt
2 tablespoons fresh lemon juice
2 teaspoons chopped fresh oregano leaves
⅛ teaspoon black pepper
2 small garlic cloves, minced
1 small red onion, cut into ½-inch-thick slices
2 tablespoons extra-virgin olive oil
Cooking spray
4 (6-inch) pitas, cut in half
2 cups arugula leaves

1. Place eggplant slices in a colander; sprinkle with 1 tablespoon salt. Toss well. Drain 30 minutes. Rinse thoroughly; pat dry with paper towels.
2. Combine remaining ½ teaspoon salt, yogurt, and next 4 ingredients in a small bowl.
3. Preheat grill to medium-high heat.
4. Brush eggplant and onion slices with oil. Place eggplant and onion slices on grill rack coated with cooking spray; grill 5 minutes on each side or until vegetables are tender and lightly browned.
5. Fill each pita half with 1½ tablespoons yogurt mixture, one-fourth of eggplant slices, one-fourth of onion slices, and ¼ cup arugula. Serves 4 (serving size: 2 pita halves).

CALORIES 311; FAT 8.2g (sat 1.6g, mono 5g, poly 1.2g); PROTEIN 12.7g; CARB 50.6g; FIBER 9.2g; CHOL 2mg; IRON 3.5mg; SODIUM 697mg; CALC 117mg

GO BEYOND SLICED BREAD

- Use wraps, lavash, hollowed-out French bread, and pitas for sandwiches with salad-type dressings since these breads will contain the spread better than sliced bread.

- Rye bread partners well with heavier meats, such as beef with horseradish spread or smoked ham with mustard.

- Flavorful, hearty-textured ciabatta, sourdough, focaccia, and multigrain breads provide a tasty contrast to milder fillings like chicken and turkey.

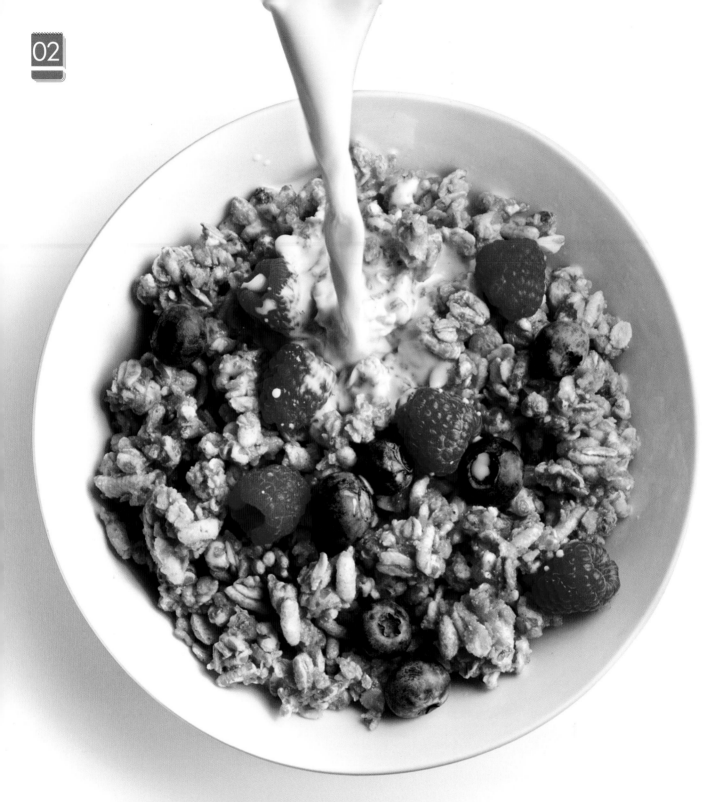

EAT BREAKFAST DAILY

MORNING BITES KEEP YOU FUELED ALL DAY.

WHAT YOUR MOTHER and teachers told you all your life, science has confirmed: Breakfast is important. It resets the body's metabolic motor after the night's long fast. Skipping breakfast sets you up for physical and mental lows and bad food choices when you pass the pastry counter at the local coffee shop. You can also use a good, satisfying breakfast to affirm your healthy-eating intentions for the day.

The modern time crunch is the worst enemy of breakfast, along with the temptation to save calories for later by skipping or skimping. But forgoing breakfast is not a smart weight-management strategy: Studies show that people who skip breakfast are twice as likely to be overweight compared to breakfast eaters (especially those who eat breakfast at home).

Plus, skipping breakfast makes it tough to make up for nutrient shortages later in the day.

Still, not just any breakfast will do. Ideally, you should include whole grains, fruits or vegetables (or both), lean protein, and low-fat dairy. Doing so incorporates two of the other 12 Healthy Habits: adding more whole grains to your diet and upping the amount of fruits and vegetables you eat daily. But if you can't pack all those good things into your morning every day, that's OK. The goal is to eat something—it can even be as simple as an apple and a piece of cheese.

This chapter offers lots of quick, make-ahead, and pick-up ideas; dispels the whole calorie-savings myth; and includes lots of nontraditional choices for the oatmeal-averse (pizza for breakfast, anyone?).

YOUR GOAL

Eat a healthy breakfast every day of the week.

The 12 Healthy Habits

| · 01 · GET COOKING | · 02 · BREAKFAST DAILY | · 03 · WHOLE GRAINS | · 04 · GET MOVING | · 05 · VEGGIE UP | · 06 · MORE SEAFOOD | · 07 · HEALTHY FATS | · 08 · GO MEATLESS | · 09 · GET STRONGER | · 10 · LESS SALT | · 11 · BE PORTION-AWARE | · 12 · EAT MINDFULLY |

Follow the Balanced Breakfast Rules

MORE THAN ANY OTHER MEAL, breakfast is an investment in good health. Eating in the morning helps you stay focused and energized and increases the likelihood that you'll get enough of the disease-fighting vitamins and minerals that are essential. And recent research makes the idea of a morning meal even more appetizing. A study in the *Journal of the American Dietetic Association* found that individuals who eat breakfast are less likely to be overweight—and more likely to exercise—than non-breakfast eaters. Here, the four cardinal rules:

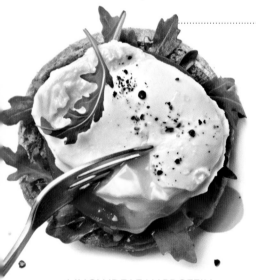

1. INCLUDE LEAN PROTEIN.
Sure, it's tempting to just grab an English muffin or bagel, but if you eat only refined carbohydrates, you'll be ravenous in two hours. Protein is digested at a slower rate than refined carbohydrates, which keeps blood sugar levels steady—and helps you feel satisfied longer. Good choices for your morning meal: fat-free milk (on cereal or in a latte or cappuccino), low-fat yogurt, soy or turkey sausage, cheese, or eggs (hard-cooked, poached, or scrambled).

2. FRONT-LOAD YOUR DAY WITH NUTRIENTS.
Breakfast offers an excellent opportunity to increase your daily vitamin and mineral intake. A recent study in the *Journal of the Academy of Nutrition and Dietetics* reported that people who ate breakfast had higher overall intakes of vitamin B_6, folic acid, vitamin C, calcium, magnesium, iron, potassium, and fiber than people who skipped their morning meal. Those nutrients help protect against a variety of diseases, ranging from heart disease to osteoporosis.

3. FILL UP WITH FIBER.
For guaranteed breakfast satisfaction, pair that lean protein with a serving of fiber-rich carbohydrates. Go for whole-grain breads and cereals that provide at least four grams of fiber per serving. These quality carbohydrates offer a long-lasting source of energy, so you continue to feel fueled several hours after eating. According to research published in the *International Journal of Food Science and Nutrition,* the energy supplied by a breakfast high in fiber-rich carbohydrates versus one that is high-fat may result in better mental focus during morning hours.

4. SAVOR YOUR FAVORITE TASTES.
If you don't like what you're eating, you won't stick with it. If your choices aren't the most nutritious, small tweaks can make them more healthful. For example, if you have a sweet tooth in the morning, try a piece of nutty whole-grain bread spread with a tablespoon each of almond butter (it's slightly sweeter than peanut butter) and fruit preserves instead of eating foods that offer sweetness but little nutritional benefit, like doughnuts.

The Empty-Stomach Warrior

"The big meal in my house was dinner, and that's how my body was conditioned."

JUNE FERESTIEN
Business Consultant

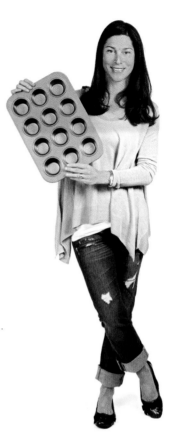

➤ **BREAKFAST CHALLENGE:** June is an athlete and has been since the age of 10, when she started competing in tennis and often headed to school without breakfast. She's now a working mom with two daughters and exercises daily—but heads to yoga on an empty stomach. She grazes during the day and saves up her calories for dinner. Despite not putting on weight, June understands the need to better balance her day. The trouble is she's not fond of traditional breakfast foods, so she needs some new ideas to draw her to the breakfast table. If you need some new morning inspirations too, read on.

OUR ADVICE

■ **Have dinner for breakfast.** If you don't like breakfast food, try savory options. Leftovers are ideal. Whole-grain sides from last night's meal (brown rice,

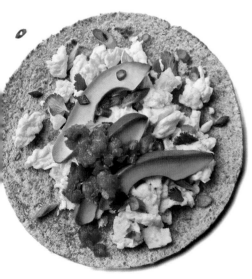

whole-wheat couscous, cold Asian sesame noodles) can become breakfast. See page 56 for more ideas.

■ **Make friends with muffins.** This ultimate make-ahead breakfast is freezer-friendly, quick to reheat, and satisfying. Pair with yogurt for a more filling meal.

■ **Build breakfast burritos.** They're quick and filling without being too heavy. Use whole-grain tortillas stuffed with scrambled eggs, avocado, and salsa, or add a smidge of sausage with leftover veggies.

■ **Poach in advance.** Try poaching eggs ahead—once they're done, shock them in cold water to stop the cooking process, drain, and store in a zip-top bag. Reheat for 30 seconds in simmering water or for about 10 seconds in the microwave, and serve over a toasted whole-wheat English muffin.

If you're not hungry in the morning, try a quick a.m. workout first to boost both your appetite and your metabolism.

Make It Mobile

EATING A SMART BREAKFAST leads to healthier choices all day long. If a rushed schedule is the issue, grab one of these 10 simple portable options as you're heading out the door.

- Single-serving bowls of whole-grain cereal combined with milk at your desk

- String cheese and whole-wheat crackers

- A hard-cooked egg and a piece of whole-wheat toast

- A six-ounce container of low-fat yogurt topped with berries and a tablespoon of nuts for added protein

- A whole-grain English muffin or apple topped with peanut butter

- A whole-wheat tortilla breakfast wrap filled with turkey and a little cheese, scrambled eggs with diced peppers and onions, or peanut butter and bananas

- A single-serving carton of low-fat, low-sodium cottage cheese paired with a piece of fruit

- A cup of plain instant oatmeal topped with a tablespoon or two of fruit preserves or chopped dried fruit to add a touch of sweetness

- A homemade yogurt parfait that you can make in a couple of minutes, like our parfaits on pages 70–71

- A slice of banana or zucchini bread smeared with cream cheese

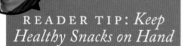

READER TIP: *Keep Healthy Snacks on Hand*

"I now keep a jar of nuts at my desk in case I did not have time to eat one of my breakfast staples: oatmeal and hard-boiled eggs (boiled the night before). It's better than munching on high-sugar snacks, which I used to do. Overall, the challenge has helped. I have put a little more variety in what I eat for breakfast without having to add additional time in the morning. I do not feel that I will stop eating breakfast now that I have a little more variety."

—*Michael Siegel,*
Healthy Habits Graduate

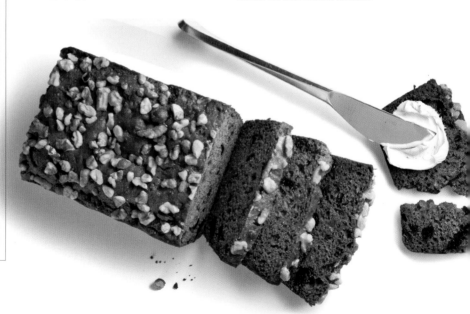

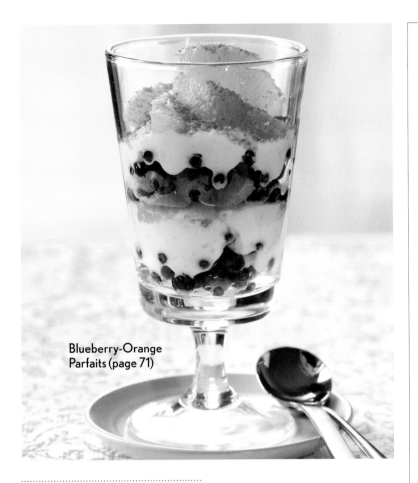

Blueberry-Orange
Parfaits (page 71)

An impressive 78% of
the 5,000-plus participants
in the National Weight
Control Registry
(an ongoing study that
tracks people's weight
loss and maintenance)
report eating a regular
breakfast and have lost an
average of 66 pounds,
maintaining that for
more than five years.

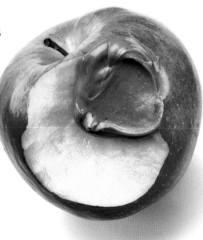

Before you order a Starbucks' bagel
or McDonald's Egg McMuffin, try one
of these healthier meals instead:

Starbucks' Protein Plate

This combo of fruit, peanut butter, a
hard-cooked egg, and a mini bagel
provides 370 calories, 5 grams of fiber,
and 17 grams of protein.

Subway's Western Egg White and Cheese Muffin Melt

This muffin, which is topped with egg
whites and fresh veggies like bell peppers and onions, has only 160 calories,
15 grams of protein, 5 grams of fiber,
and as much calcium as a glass of milk.

McDonald's Scrambled Eggs and English Muffin

A side of scrambled eggs, an English
muffin, strawberry preserves, and a
large coffee—all ordered individually—
are only 365 calories.

Jamba Juice Mango Peach Topper

This smoothie combines bananas,
peaches, mangos, soymilk, and fat-free
yogurt with a crunchy organic pumpkin flaxseed granola topping. One
12-ounce serving has 340 calories,
5 grams of fat, 6 grams of fiber, and at
least half your daily dose of vitamins A
and C. Order yours with an extra Whey
Protein Superboost for a total of 19
grams of satiating protein.

Get Motivated in the Morning

NOT BEING HUNGRY IN THE MORNING and a lack of time were the two top reasons cited in the *Cooking Light* community for skipping breakfast. *Cooking Light* 12HH coach Allison Fishman shares her four motivating strategies:

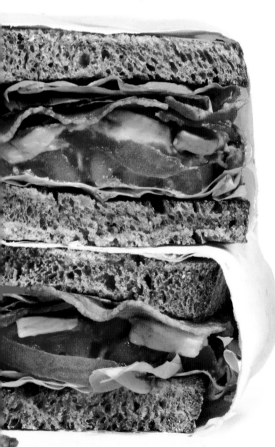

CHANGE YOUR EVENING ROUTINE.

Are you consistently going to bed on a full stomach? Try curtailing late-night eating, and you may find that you'll wake up with a better appetite for breakfast.

EAT YOUR BREAKFAST IN STAGES.

If you can't handle a meal first thing in the morning, it's OK to ease into your day. Grab a handful of nuts and an apple as you're leaving the house, and have a larger breakfast, like a scrambled egg wrap, at the office.

GET UP EARLIER.

You may need some extra time in the morning to feel hungry. Set your alarm 15 minutes earlier to help kick-start your appetite for breakfast before you leave the house.

FIND SOME NEW FAVORITES.

You're more likely to eat breakfast if it's something you really enjoy. Experiment with different smoothies, explore new nut butters to spread on your toast, or make tasty muffins and quick breakfast breads in advance. That way you can freeze them and pop them in the toaster while you're getting ready.

CONSIDER DINNER FOR BREAKFAST

Breakfast foods like oatmeal and eggs aren't for everyone. If you find that your dislike of traditional morning fare is why you turn up your nose to this meal, try one of these leftover lunch or dinner staples:

1. Chicken, tuna, or egg salad paired with whole-grain crackers

2. Veggie soup or chili spooned over scrambled eggs

3. Leftover steak topped with salsa and wrapped in a flour tortilla

4. Last night's cold pizza. It contains antioxidant-filled tomato sauce, calcium-rich cheese, and veggies.

5. A breakfast BLT. Add avocado for a dose of healthy fats.

Consider Eggs When Eating Out

THERE'S NO NEED TO SHY AWAY FROM EGGS FOR BREAKFAST—at 70 calories each, they're a compact, nutrient-rich source of high-quality protein, vitamin D, and brain- and eye-boosting choline, lutein, and zeaxanthin. In fact, one study published in the journal *Nutrition Research* found that men who consumed an egg-based breakfast ate about 400 calories less over a 24-hour period than when they consumed a carb-based one. But while eggs are delicious and nutritious when simply prepared (think poached or scrambled and paired with whole-wheat toast topped with homemade fruit preserves), when they cross the road to get to the restaurant side, they tend to pick up a fair amount of fat and calories on the way. Here's a look at the best (and splurge-only) choices for eggs on the menu.

HEALTHY CHOICES:

Two eggs: *173 calories*
Most restaurants use a little butter or oil to scramble or fry their eggs. That's fine; just swap traditional sides, like bacon and buttered toast, for smarter options, such as whole-wheat toast and fruit.

Veggie omelet: *537 calories*
A good choice, but quiz the server: Is this more egg and cheese than vegetables? If so, ask the kitchen to double the veggies and halve the cheese. You'll still get a deliciously satisfying breakfast.

POSSIBLE OPTIONS:

Frittata: *594 calories*
The light and fluffy cousin to the quiche can be packed with delicious seasonal veggies (asparagus = yum). But hold or halve the starchy sides, and ask about creamy sauces on top.

Egg sandwich: *648 calories*
Options range from 500 to nearly 1,000 calories, depending on fillings and the type of bread used (mega-bagel vs. English muffin). Pull out some meat or cheese if it looks overloaded.

SAVE FOR A SPLURGE ONLY:

Eggs Benedict: *669 calories*
Who doesn't love the decadence of poached eggs on an English muffin with salty smoked meat smothered in hollandaise? But save and share for a splurge. It's as high in fat (18g sat fat) and sodium (2,196mg) as it sounds.

Huevos rancheros: *1,097 calories*
The eggs, beans, and salsa here start out virtuous, then party with cheese, sour cream, and a tortilla, resulting in half your daily calories and nearly all your sodium.

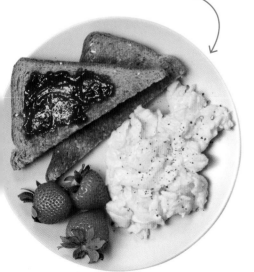

The Saving-My-Calories-for-Later Mom

"I make my kids anything in the morning, because ironically, I know how important it is to eat breakfast."

DANA BACARDI
Nonprofit Development Director

➤ **BREAKFAST CHALLENGE:** Over the years, Dana has seen some pounds creep on, so now that she's watching her intake, breakfast has gone on the back burner. But she's open to the idea: "Bowl and spoon is preferable—so I can eat quickly, throw the bowl in the sink, and head out."

OUR ADVICE

■ **Don't deprive yourself as a weight-control tactic.** Skipping breakfast can cause your body to increase fat storage and lead to weight gain. Studies show that people who eat breakfast regularly tend to weigh less than those who skip the morning meal.

■ **Have a breakfast sandwich.** Dana makes lunch for her kids every day, so it should be easy to keep the sandwich assembly line going for herself: a pita stuffed with peanut butter, banana, and honey; ham and cheddar on whole-grain bread; or hummus and cucumber slices on a tortilla.

■ **Choose cereals wisely.** The simplest breakfast is, of course, cereal—but look for one with a whole grain as the first ingredient, and one that contains at least 4 grams of fiber and offers at least 5 grams of protein per serving. Good examples are Kashi GoLean cereals, Post Shredded Wheat, and Müeslix.

■ **Make homemade fro-yo.** Mix a teaspoon of vanilla extract and a drizzle of honey into a large carton of plain fat-free or low-fat plain Greek yogurt, and freeze in an ice-cream maker. Enjoy a scoop for breakfast with fresh or frozen berries. Or stir in chunked or pureed fruit before freezing for fruity frozen yogurt.

FOLLOW UP: *Make Healthy Options Convenient*

"I haven't just changed my habits, my entire family now enjoys the upgraded cereals we have in our cupboards, and everyone (including my husband) likes to grab a quick bowl in the morning, sometimes with a little fruit on top. We put cereal, milk, bowls, and some fruit on the island counter for self-service breakfast. I make sure our new fruit bowl (which I always keep stocked) is in a convenient location—on the kitchen counter—so that we can all eat more fruit throughout the day, too."

—*Dana Bacardi*

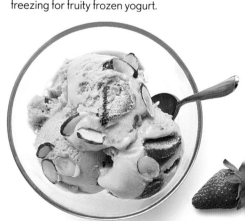

Suggested pour (1 cup) = 120 calories

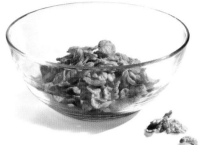

Average pour (1²/₅ cups) = 168 calories

Largest pour (3²/₃ cups) = 440 calories

It's hard to tell by looking, but this is 267% more than the suggested pour.

AVOID THE OVER-POUR

Cereal's a simple and healthy low-calorie breakfast choice, but not if you pour half the container into your cereal bowl. When we had 100 people show us their typical cereal pour, only one in ten poured close to the recommended portion. Our advice: Read labels, then practice with a measuring cup until you're able to eyeball the desired serving easily. If you change cereals, start over. Don't use a large cereal bowl that begs to be filled. And remember, some cereals, especially granola, have way more calories by volume than others.

 What are your a.m. solutions?

"I have instant oatmeal with fresh blueberries or strawberries every day for breakfast. I make my oatmeal with fat-free milk. I also make the kids' breakfast before the bus comes: eggs, whole-wheat toast, orange juice...or sometimes they have oatmeal with fruit and a bagel. You just make time for things that are important."

—*Janis Nunez*

"I hard-cook my eggs for the week on Sunday. For a quick breakfast, I top a whole-wheat bagel with a couple of preboiled egg whites and reduced-fat cheese and pop it in the toaster oven. I usually enjoy it with a side of berries or banana. Breakfast energizes me, so I wake up early and eat before I even get dressed for the day...I can never say I don't have time!"

—*Sonja Wilson*

"I don't limit breakfast to 'breakfast' foods. Yesterday, I had black bean soup for breakfast. Another day, it was red beans and rice. Sometimes I quickly sauté some kale and eat it with an egg."

—*Sherlonya Turner*

A study in the *American Journal of Clinical Nutrition* found that women who skipped breakfast consumed about 100 more calories and had higher LDL ("bad") and total cholesterol levels than women who ate breakfast. The breakfast eaters also had a better insulin response to eating, suggesting a lower risk of diabetes.

Keep Your Oats Interesting

HOT CEREAL MAKES FOR A NOURISHING, SATISFYING START to your day. Whether you choose old-fashioned rolled or steel-cut oats, or some other whole grain, a bowl of hot cereal is a superb base for layering on fruit, nuts, and low-fat milk.

Rise and Shine Oatmeal

Almonds help boost the protein in your bowl. You can also use chopped walnuts or pecans as well as any dried fruit you'd like, such as cranberries or cherries.

2 cups 1% low-fat milk
2 cups old-fashioned rolled oats
½ cup golden raisins
2 tablespoons honey
½ teaspoon kosher salt
½ teaspoon vanilla extract
½ teaspoon ground cinnamon
6 tablespoons sliced almonds, toasted
2 tablespoons brown sugar

1. Bring milk to a boil over medium heat. Stir in oats; cook 5 minutes. Remove from heat; stir in raisins and next 4 ingredients. Serve with nuts and sugar. Serves 4 (serving size: 1 cup oatmeal mixture, 1½ tablespoons almonds, and 1½ teaspoons sugar).

CALORIES 380; FAT 8.4g (sat 1.6g, mono 4g. poly 2.1g); PROTEIN 13g; CARB 66.3g; FIBER 6.1g; CHOL 5mg; IRON 2.4mg; SODIUM 304mg; CALC 216mg

KNOW YOUR OAT OPTIONS

Oats are rich in soluble fiber, which can improve heart health, lower your risk for type 2 diabetes, and help with weight control by keeping you feeling full longer. Here's a guide to all your oat options:

■ **Old-Fashioned Rolled Oats (Regular):** What most of us know as oatmeal is made of whole groats that have been steamed, then flattened by larger rollers. They're ready in 5 minutes.

■ **Oat Groats:** Oats as nature intended. You'll need about 45 minutes of stove-top simmering before they're tender.

■ **Steel-Cut (Irish):** These are whole-oat groats that have been halved or cut into three pieces so they cook faster (about 20 minutes), and the finished dish is chewier.

■ **Quick-Cooking Instant:** Regular rolled oats that are flattened even more, then cooked and dried. (Not to be confused with sugary pulverized instant oat packets.)

ROLLED   **OAT GROATS**   **STEEL-CUT**   **INSTANT**

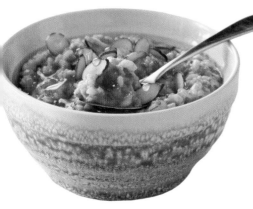

Overnight Honey-Almond Multigrain Cereal

Steel-cut oats and barley soak up water overnight so they're ready to go in the morning. Use a big bowl for cooking, because the grains will expand.

⅓ cup steel-cut oats
2 tablespoons uncooked pearl barley
1¼ cups water
⅛ teaspoon salt
¼ teaspoon ground cinnamon
⅛ teaspoon ground nutmeg
1 tablespoon sliced almonds, toasted
1 tablespoon honey

1. Combine oats, barley, and 1¼ cups water in a large microwave-safe bowl. Cover and refrigerate 4 hours or overnight.
2. Uncover bowl, and stir in salt. Microwave, uncovered, at HIGH 6 minutes or until most of liquid is absorbed, stirring well after 3 minutes. Stir in cinnamon and nutmeg. Top with almonds and honey. Serves 1 (serving size: 1 bowl).

CALORIES 388; FAT 7.1g (sat 0.9g, mono 3g, poly 2g); PROTEIN 11.2g; CARB 75g; FIBER 10g; CHOL 0mg; IRON 3.7mg; SODIUM 300mg; CALC 56mg

Muesli with Cranberries and Flaxseed

Oats do not always need to be served hot. Try this chilled version of muesli, the German word for "mixture" that's full of heart-healthy fats, whole grains, dried fruit, and calcium- and protein-rich yogurt.

2 cups old-fashioned rolled oats
½ cup dried cranberries
⅓ cup wheat germ
⅓ cup ground flaxseed
¼ cup maple syrup
½ teaspoon ground cinnamon
½ teaspoon vanilla extract
3 cups 1% low-fat milk
3 tablespoons slivered almonds, toasted
3 tablespoons chopped pecans, toasted
3 tablespoons pumpkinseed kernels, toasted
3 cups plain fat-free yogurt
2 tablespoons maple syrup

1. Combine first 7 ingredients in a large bowl, and pour milk over mixture, stirring to combine. Cover and chill 3 hours or overnight.
2. Combine nuts and pumpkinseed kernels in a small bowl. Spoon ¾ cup oat mixture into each of 6 bowls. Top each serving with ½ cup yogurt; sprinkle each serving with 1½ tablespoons nut mixture, and drizzle with 1 teaspoon maple syrup. Serves 6.

CALORIES 421; FAT 12.4g (sat 2.2g, mono 4.8g, poly 4.3g); PROTEIN 19.5g; CARB 62.4g; FIBER 6.6g; CHOL 7mg; IRON 3.5mg; SODIUM 162mg; CALC 457mg

Experiment to find the kind of breakfast that makes you feel the best and supports good choices the rest of the day. Ideally, your breakfast should include whole grains, a serving of fruits or vegetables, some lean protein, and low-fat dairy. This mix of foods gives you what you need to jump-start your day.

> ### READER TIP:
> *Make Breakfast Ahead*
>
> "I make a big batch of steel-cut oatmeal and portion it out for a few days' worth of breakfasts. Every morning I add fresh berries, flaxseed meal, and soy milk. If you microwave the berries with the oatmeal, it tastes like blueberry pie."
>
> —*Cathy Kessler*

Try New Oatmeal Toppings

THINK BEYOND BROWN SUGAR to kick up the flavor and texture of your bowl. Start with a bowl of hot cooked oatmeal made with ½ cup of dry oats and water, which has 150 calories, and then swirl, sprinkle, or top with any one of these 18 options. All clock in at 50 calories each or less—except the peanut butter, which comes in at right around 100 calories for 1 tablespoon.

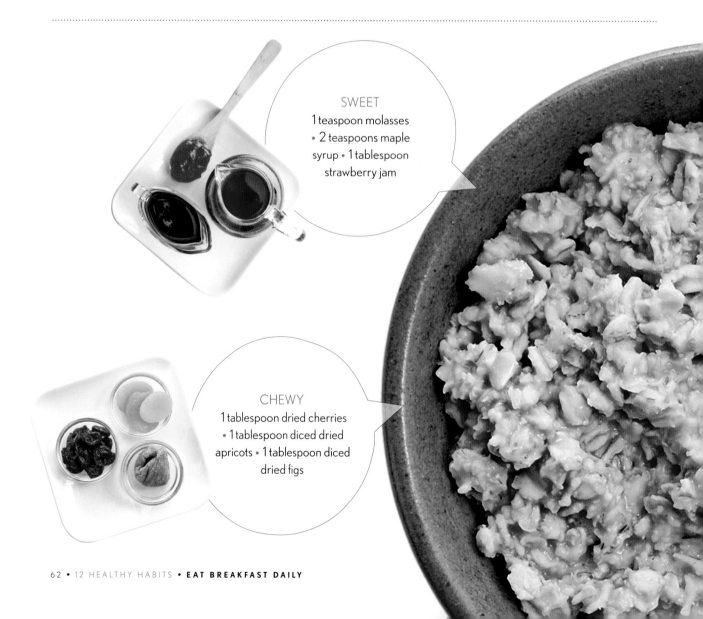

SWEET
1 teaspoon molasses • 2 teaspoons maple syrup • 1 tablespoon strawberry jam

CHEWY
1 tablespoon dried cherries • 1 tablespoon diced dried apricots • 1 tablespoon diced dried figs

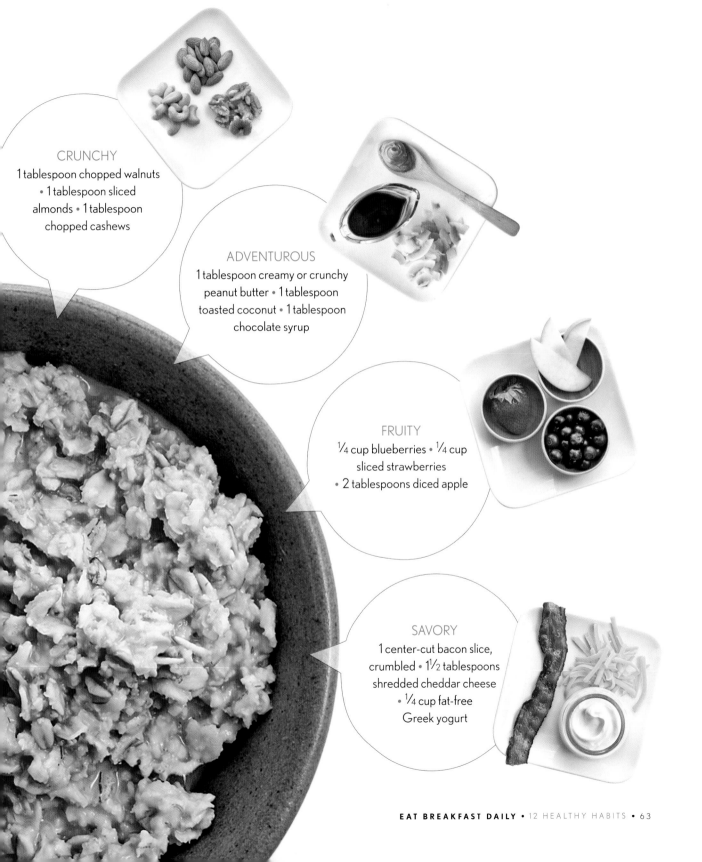

CRUNCHY
1 tablespoon chopped walnuts • 1 tablespoon sliced almonds • 1 tablespoon chopped cashews

ADVENTUROUS
1 tablespoon creamy or crunchy peanut butter • 1 tablespoon toasted coconut • 1 tablespoon chocolate syrup

FRUITY
¼ cup blueberries • ¼ cup sliced strawberries • 2 tablespoons diced apple

SAVORY
1 center-cut bacon slice, crumbled • 1½ tablespoons shredded cheddar cheese • ¼ cup fat-free Greek yogurt

Go For Whole Grains on the Griddle

WHEN YOU HAVE A LITTLE MORE TIME in the morning, these pancakes and French toast recipes are worth the effort. Plus, they're a delicious way to work in more whole grains.

Whole-Wheat Buttermilk Pancakes

Mixing whole-wheat flour with all-purpose adds whole grains while still keeping these pancakes light and fluffy.

3.6 ounces whole-wheat flour
  (about $3/4$ cup)
3.4 ounces all-purpose flour
  (about $3/4$ cup)
3 tablespoons sugar
$1\frac{1}{2}$ teaspoons baking powder
$\frac{1}{2}$ teaspoon baking soda
$\frac{1}{8}$ teaspoon salt
$1\frac{1}{2}$ cups low-fat buttermilk
1 tablespoon canola oil
1 large egg
1 large egg white
$3/4$ cup maple syrup
3 tablespoons butter

1. Weigh or lightly spoon flours into dry measuring cups; level with a knife. Combine flours and next 4 ingredients in a large bowl, stirring with a whisk. Combine buttermilk and next 3 ingredients, stirring with a whisk. Add buttermilk mixture to flour mixture, stirring just until moist.

2. Heat a nonstick griddle or large nonstick skillet over medium heat. Spoon about ¼ cup batter per pancake onto griddle. Turn pancakes over when tops are covered with bubbles and edges look cooked. Serve with syrup and butter. Serves 6 (serving size: 2 pancakes, 2 tablespoons syrup, and 1½ teaspoons butter).

CALORIES 347; FAT 9.9g (sat 4.4g, mono 3.4g, poly 1.3g); PROTEIN 7.4g; CARB 59.2g; FIBER 2.3g; CHOL 53mg; IRON 2.1mg; SODIUM 375mg; CALC 197mg

A recent Israeli study found that subjects who ate a 600-calorie breakfast high in protein and carbs that also included dessert lost on average 40 pounds more than those who ate a smaller 300-calorie breakfast.

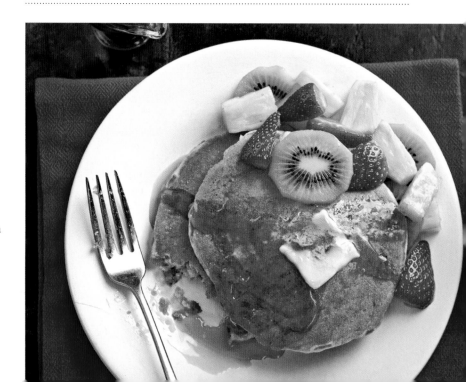

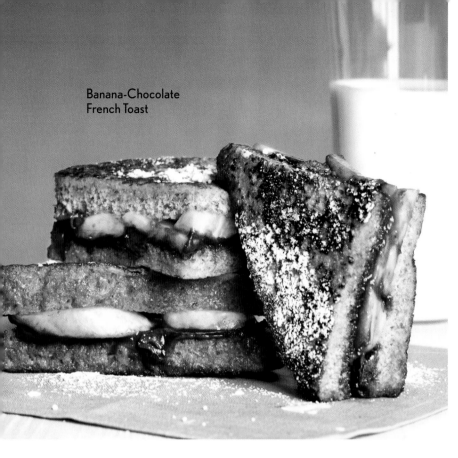

Banana-Chocolate
French Toast

Banana-Chocolate French Toast

¼ cup 1% low-fat milk
¾ teaspoon vanilla extract
½ teaspoon sugar
⅛ teaspoon salt
2 large eggs, lightly beaten
6 (1½-ounce) slices whole-grain bread
4½ tablespoons chocolate-hazelnut spread (such as Nutella)
1 cup thinly sliced banana (about 8 ounces)
2 teaspoons canola oil
1½ teaspoons powdered sugar

1. Combine first 5 ingredients in a shallow dish.
2. Spread each of 3 bread slices with 1½ tablespoons chocolate-hazelnut spread; arrange ⅓ cup banana slices over each bread slice. Top sandwiches with remaining 3 bread slices.
3. Heat a large nonstick skillet over medium-high heat. Add oil to pan; swirl to coat. Working with 1 sandwich at a time, place into milk mixture, turning gently to coat both sides. Carefully place coated sandwiches in pan. Cook 2 minutes on each side or until lightly browned. Cut each sandwich into 4 triangles. Sprinkle evenly with powdered sugar. Serves 4 (serving size: 3 triangles).

CALORIES 390; FAT 13.8g (sat 3.6g, mono 6.8g, poly 3.2g); PROTEIN 11.7g; CARB 53.6g; FIBER 6g; CHOL 91mg; IRON 2.6mg; SODIUM 391mg; CALC 115mg

Oatmeal Pancakes

1.1 ounces all-purpose flour (about ¼ cup)
1 cup quick-cooking oats
1 tablespoon sugar
½ teaspoon baking powder
½ teaspoon baking soda
¼ teaspoon ground cinnamon
1 cup nonfat buttermilk
2 tablespoons unsalted butter, melted
1 large egg

1. Weigh or lightly spoon flour into a dry measuring cup; level with a knife. Combine flour and next 5 ingredients in a medium bowl, stirring with a whisk.
2. Combine buttermilk, butter, and egg in a small bowl. Add to flour mixture, stirring just until moist.
3. Heat a nonstick griddle or large nonstick skillet over medium heat. Spoon about 2½ tablespoons batter per pancake onto griddle. Turn pancakes over when tops are covered with bubbles; cook until bottoms are lightly browned. Serves 3 (serving size: 4 pancakes).

CALORIES 273; FAT 11.2g (sat 5.7g, mono 3.3g, poly 1.3g); PROTEIN 10g; CARB 34.7g; FIBER 2.8g; CHOL 91mg; IRON 2.1mg; SODIUM 375mg; CALC 184mg

Make Friends with Muffins

EASY-TO-MAKE MUFFINS are an ideal grab-and-go breakfast or midmorning snack. Make a batch and freeze so they're always at the ready when you need a quick morning meal.

Cherry-Wheat Germ Muffins

6.75 ounces all-purpose flour (about 1½ cups)
¾ cup dried cherries, coarsely chopped
½ cup toasted wheat germ
½ cup packed dark brown sugar
1 teaspoon baking powder
1 teaspoon baking soda
½ teaspoon salt
¼ teaspoon ground allspice
1 cup low-fat buttermilk
¼ cup canola oil
1 large egg, lightly beaten
Cooking spray

1. Preheat oven to 400°.
2. Weigh or lightly spoon flour into dry measuring cups; level with a knife. Combine flour and next 7 ingredients in a large bowl, stirring with a whisk. Make a well in center of mixture. Combine buttermilk, oil, and egg in a bowl, stirring well with a whisk. Add buttermilk mixture to flour mixture, stirring just until moist.
3. Place 12 muffin-cup liners in muffin cups; coat liners with cooking spray. Divide batter evenly among prepared muffin cups. Bake at 400° for 15 minutes or until a wooden pick inserted in center comes out clean. Cool 5 minutes in pan on a wire rack. Serves 12 (serving size: 1 muffin).

CALORIES 202; FAT 5.9g (sat 0.7g, mono 3.3g, poly 1.8g); PROTEIN 4.5g; CARB 32.4g; FIBER 2.2g; CHOL 16mg; IRON 1.5mg; SODIUM 268mg; CALC 68mg

Blueberry Oatmeal Muffins

1⅔ cups quick-cooking oats
3 ounces all-purpose flour (about ⅔ cup)
2.33 ounces whole-wheat flour (about ½ cup)
¾ cup packed brown sugar
2 teaspoons ground cinnamon
1 teaspoon baking powder
1 teaspoon baking soda
¾ teaspoon salt
1½ cups low-fat buttermilk
¼ cup canola oil
2 teaspoons grated lemon rind
2 large eggs
2 cups frozen blueberries
2 tablespoons all-purpose flour
Cooking spray
2 tablespoons granulated sugar

1. Preheat oven to 400°.
2. Place oats in a food processor; pulse 5 to 6 times or until oats resemble coarse meal. Place in a bowl.
3. Weigh or lightly spoon flours into dry measuring cups; level with a knife. Add flours and next 5 ingredients to oats; stir well. Make a well in center of mixture. Combine buttermilk and next 3 ingredients. Add to flour mixture; stir just until moist.

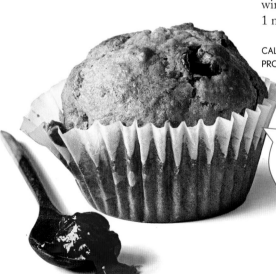

Vary the flavor with dried apricots or blueberries.

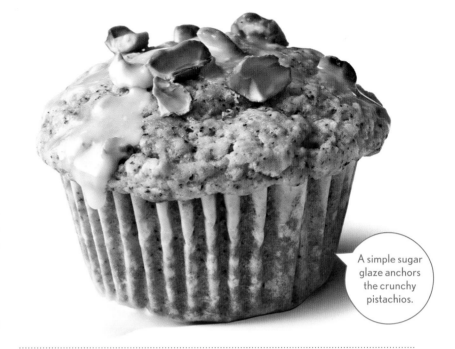

4. Toss berries with 2 tablespoons flour; gently fold into batter. Spoon batter into 16 muffin cups coated with cooking spray; sprinkle granulated sugar evenly over batter. Bake at 400° for 20 minutes or until muffins spring back when touched lightly in center. Remove from pans immediately; cool on a wire rack. Serves 16 (serving size: 1 muffin).

CALORIES 190; FAT 5g (sat 0.6g, mono 2.4g, poly 1.2g); PROTEIN 4.2g; CARB 33.3g; FIBER 2.4g; CHOL 23mg; IRON 1.6mg; SODIUM 248mg; CALC 74mg

A simple sugar glaze anchors the crunchy pistachios.

Pistachio-Chai Muffins

7.9 ounces all-purpose flour (about 1¾ cups)
½ cup packed brown sugar
1 teaspoon baking powder
1 teaspoon baking soda
¼ teaspoon salt
2 chai blend tea bags, opened
1 cup low-fat buttermilk
¼ cup butter, melted
1½ teaspoons vanilla extract, divided
1 large egg, lightly beaten
Cooking spray
⅓ cup shelled dry-roasted pistachios, chopped
½ cup powdered sugar
1 tablespoon water

1. Preheat oven to 375°.
2. Weigh or lightly spoon flour into dry measuring cups; level with a knife. Combine flour and next 4 ingredients in a large bowl, stirring with a whisk. Add tea to flour mixture, stirring well. Make a well in center of mixture. Combine buttermilk, butter, 1 teaspoon vanilla, and egg in a bowl, stirring well with a whisk. Add buttermilk mixture to flour mixture, stirring just until moist.
3. Place 12 muffin-cup liners in muffin cups; coat liners with cooking spray. Divide batter evenly among prepared muffin cups. Sprinkle nuts evenly over batter. Bake at 375° for 15 minutes or until a wooden pick inserted in center comes out clean. Cool 5 minutes in pan on a wire rack.
4. Combine remaining ½ teaspoon vanilla, powdered sugar, and 1 tablespoon water, stirring until smooth. Drizzle evenly over muffins. Serves 12 (serving size: 1 muffin).

CALORIES 192; FAT 6.2g (sat 2.8g, mono 2.1g, poly 0.8g); PROTEIN 3.9g; CARB 30.5g; FIBER 0.9g; CHOL 26mg; IRON 1.2mg; SODIUM 259mg; CALC 61mg

FIVE TIPS FOR PERFECT MUFFINS

1. Leave a few lumps. Over-stirring can toughen a muffin.

2. Spray the liners with cooking spray before adding the batter.

3. Check for doneness early (about 5 minutes before specified time), as ovens can vary.

4. Cool 5 minutes in the pan, then eat warm or remove to a rack so muffins don't get soggy.

5. Store correctly so muffins stay fresh. Keep in an airtight container for a day or two. Or wrap individually in plastic wrap, place all in a zip-top bag, and freeze up to one month. Thaw at room temperature or in the microwave for 10 to 30 seconds.

Bake a Better Breakfast

WAKE UP TO A HEARTY QUICK BREAD. It's a satisfying breakfast that's a snap to prepare. These loaves are chock-full of nutrient-rich ingredients like nuts, fruits, and dairy. For more whole grains, use whole-wheat flour in place of half of the all-purpose flour. A warm slice (even with a small pat of butter or smear of cream cheese and jam) is a much better choice than a glazed doughnut or scone that you might grab once you head out the door.

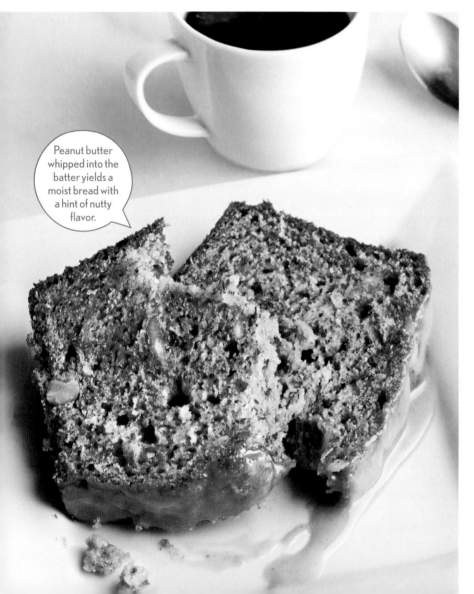

Peanut butter whipped into the batter yields a moist bread with a hint of nutty flavor.

Peanut Butter Banana Bread

Bread:
1½ cups mashed ripe banana
⅓ cup plain fat-free yogurt
⅓ cup creamy peanut butter
3 tablespoons butter, melted
2 large eggs
½ cup granulated sugar
½ cup packed brown sugar
6.75 ounces all-purpose flour
    (about 1½ cups)
¼ cup ground flaxseed
¾ teaspoon baking soda
½ teaspoon salt
½ teaspoon ground cinnamon
⅛ teaspoon ground allspice
2 tablespoons chopped dry-roasted
    peanuts
Cooking spray

Glaze:
⅓ cup powdered sugar
1 tablespoon 1% low-fat milk
1 tablespoon creamy peanut butter

1. Preheat oven to 350°.
2. To prepare bread, place first 5 ingredients in a bowl; beat with a mixer at medium speed. Add granulated and brown sugars; beat until blended.

3. Weigh or lightly spoon flour into dry measuring cups; level with a knife. Combine flour and next 5 ingredients in a small bowl. Add flour mixture to banana mixture; beat just until blended. Stir in nuts. Pour batter into a 9 x 5–inch loaf pan coated with cooking spray. Bake at 350° for 1 hour and 5 minutes or until a wooden pick inserted in center comes out clean. Remove from oven; cool 10 minutes in pan on a wire rack. Remove bread from pan; cool.

4. To prepare glaze, combine powdered sugar, milk, and 1 tablespoon peanut butter in a small bowl, stirring with a whisk. Drizzle glaze over bread. Serves 16 (serving size: 1 slice).

CALORIES 198; FAT 7.4g (sat 2.3g; mono 2.7g, poly 1.8g); PROTEIN 4.7g; CARB 29.7g; FIBER 1.9g; CHOL 28mg; IRON 1.1mg; SODIUM 200mg; CALC 27mg

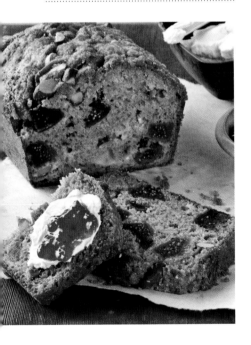

Fig, Applesauce, and Almond Breakfast Loaf

1 cup dried figs
1/2 cup boiling water
Cooking spray
1 tablespoon all-purpose flour
2 1/2 tablespoons brown sugar
2 tablespoons all-purpose flour
1 1/2 tablespoons coarsely chopped almonds
1 tablespoon chilled butter, cut into small pieces
1/8 teaspoon ground cinnamon
2 large egg whites
1 large egg
3/4 cup applesauce
1/3 cup plain fat-free yogurt
1/4 cup canola oil
1/2 teaspoon almond extract
3/4 cup granulated sugar
6.75 ounces all-purpose flour (about 1 1/2 cups)
2.5 ounces whole-wheat flour (about 1/2 cup)
1/3 cup chopped almonds, toasted
1 teaspoon baking powder
1 teaspoon ground cinnamon
1/2 teaspoon salt
1/2 teaspoon baking soda

1. Combine figs and 1/2 cup boiling water in a small bowl; let stand 30 minutes.
2. Preheat oven to 350°. Coat 2 (8-inch) loaf pans with cooking spray; dust with 1 tablespoon flour.
3. Combine brown sugar and next 4 ingredients in a small bowl, stirring with a fork until crumbly; set aside.
4. Place egg whites and egg in a medium bowl; stir well with a whisk. Add applesauce, yogurt, oil, and almond extract; stir well. Add granulated sugar; stir well.

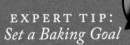
5. Weigh or lightly spoon 6.75 ounces all-purpose flour and 2.5 ounces whole-wheat flour into dry measuring cups; level with a knife. Combine flours and remaining ingredients in a large bowl, stirring with a whisk. Drain figs, and coarsely chop. Add figs and applesauce mixture to flour mixture, stirring just until combined. Divide batter between prepared pans. Sprinkle streusel over batter. Bake at 350° for 55 minutes or until a wooden pick inserted in center comes out clean. Cool 15 minutes in pans on a wire rack; remove from pans. Cool completely on wire rack. Serves 18 (serving size: 1 slice).

CALORIES 185; FAT 5.9 (sat 0.9g; mono 3.1g, poly 1.5g); PROTEIN 3.8g; CARB 30.9g; FIBER 2.5g; CHOL 14mg; IRON 1.2mg; SODIUM 140mg; CALC 58mg

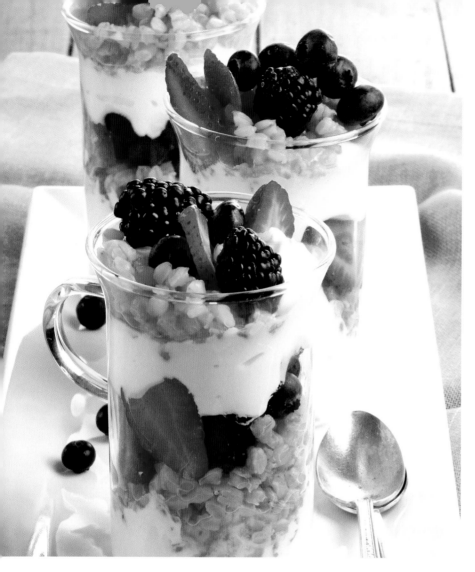

Greek Yogurt Parfaits

Grano, which means "grains" in Italian, are the polished whole berries from durum semolina wheat.

1 cup uncooked grano
12 cups water, divided
¼ cup orange blossom honey
¼ teaspoon kosher salt
4 cups plain 2% reduced-fat Greek yogurt
2 cups fresh berries (such as blackberries, blueberries, or sliced strawberries)

1. Soak grano in 6 cups water overnight. Drain. Place in a medium saucepan with remaining 6 cups water over medium-high heat; bring to a boil. Reduce heat, and simmer 20 minutes or until grano is just tender. Drain well. Stir in honey and salt. Cool to room temperature.
2. Spoon ¼ cup yogurt into each of 8 parfait glasses. Top yogurt with 3 tablespoons grano and 2 tablespoons berries. Repeat layers with remaining ingredients. Serves 8 (serving size: 1 parfait).

CALORIES 228; FAT 3.1g (sat 2.1g, mono 0.1g, poly 0.2g); PROTEIN 14.1g; CARB 38.9g; FIBER 4.8g; CHOL 7mg; IRON 0.8mg; SODIUM 106mg; CALC 130mg

Make Your Own Yogurt Parfaits

YOGURT PARFAITS are popping up at coffee shops and fast food outlets, but try making your own at home so you can control the quality of ingredients and the amount of added sugar. They're a tasty (and portable) way to get a serving of low-fat dairy, whole grains, and fruit.

Slow-Roasted Grape and Yogurt Parfaits

The roasting process softens the grapes slightly and heightens their flavor.

Cooking spray
2 cups seedless black grapes
2 cups seedless red grapes
3 tablespoons sugar
2 cups plain fat-free Greek yogurt, divided
¼ cup walnut halves, toasted and coarsely chopped
8 teaspoons honey
Thinly sliced fresh mint (optional)

1. Preheat oven to 200°. Coat a jelly-roll pan with cooking spray.
2. Rinse grapes; drain well, leaving slightly moist. Combine grapes and sugar in a large bowl; toss to coat. Arrange grapes on prepared jelly-roll pan. Bake at 200° for 3 hours or until grapes are softened but still hold their shape. Remove from oven; cool completely.
3. Spoon ¼ cup yogurt into bottom of each of 4 parfait glasses. Top each serving with about ⅓ cup grapes, 1½ teaspoons walnuts, and 1 teaspoon honey. Repeat layers; garnish with sliced mint, if desired. Serves 4 (serving size: 1 parfait).

CALORIES 298; FAT 5g (sat 0.5g, mono 0.7g, poly 3.5g); PROTEIN 12.2g; CARB 55.5g; FIBER 2g; CHOL 0mg; IRON 0.9mg; SODIUM 46mg; CALC 100mg

Blueberry-Orange Parfaits

The parfaits come together in a few minutes if you purchase orange sections from the refrigerated produce section of your grocery store.

1½ tablespoons Demerara or turbinado sugar
½ teaspoon grated orange rind
2 (7-ounce) cartons plain 2% reduced-fat Greek yogurt
2 cups fresh blueberries
2 cups orange sections (about 2 large)
¼ cup wheat germ

1. Combine first 3 ingredients in a small bowl, stirring until blended. Spoon ¼ cup blueberries into each of 4 tall glasses. Spoon about 2½ tablespoons yogurt mixture over blueberries in each glass. Add ¼ cup orange to each serving. Repeat layers with remaining blueberries, yogurt mixture, and orange. Sprinkle 1 tablespoon wheat germ over each serving; serve immediately. Serves 4 (serving size: 1 parfait).

CALORIES 186; FAT 3g (sat 1.6g, mono 0.1g, poly 0.5g); PROTEIN 11.8g; CARB 31.9g; FIBER 4.2g; CHOL 5mg; IRON 1mg; SODIUM 34mg; CALC 125mg

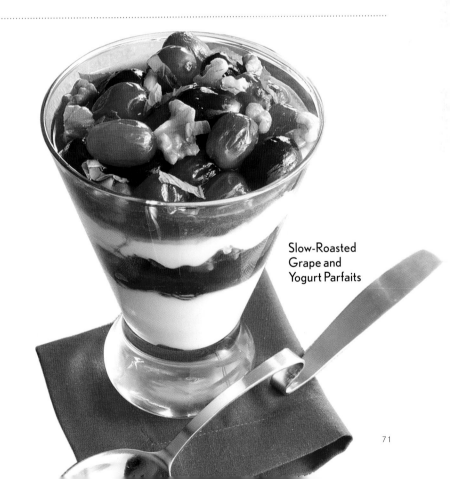

Slow-Roasted Grape and Yogurt Parfaits

Opt for Eggs More Often

EGGS HAVE BEEN REDEEMED of their rotten reputation. Now pretty much everyone knows that the bad rap eggs got over their cholesterol content was unfair—cholesterol in food isn't the heart disease culprit (attention has turned to saturated fat). The news about eggs keeps getting better. Updated USDA data shows that eggs are higher in vitamin D and lower in cholesterol (185mg down from 215mg) than previously recorded.

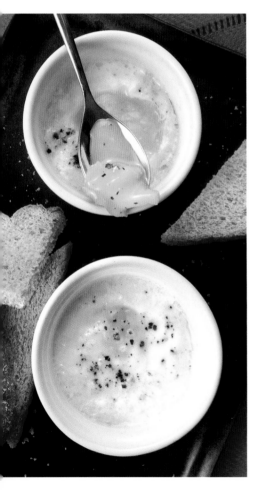

Simple Baked Eggs

This is an easy way to cook individual servings of eggs at one time. They can bake while you're getting dressed for work.

1 tablespoon butter
6 large eggs
1 teaspoon freshly ground black pepper
3/4 teaspoon salt
2 tablespoons whipping cream

1. Preheat oven to 350°.
2. Coat each of 6 (3-ounce) ramekins or custard cups with 1/2 teaspoon butter. Break 1 egg into each prepared ramekin. Sprinkle eggs evenly with pepper and salt; spoon 1 teaspoon cream over each egg. Place ramekins in a 13 x 9–inch glass or ceramic baking dish; add hot water to pan to a depth of 1 1/4 inches. Bake at 350° for 15 minutes or until egg whites are set. Serves 6 (serving size: 1 egg).

CALORIES 109; FAT 8.7g (sat 3.9g, mono 2.9g, poly 0.8g); PROTEIN 6.5g; CARB 0.8g; FIBER 0.1g; CHOL 223mg; IRON 0.9mg; SODIUM 380mg; CALC 32mg

Quick Garden Omelet

1/2 (20-ounce) package refrigerated red potato wedges, coarsely chopped
6 ounces presliced cremini mushrooms
1/2 teaspoon salt, divided
4 teaspoons butter, divided
8 large eggs
1/2 teaspoon freshly ground black pepper
1 cup bagged baby spinach leaves, coarsely chopped
1/2 cup (2 ounces) crumbled goat cheese

1. Heat a 12-inch nonstick skillet over medium-high heat. Add potatoes to pan; sauté 10 minutes, stirring occasionally. Stir in mushrooms and 1/4 teaspoon salt; sauté 8 minutes or until potatoes are tender, stirring occasionally. Remove from pan; set aside.
2. Wipe pan clean with paper towels. Melt 2 teaspoons butter in pan over medium-high heat. Combine eggs, remaining 1/4 teaspoon salt, and pepper in a bowl, stirring with a whisk until eggs are frothy. Pour half

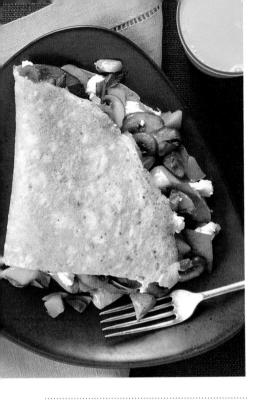

of egg mixture into pan; stir briskly with a heatproof spatula for about 10 seconds or until egg starts to thicken. Carefully loosen set edges of omelet with spatula, tipping pan to pour uncooked egg to sides. Continue this procedure 10 to 15 seconds or until almost no runny egg remains.

3. Remove pan from heat; arrange half of potato mixture, ½ cup spinach, and ¼ cup cheese over omelet in pan. Run spatula around edges and under omelet to loosen it from pan. Fold omelet in half. Slide omelet from pan onto a platter. Cut in half crosswise. Repeat procedure with remaining butter, egg mixture, potato mixture, spinach, and cheese. Serves 4 (serving size: 1 omelet half).

CALORIES 277; FAT 14.9g (sat 6.8g, mono 5.5g, poly 1.7g); PROTEIN 18.3g; CARB 13.7g; FIBER 2.2g; CHOL 377mg; IRON 2.8mg; SODIUM 596mg; CALC 89mg

HOW TO MAKE A GREAT OMELET

Omelets are easy to make and fun to fill. Dress one up with leftover vegetables, such as mushrooms, cherry tomatoes, and green onions or add ham or turkey, plus a little cheese for calcium. Precook meats and dice vegetables beforehand, because you'll have to work quickly and stay with the omelet as it cooks swiftly. Before beginning, preheat a nonstick pan over medium-high heat. It's important that the pan be hot. To test, add a few drops of water; they should sizzle.

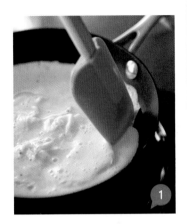

1. Whisk eggs until slightly frothy, about 20 to 30 seconds, and pour eggs into pan. Working quickly, stir the egg that coagulates around the sides back into the runny, uncooked center. Continue cooking and stirring as you tip the pan, allowing the uncooked egg to run out to the sides. Repeat this procedure until eggs are cooked to desired consistency.

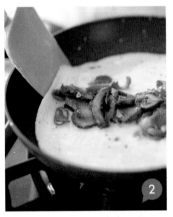

2. Sprinkle filling over the omelet. Remove pan from heat. Run the spatula around the eggs and under the omelet to loosen it from the pan.

3. Hold the pan over the plate, and tip it up and away, sliding the omelet from the pan onto the plate. Serve immediately.

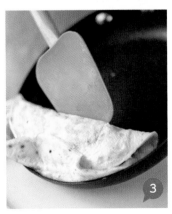

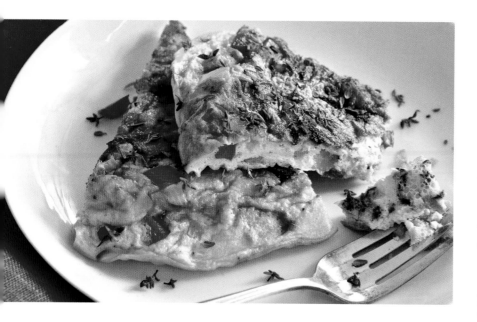

Summer Vegetable Frittata

1½ tablespoons olive oil
1 cup diced zucchini
½ cup chopped red bell pepper
⅓ cup chopped onion
1 tablespoon chopped fresh thyme
½ teaspoon salt, divided
¼ teaspoon freshly ground black
   pepper, divided
2 garlic cloves, minced
½ cup chopped seeded tomato
9 large eggs

1. Heat a 10-inch nonstick broiler-proof skillet over medium heat. Add oil to pan; swirl to coat. Add zucchini, bell pepper, onion, thyme, ¼ teaspoon salt, ⅛ teaspoon black pepper, and garlic. Cover and cook 7 minutes or until vegetables are tender, stirring occasionally. Stir in tomato. Cook, uncovered, 5 minutes or until liquid evaporates.
2. Combine eggs, remaining ¼ teaspoon salt, and remaining ⅛ teaspoon black pepper in a medium bowl; stir with a whisk until frothy. Pour egg mixture into pan over vegetables, stirring gently. Cover, reduce heat, and cook 15 minutes or until almost set in center.
3. Preheat broiler.
4. Broil frittata 3 minutes or until set. Invert onto a serving platter; cut into 8 wedges. Serves 4 (serving size: 2 wedges).

CALORIES 227; FAT 16.4g (sat 4.2g, mono 8g, poly 2.1g); PROTEIN 15.1g; CARB 5.5g; FIBER 1.1g; CHOL 476mg; IRON 2.4mg; SODIUM 458mg; CALC 80mg

WHITE VS. BROWN EGGS

In the era of fancy omega-3 eggs, brown eggs retain a certain rustic allure, but they're no more nutritious than their white counterparts. A large brown egg contains the same proportion of white and yolk, and the same nutrients, as a white egg. Brown eggs simply come from a different breed of hens, which are often bigger birds and require more feed than standard white-egg-laying Leghorn chickens. Those costs are usually passed on, resulting in a 25% price premium paid for what is basically an aesthetic choice. What to do: Choose by wallet or style sensibility. Either way, you'll pick a good egg.

DECODING EGG CARTONS

Egg cartons are dotted with claims these days. Here's help in translating the callouts.

■ **Omega-3:** Hens that eat flaxseeds lay eggs that can be higher in these heart-healthy fatty acids.

■ **Vegetarian-fed:** No nutritional difference, but perhaps more appealing to egg-eating vegetarians.

■ **Hormone-free:** Nice to know, but there are no hormone products approved for egg production.

■ **Cage-free:** Implies more humane treatment than battery crowding, but the claim is lightly regulated.

Open-Faced Sandwiches with Ricotta, Arugula, and Fried Egg

4 (2-ounce) slices whole-wheat country bread
Cooking spray
2 cups arugula
1 tablespoon extra-virgin olive oil, divided
1 1/2 teaspoons fresh lemon juice
1/2 teaspoon salt, divided
1/2 teaspoon freshly ground black pepper, divided
4 large eggs
3/4 cup part-skim ricotta cheese
1/4 cup (1 ounce) grated fresh Parmigiano-Reggiano cheese
1 teaspoon chopped fresh thyme

1. Preheat broiler.
2. Coat both sides of bread with cooking spray. Broil 2 minutes on each side or until lightly toasted.
3. Combine arugula, 2 teaspoons oil, juice, 1/8 teaspoon salt, and 1/4 teaspoon pepper; toss gently.
4. Heat a large nonstick skillet over medium heat. Add remaining 1 teaspoon oil; swirl to coat. Crack eggs into pan; cook 2 minutes. Cover and cook 2 minutes or until whites are set. Remove from heat.
5. Combine 1/4 teaspoon salt, ricotta, Parmigiano-Reggiano, and thyme; spread over bread slices. Divide salad and eggs evenly over bread. Sprinkle with remaining 1/8 teaspoon salt and remaining 1/4 teaspoon pepper. Serves 4 (serving size: 1 sandwich).

CALORIES 337; FAT 15.8g (sat 5.9g; mono 6.9g; poly 1.6g); PROTEIN 21.8g; CARB 27.2g; FIBER 4.1g; CHOL 231mg; IRON 2.8mg; SODIUM 807mg; CALC 316mg

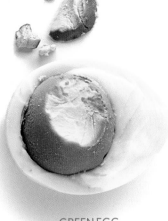

GOOD EGG

GREEN EGG

PERFECTING THE HARD-COOKED EGG

If your hard-cooked eggs often turn out with a green ring around the yolk, here's the fix: The key is to heat them slowly and cool them quickly. Place eggs in a saucepan, cover with water to 1 inch above eggs, and bring to a boil. Immediately remove from heat; cover and let stand 10 minutes (for small eggs) or 15 (for large). Peel the eggs immediately; or, if you're not using them right away, allow the eggs to cool in ice water. To peel, crack the top of each egg with a spoon, and roll the egg gently on a flat surface to break up the shell. Peel under cold running water.

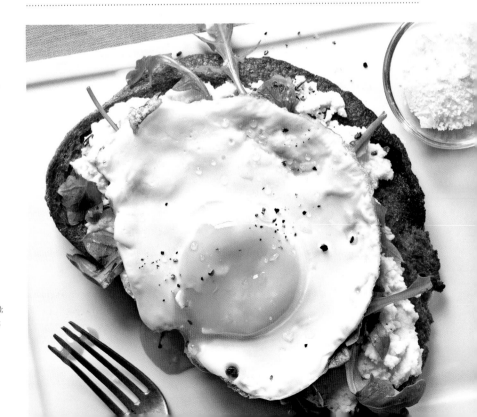

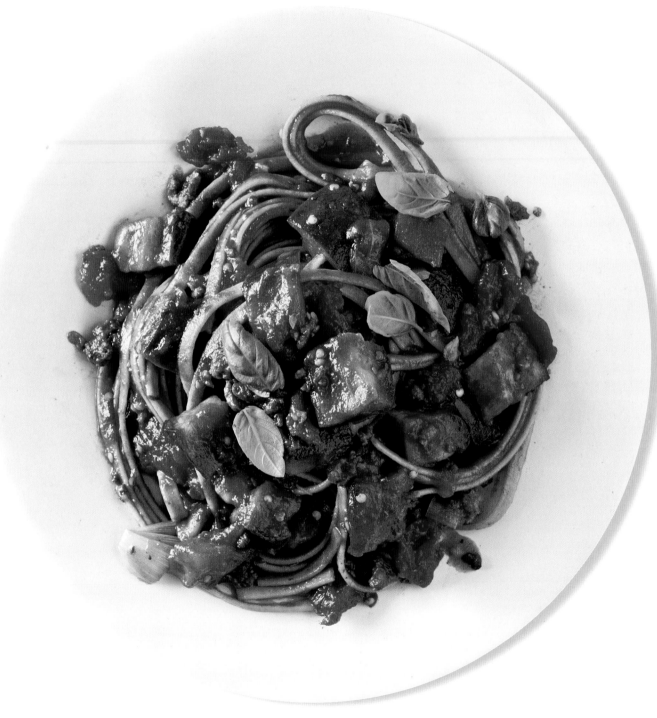

GO FOR WHOLE GRAINS

CHOOSE WHOLE, AND YOU WON'T FEEL HALF-FULL.

THE ERA OF CARB PHOBIA IS PASSING, and public taste is rebounding toward simpler foods. Whole grains are definitely back in the spotlight, the soul of the health-food ideal. Today's "it" food is one of mankind's oldest foods—only in the last century, in fact, have refined grains become more popular than whole grains, thanks to the introduction of white flour at the industrial level.

When left whole, grains are full of protein, fiber, complex carbohydrates, vitamins, and antioxidants, many of which are stripped away during the refining process. A diet rich in whole grains is associated with a lower risk of heart disease, stroke, and type 2 diabetes, and whole grains in the diet seem to help with weight control.

Problem is, getting whole grains into a modern diet isn't simple at all. Only half of you say you're regularly eating three servings of whole grains a day, and no wonder: The whole-grain landscape is confusing. There is no simple standard for a serving. Food labels are unreliable. Definitions are tricky. The goal of this habit is to help you figure out the maze of information by taking a simple approach to servings, decoding the labels, and then getting three servings of whole grains into your diet each day, without a lot of fuss. It can be as simple as having a serving at breakfast, lunch, and snack time or dinner.

YOUR GOAL

Eat three servings of whole grains each day.

The 12 Healthy Habits

| · 01 · GET COOKING | · 02 · BREAKFAST DAILY | · 03 · WHOLE GRAINS | · 04 · GET MOVING | · 05 · VEGGIE UP | · 06 · MORE SEAFOOD | · 07 · HEALTHY FATS | · 08 · GO MEATLESS | · 09 · GET STRONGER | · 10 · LESS SALT | · 11 · BE PORTION-AWARE | · 12 · EAT MINDFULLY |

Make Simple Swaps

SOMETIMES JUST A LITTLE SWITCH in meals or snacks or the ingredients you typically use can translate into huge gains for your whole-grain goals.

WHEN MAKING SANDWICHES...

Use whole-wheat bread, pitas, or tortillas. All count as up to two of your three recommended daily servings of whole grain. Typically, two slices of whole-wheat bread contain fewer calories and a bit more fiber than one whole-wheat pita, which has less sodium. Just check the label to make sure it says 100% whole wheat.

WHEN BAKING...

Sub half of your all-purpose flour with whole-wheat flour. But don't just dive into your favorite recipes for muffins, breads, and cookies and replace all the flour with whole-wheat. There are definite texture and flavor differences. Starting out, you may seek recipes using a mix of flours to get your palate used to the differences.

WHEN BUYING CEREAL...

Make sure you see the words "whole grain" as the first ingredient, such as whole-wheat, whole oats, or whole corn. Instant oatmeal is also a quick and easy choice (just make sure sugar and salt aren't also listed as top ingredients).

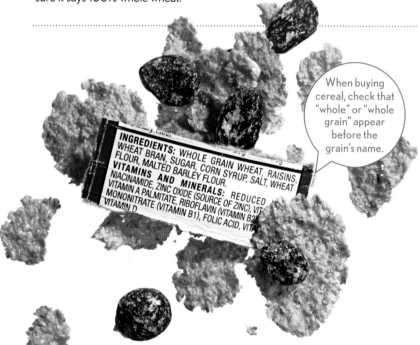

When buying cereal, check that "whole" or "whole grain" appear before the grain's name.

INGREDIENTS: WHOLE GRAIN WHEAT, RAISINS, WHEAT BRAN, SUGAR, CORN SYRUP, SALT, WHEAT FLOUR, MALTED BARLEY FLOUR.
VITAMINS AND MINERALS: REDUCED
NIACINAMIDE, ZINC OXIDE (SOURCE OF ZINC), VIT
VITAMIN A PALMITATE, RIBOFLAVIN (VITAMIN B2
MONONITRATE (VITAMIN B1), FOLIC ACID, VITA
VITAMIN D

EXPERT TIP:
Get Started Early

"If you don't get your whole grains at breakfast, your odds of eating at least three servings go down as the day goes on. You may think that you're getting fiber in other ways, like fruits and vegetables, but studies indicate that grain fiber is the most protective of our health. It may take a little planning, and eating more often at home, but it's not that difficult to do."

—*Joanne Slavin, PhD, RD, professor in the Department of Food Science and Nutrition, University of Minnesota*

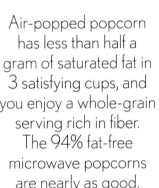

WHEN COOKING PASTA...

Opt for the whole-grain variety. There are also brown rice, Kamut berries, rye, spelt, or pastas that you can try to add variety. Their flavor can range from slight to very pronounced, so plan to serve with bold-flavored sauces, such as a garlicky-herby marinara or a robust mushroom sauce.

WHEN SNACKING...

Go for popcorn instead of pretzels. Three cups of air-popped popcorn count as a fiber-rich whole-grain serving. If choosing the bagged variety, read the ingredient list: Many of the brand names have added salt, butter, and sugar.

MAKE YOUR SNACKS WHOLE. Spread peanut butter on a slice of whole-wheat bread and top with sliced banana and almonds.

Air-popped popcorn has less than half a gram of saturated fat in 3 satisfying cups, and you enjoy a whole-grain serving rich in fiber. The 94% fat-free microwave popcorns are nearly as good.

THE DISH ON WHOLE GRAINS

Here are four reasons why enjoying more whole-grain foods can help keep you healthy and trim.

1. It lowers risk of heart disease. In a 2008 meta-analysis, which compiles data from several studies, researchers concluded that whole-grain consumption not only made heart disease less likely, but less serious if it does occur.
2. It reduces risk of insulin resistance and metabolic syndrome. Research from the Harvard School of Public Health has found that three or more servings of whole grains daily reduces your risk of developing these two precursors to type 2 diabetes.
3. It lowers chances of colon cancer. It may cut your risk by about 20%, according to a meta-analysis published in the *British Medical Journal.*
4. It helps you stay at a healthy weight. Women who consume more whole grains weigh less than those who don't, according to the Harvard Nurses' Health Study, which tracks the health of thousands of nurses.

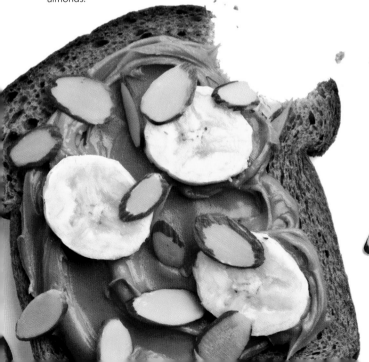

Fortify Your Favorite Foods

UPPING YOUR WHOLE-GRAIN INTAKE becomes a whole lot easier when you add whole grains to some of your best-loved meals.

AT BREAKFAST...

- Stir a handful of rolled oats, wheat berries, or whole-grain granola into your yogurt.
- Toss toasted amaranth seeds into the batter for pancakes, muffins, and breads.
- Use last night's leftover quinoa or bulgur as a base for hot cereal. Reheat and top with cinnamon, brown sugar, or any of the toppings on page 62-63.

AT LUNCH...

- Use wheat berries, spelt, or millet for a pasta-like salad with chopped veggies and fresh herbs, like Wheat Berry Salad with Raisins and Pistachios on page 107.
- Add brown rice or barley to home-made or canned soup.
- Go for 100% whole-wheat flour tortillas when making quesadillas, tacos, and chips.

AT DINNER...

- Stir bulgur or oats into ground beef or turkey when making meatballs, burgers, or meat loaf.
- Toss a cup of wheat berries or wild rice into your favorite slow-cooker chili.
- Serve entrées (like chicken in a sauce or braised meat) on top of brown rice, whole-wheat noodles, or whole-grain polenta.

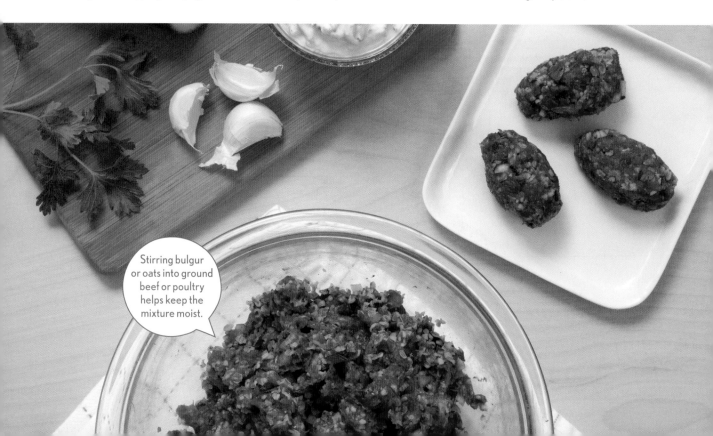

Stirring bulgur or oats into ground beef or poultry helps keep the mixture moist.

The Whole-Grain Newbie

"I don't really pay attention to whole grains, but this is a chance to get healthier."

L'ANNE GILMAN
Gallery Owner

➤ **WHOLE-GRAIN CHALLENGE:** L'Anne loves to cook, but she worries that her heavy Southern cooking—fried chicken, dumplings, and meat loaf—will eventually take its toll on her health. She also wants to set a healthier example for her three kids.

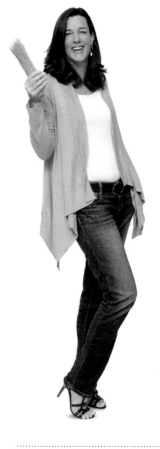

OUR ADVICE

■ **Find a whole-grain baking mix.** There are a variety of whole-grain baking mixes out there for convenient pancakes, biscuits, even chicken and dumplings. Look in your supermarket, or buy online.

■ **Add whole grains gradually.** You don't have to go whole-hog right away—it might backfire with picky eaters. Try a combo of half regular pasta with half whole-wheat at first to help your family gradually adjust to the differences in taste and texture.

■ **Use whole-wheat breadcrumbs.** Pulse 100% whole-wheat bread in a food processor to make breadcrumbs (1 slice will produce about ½ cup crumbs). Use as breading for chicken cutlets, a binder for meat loaf, or a topping for casseroles like mac and cheese. To complement the nutty flavor (or mask it, if some don't enjoy it), toss with olive oil, garlic, and herbs.

■ **Use whole-wheat flour in cookies, muffins, and breads.** But start with half all-purpose flour and half whole-wheat flour since whole-wheat flour affects texture and flavor.

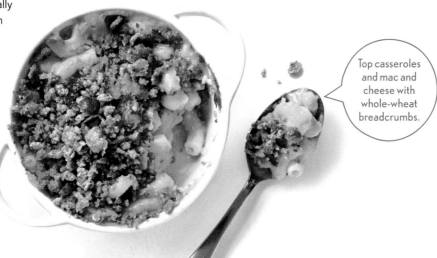

Top casseroles and mac and cheese with whole-wheat breadcrumbs.

Meet the Whole Grain!

A GRAIN IS A SEED, WITH THREE PARTS: the germ, the endosperm, and the bran. Refined grains consist of only one part of the seed: the starchy endosperm, which lacks some valuable nutrients.

Germ: The inner embryo of the grain is the nutrient storehouse and sprouts into a new plant when fertilized by pollen.
Provides: healthy fats, vitamin E, B vitamins, phytonutrients, and minerals

Endosperm: The starchy, thick middle layer serves as the energy supply for the growing plant.
Provides: protein and carbohydrates

Bran: The tough outer shell helps protect the other two parts of the kernel from assault by sunlight, pests, water, and disease.
Provides: antioxidants, fiber, B vitamins, and minerals

COUNTING ON WHOLE GRAINS

Certain foods are always whole grain, such as oatmeal, brown rice, and quinoa, while others are sometimes whole grain depending on how they've been processed. It gets even trickier when it comes to breads, cereals, crackers, and other processed grain foods. Many of these products contain a mixture of whole and refined grains.

A product can only be called "whole grain" if it includes at least 51% whole-grain ingredients or 8 grams of whole grains per serving. A full serving is 16 grams of whole grains, which is the amount you'll find in foods labeled 100% whole-grain or those that list whole wheat or another whole grain as the first ingredient.

Keep in mind that a serving of grains may not be equal to a serving of whole grains. You need 16 grams of *whole grains* before it's a full serving of the good stuff. For instance, a cracker that touts "made with whole grains" may provide only 5 grams of whole grain per serving, which means you'd need to eat more than 3 servings, or 48 crackers (more than 200 calories), to get a single whole-grain serving. That's why checking the ingredient list is so important.

Focus on 48: The daily goal is 48 grams of whole grains, or three servings that each provide 16 grams of whole-grain ingredients.

16 GRAMS + 16 GRAMS + 16 GRAMS = 48 GRAMS

The Whole-Grain Seeker on a Budget

"I'm confused about what I'm getting—or not getting—when I read labels."

ADAM HICKMAN
Cooking Light *Recipe Developer*

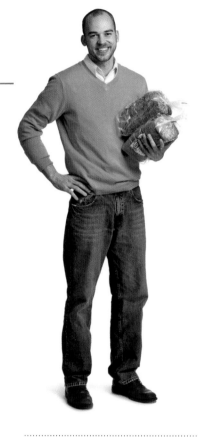

➤ **WHOLE-GRAIN CHALLENGE:** "I eat raisin bran and feel proud, but I'm not even sure it's whole grain," says Adam. "I need help translating what the marketing people put on packages. Whole grains can be expensive, and I want to make sure what I'm buying is genuine, and that I'm eating the right amount of it."

OUR ADVICE

■ **Read front-of-box claims.** Look for "100% whole grain" or "whole grain." The 100% claim means all grains in the product are whole, and you'll get at least 16 grams per serving. Labeling, particularly for products that say "made with whole grains" can be confusing. Check out "Counting On Whole Grains" on the opposite page for more tips.

■ **Look for other claims and stamps.** If you see a claim or stamp (like the Whole Grains Council stamp), use this as a starting point. Still check for "100% whole-wheat" or "whole grain," and avoid products with a long list of ingredients. Also know that the absence of a stamp doesn't mean much: It's a voluntary program, so not every whole-grain product will have the WGC stamp.

■ **Study the ingredient list.** If the product lists "100% whole-wheat" or "whole-grain" wheat, corn, or other whole grain first, you've found the real thing.

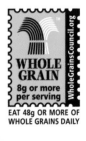

WHOLE GRAIN
8g or more per serving
WholeGrainsCouncil.org
EAT 48g OR MORE OF WHOLE GRAINS DAILY

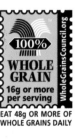

100%
WHOLE GRAIN
16g or more per serving
WholeGrainsCouncil.org
EAT 48g OR MORE OF WHOLE GRAINS DAILY

Avoid the Imposters: What *Isn't* a Whole Grain

WALK THROUGH ANY SUPERMARKET and you'll find an array of whole-grain and health claims on packages. But how can you tell if a product is really a whole-grain food? Here are foods that might seem to be whole grains—but really aren't.

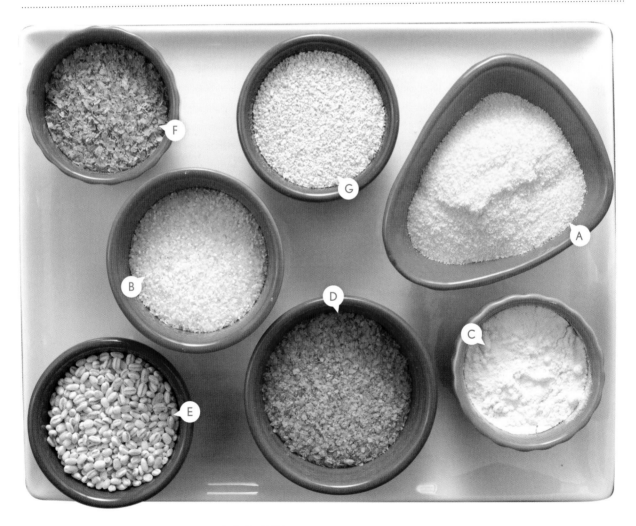

A. DEGERMINATED CORNMEAL

Degermination involves the removal of the oil-rich and vitamin-packed germ from the whole grain. It yields a more shelf-stable product, which is desirable for food manufacturers but not for your whole-grain goals.

B. GRITS

Most commercial quick-cooking grits are made from white hominy, which is a form of corn that has had the hull and germ removed, and therefore is not a whole grain. Though often difficult to find, whole-grain grits are slowly becoming more widely available, especially from local stone-grinding mills. Just remember: If the grits are made from hominy, they're not a true whole grain.

C. UNBLEACHED OR ENRICHED FLOUR

While both the unbleached and enriched aspects of flour are good qualities, they do not indicate a whole grain. Unbleached flour is allowed to "bleach" naturally with age, while bleached flour is chemically treated to speed up the whitening process.

Enriched flour is nutritionally enhanced with B vitamins, iron, and folic acid.

D. WHEAT GERM

While this is a great source of B vitamins, minerals, healthy fats, and protein, wheat germ is not a true whole grain. As the name imparts, the germ stands alone, in its unnatural state without the bran and endosperm. For bonus nutrition, use this product as a healthy addition—but not a substitution for—whole-grain breads, muffins, cereals, and cookies.

E. PEARLED BARLEY

Though extremely healthy and full of fiber, when barley is "pearled" it can no longer claim itself as a whole grain, as most of the bran has been stripped from the grain.

F. WHEAT BRAN OR G. OAT BRAN

They're a high-fiber option, but are not whole grains—the bran has been stripped from the germ and endosperm. Don't scratch this choice off your grocery list, though: You can mix either type into a 100% whole-grain cereal for a healthy fiber boost.

When buying whole grains, watch for added sugars and salt that can add unwanted calories and sodium.

EXPERT TIP:
Read the Fine Print

"Many products are labeled 'whole grain' on the front, but you'll find that 'unbleached enriched wheat flour' is listed as the first ingredient. Neither 'unbleached' nor 'enriched' indicates a whole grain. Likewise, if a product claims it's made from 'whole white wheat flour,' but it isn't the first ingredient on the list, it's a less reliable source for whole grains."

—*Sidney Fry, MS, RD,*
Cooking Light
Nutrition Editor

WHAT YOU MIGHT SEE	WHAT THE WORDS MEAN
100% wheat ⟶	Only wheat was used, but there's no indication if the grain is whole. You need to see "100% whole wheat" to be sure it's whole grain.
Multigrain ⟶	The product includes several grains, but there's no way to know if they're whole or refined.
Seven-grain ⟶	Made with seven different grains, but some parts of the grain may be missing.
Durum wheat ⟶	Durum is a type of wheat with a high protein content, but the germ and bran have been removed. Only "whole durum flour" is a whole grain.
Organic flour with whole grains ⟶	The flour may be organic, but that has nothing to do with whole or refined grains.
Made with whole grains ⟶	Some of the grains inside may be whole, but it could be as little as 5%. Look for "100% whole grain."

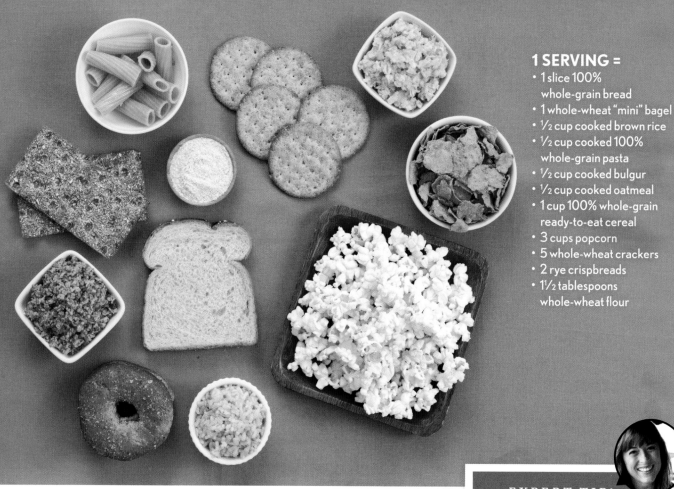

What Is a Serving?

THE U.S. DIETARY GUIDELINES RECOMMEND that Americans consume a total of 6 ounces of grains per day with at least half of those being whole grains. A bowl of cooked brown rice or oatmeal is perhaps the simplest example of a whole-grain food—half a cup of either is the government's definition of a serving, as is a half-cup of whole-grain pasta. Things get trickier with whole-grain products, though, because you have to ask how much whole grain is in the food.

EXPERT TIP:
Consider Crispy Options

"I'm really into crispbread—a thick, hearty cracker that can stand up to whatever you put on it. They're only 40 calories per serving, and they're positively vibrant with whole grains and fiber. I treat them as I would a bagel, with a sliced hard-cooked egg, a sprinkle of salt and pepper, and a drizzle of olive oil."

—*Allison Fishman, 12HH coach and author of* You Can Trust a Skinny Cook

The Busy Young Mom

"My family doesn't love whole grains."

SARAH SORENSEN
Stay-at-Home Mom

➤ **WHOLE-GRAIN CHALLENGE:** Sarah tries to get as much healthy food into meals as she can, but neither her son Ben nor her husband Tyler are crazy about whole grains. Her small family loves pizza and Asian food, but it's tricky to incorporate whole grains into those. Sarah likes to cook, but nap time is her only window for doing it.

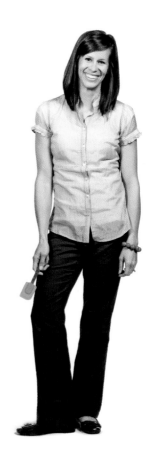

OUR ADVICE

■ **Try white whole-wheat bread and other white whole-wheat products.** This isn't a bait-and-switch gimmick; white whole-wheat flour is made from an albino variety of wheat that contains all the nutrients of its darker counterpart. Bread is the most common product made from it, but you can also find crackers and baking mixes.

■ **Cook in bulk.** Make whole-grain salads in advance, chill, and enjoy for easy, quick-to-pack lunches. Try recipes with lots of herbs and vegetables, like Chicken Tabbouleh with Tahini Drizzle on page 106. Substitute leftover shrimp or stir in rotisserie chicken to vary the flavor.

■ **Make a whole-grain bed for Asian dishes.** Boil-in-bag brown rice is a fast partner for stir-fries. Or try 100% buckwheat soba noodles, which cook in less than 10 minutes. Other quick options are bulgur (cracked wheat) and 100% whole-wheat couscous, ready in minutes and great with saucy curries or stir-fries.

■ **Make whole-wheat pizza crust** from either whole-wheat flour or white whole-wheat flour. Either way, once you add toppings, the whole-graininess is barely detectable. Make a big batch, and freeze in one-pizza quantities.

■ **Trade in your crackers for whole-grain options.** Try reduced-fat Triscuits or Wheat Thins—an easy lunch with chicken salad, packable for Tyler.

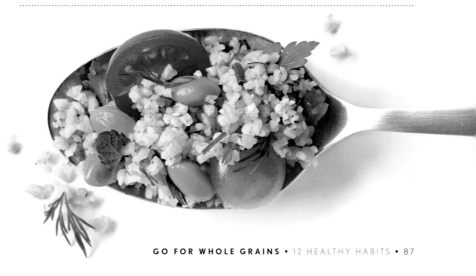

Get to Know Whole Grains

MOST OF US KNOW THAT GRAINS ARE GOOD FOR US but have difficulty naming more than two or three. Here's an A-Z guide to fifteen of the most versatile—from amaranth to wheat berries.

AMARANTH

This tiny ancient grain (it's about the size of a poppy seed) was once a sacred food of the Aztecs. It has a slightly peppery, molasses-like flavor with a faint nuttiness and pleasingly crunchy texture.

WAYS TO ENJOY: It's good as a thickener in soups because when cooked, it has a slightly gelatinous texture. Toss amaranth or amaranth flour into breads, muffins, and pancakes.

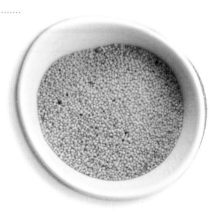

BROWN RICE

Brown rice is the unrefined version of white rice. Other whole-grain options include the exotic red, purple, and black rices. Wild rice is also a whole grain, even though it's not technically a rice—it's harvested from wild aquatic water grasses.

WAYS TO ENJOY: Reach for these whole-grain rices instead of white rice when making stir-fries, casseroles, soups, and salads.

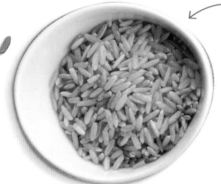

BARLEY

Barley, best known as an ingredient in beer and soup, is a great source of fiber: 1/2 cup offers more than 15 grams. Most barley is pearled to remove some of the bran, so it's not technically a whole grain. Dehulled barley is considered whole because only the hull (not the bran layer) is removed.

WAYS TO ENJOY: Since barley is so starchy, it can be treated just like Arborio rice for risottto. With its neutral flavor and ability to readily absorb flavors, it's a chameleon among grains. Add cooked barley to soups and stews or use as a base for pilafs or cold salads.

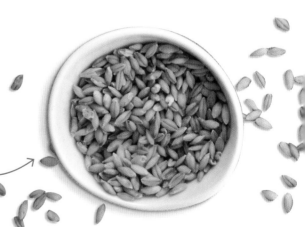

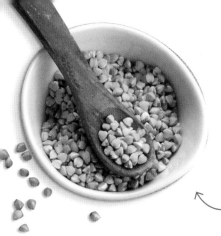

BUCKWHEAT

Despite its name, buckwheat isn't technically wheat or even a grain at all. It's a seed related to rhubarb. The whole form minus the hull is known as groats. When dry roasted or toasted, it's called kasha, the Russian name for cereal.
WAYS TO ENJOY: Try roasted buckwheat grains (kasha) for a hot breakfast cereal or as the base for vegetable stuffing. Buckwheat grits make for a great whole-grain polenta. Use buckwheat flour to make hearty whole-grain pancakes and waffles.

BULGUR

Bulgur, familiar to many of us through the Middle Eastern dishes tabbouleh and kibbeh, is wheat that has been steamed whole, dried, then cracked.
WAYS TO ENJOY: Bulgur comes in three grinds—fine (#1), medium (#2), and coarse (#3). Fine and medium bulgurs are used for tabbouleh and kibbeh, and the coarse is good in pilafs and other rice-like dishes. Try Bulgur with Dried Cranberries on page 104.

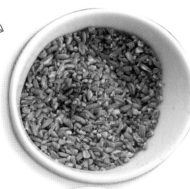

FREEKEH

Dating back to the ancient Middle East, freekeh is a roasted wheat that is harvested young when the grain is still green, soft, and full of moisture. Look for it in Middle Eastern markets and large super-markets.
WAYS TO ENJOY: Similar to bulgur, farro, and spelt, freekeh can be used to make deliciously woodsy pilafs and other rice-like dishes. It pairs well with smoky flavors, such as smoked paprika and cumin, or Middle Eastern ingredients like mint and toasted pine nuts. The smokiness of freekeh makes it an ideal base for vegetarian burgers.

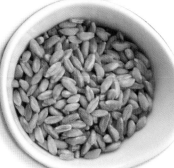

FARRO

This ancient strain of wheat once fueled the Roman legions. Look for whole farro instead of "pearled" to get more whole-grain goodness.
WAYS TO ENJOY: Farro's hearty flavor pairs well with mushrooms, sausage, beans, olives, and vegetables of all kinds, whether it's cooked like a risotto (like our Farro Risotto with Mushrooms on page 100) or served cold in salads.

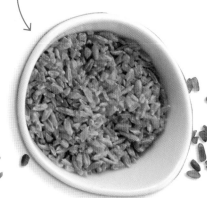

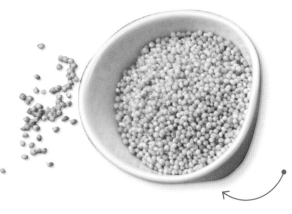

MILLET

Poor millet once was dismissed as bird seed, which is where most of it turns up in the United States, but now it's finding a new audience due to its whole-grain status and heirloom pedigree. This small, round, yellow grain is a staple in Africa and Asia.

WAYS TO ENJOY: You can toss toasted millet in salads and baked goods for a nutty crunch, or simmer and serve it with Parmesan and herbs as a side dish similar to polenta.

KAMUT® BERRIES

It's a primitive high-protein variety of wheat and takes its name from the ancient Egyptian word for wheat. Kamut berries are about twice the size of wheat berries but are similar in flavor and texture.

WAYS TO ENJOY: Use whole Kamut berries in salads, pilafs, soups, and stews. Try Kamut pasta or couscous as a base for a veggie-studded sauce.

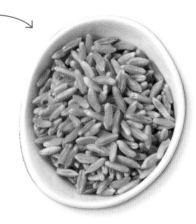

QUINOA

These tiny grains have a mild, sweet flavor with a unique texture that's both fluffy and slightly crunchy.

WAYS TO ENJOY: Most quinoa needs to be rinsed to remove the natural coating called saponins, a bitter substance that protects the plant in the wild. It goes well with all kinds of vegetables, herbs, dried fruits, and nuts. Try Quinoa with Roasted Garlic, Tomato, and Spinach on page 105.

OATS

Oats are unique among grains because they almost never have the bran or germ removed. Virtually all forms, even quick-cooking varieties and instant, are whole grains.

WAYS TO ENJOY: A steaming bowl of oatmeal is a classic breakfast; if you prefer a chewier, nuttier texture, consider steel-cut oats, also called Irish or Scottish oats. They can also be added to salads (like Waldorf Salad with Steel-Cut Oats on page 107). Try adding rolled oats to baked goods for added texture and nutrition.

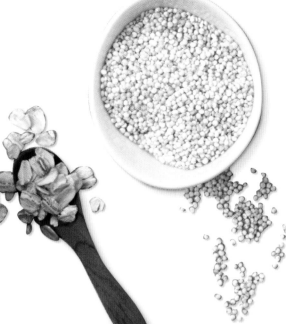

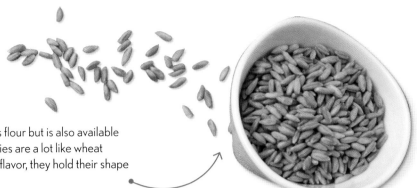

RYE

Rye is most commonly seen as flour but is also available as whole rye berries. Rye berries are a lot like wheat berries—chewy and neutral in flavor, they hold their shape when cooked.

WAYS TO ENJOY: Rye berries can be added to breads, or rolled rye can be quickly cooked for a tasty breakfast cereal. When buying rye bread, look for "whole rye" on the label to make sure it's whole grain.

WHEAT BERRIES

Wheat berries are the whole-grain kernels of wheat with only the inedible hull removed.

WAYS TO ENJOY: They take about an hour to cook but are worth the wait. Try as a main-dish salad tossed with beans and roasted vegetables or stirred into oatmeal as a chewy contrast to oats.

SPELT

Another primitive form of wheat similar to Kamut berries, spelt is a good source of fiber and is higher in protein yet lower in gluten than durum wheat.

WAYS TO ENJOY: Spelt takes longer to cook than other grains, although the kernels can be soaked overnight to shorten cook time. Try cooked spelt berries as a hot cereal with dried fruit and maple syrup, or use as a foundation for hearty salads.

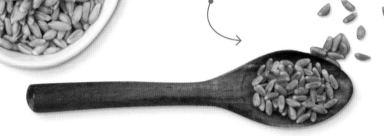

TEFF

The world's tiniest grain, teff is believed to have originated in Ethiopia thousands of years ago. The grain's name comes from *teffa,* meaning "lost" in Amharic. Teff can be ivory, light tan, brown, red, or purple.

WAYS TO ENJOY: Whole teff can be cooked like polenta and used to thicken soups, stews, and casseroles. Substitute teff flour for part of the all-purpose flour in baked goods.

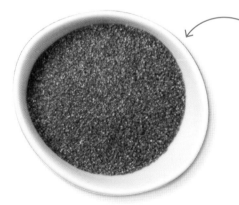

How to Cook Whole Grains

WHOLE GRAINS MAY SEEM INTIMIDATING, but they're extremely easy to prepare. If you can boil water, you can cook whole grains. The cooking method is essentially the same for all of them, except for bulgur, which has been precooked, and couscous, which is a quick-cooking pasta. Here's our guide:

- When cooking grains, bring them to a boil, lower the heat, cover the pot with a tight-fitting lid, and then cook until the liquid is absorbed. Most whole grains can be cooked just like rice with the standard ratio of two parts liquid to one part grain, although sturdier grains like spelt, wheat berries, steel-cut oats, Kamut berries, and rye berries are cooked at a ratio of four parts liquid to one part grain.
- If the grains are sticking to the bottom of the pan, turn off the heat, add a small amount of liquid, cover the pan, and let it sit for a few minutes.

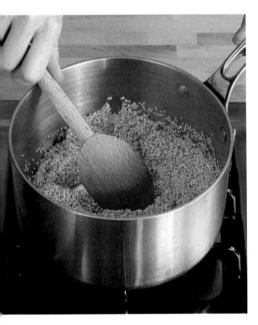

A FEW THINGS TO CONSIDER

- Use the right proportion of liquid. Be sure to check package directions or recipes, as too much liquid can result in gummy grains.
- Try a flavorful liquid instead of water (or a combination of the two). Boost flavor with chicken stock, vegetable broth, juice, or wine.
- Toast the grains before cooking. A quick toasting in oil helps build flavor and brings out the sweet nuttiness of the grains.

BUYING AND STORING GRAINS

Whole grains were once tucked away on the shelves of health-food stores, but you can now find many of them at your local supermarket. Brown rice, bulgur, wild rice, barley, and oats are widely available. Some of the more exotic grains can be a little harder to find. Look for them in bulk bins or on natural food aisles. You may have to visit a specialty food store or order them online.

Keep in mind, whole grains contain oils that eventually turn rancid, so shop at stores where the turnover seems high, and buy only what you plan to use within a few months. If you have space, it's best to refrigerate grains, but you still can't keep them forever. You can tell if they've lost their freshness by their smell: Old grains, including flours, will have a stale odor.

> Toast the grains before cooking. It helps build flavor and brings out the sweet nuttiness of the grains.

Healthy Habits Graduate

"Anything you would serve over rice also works with quinoa."

HEATHER JOHNSON
Advertising Agency Project Manager

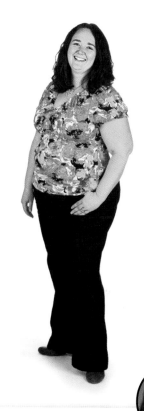

➤ **WHOLE-GRAIN CHALLENGE:** Heather Johnson is not at all shy about the fact that eating three servings of whole grains a day presented a massive challenge to her. "The only experience I had with whole grains was when an ex-boyfriend made me try kasha, the hot kind," says Heather. With some coaching and enlightening from *Cooking Light*'s Healthy Habits coach Allison Fishman, Heather has now tasted victory—and a whole lot of whole grains. Here's how she did it:

HER ADVICE

- **Substitute whole grains for pasta or white rice.** "I buy pasta that's made from quinoa, which I've found I really love. It cooks like rice, but it tastes better—I boil it with chicken broth instead of water to give it a little extra flavor."

Keep frozen corn on hand for a whole-grain side the whole family can enjoy.

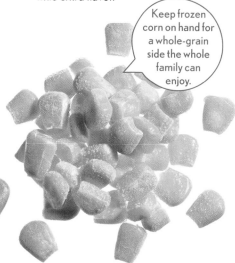

- **Do some bread-aisle research.** "Allison suggested a couple of whole-grain breads, but I discovered Aunt Mille's (available in the Midwest). Their Indian Grain is my favorite; one slice has 22 grams of whole grains! I love toast in the morning, and if all else fails, I'll have a sandwich at lunch, so finding an awesome whole-grain bread was my savior."
- **Keep corn in the freezer.** "It's a whole grain, and I absolutely love it. My husband is a meat guy, so if I'm making a meat main course, I'll just serve up some corn on the side."
- **Make snacks count.** "I've found a few snacks with whole grains that I really like: Kashi's granola bars are really crunchy, and SunChips are a whole grain, too. I have the Harvest Cheddar kind in the cupboard, and when I'm really hungry, I think, 'I'm going to eat my SunChips and get my whole grain in!'"

EXPERT TIP:
Rethink Your Cereal Bowl

"We often think of oatmeal as a healthy breakfast choice, but grains like quinoa and bulgur are amazingly delicious in the morning, too. Make extra when preparing whole grains for dinner and reserve an unseasoned portion for breakfast. In the morning, warm a little, and top with brown sugar, cinnamon, fruit, a splash of milk, and grated orange rind."

—*Regan Jones, RD, blogger,*
The Professional Palate

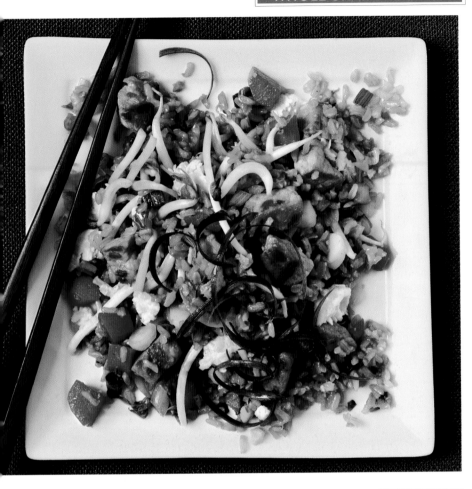

"This is the only authentic-tasting fried rice recipe I have ever had," said SoonerSinger on CookingLight.com. "It was just like take-out minus the grease!"

Almost Classic Pork Fried Rice

2 tablespoons peanut oil or olive oil, divided

½ teaspoon kosher salt, divided

½ pound boneless loin pork chop, cut into ½-inch pieces

½ cup chopped carrot

½ cup chopped celery

½ cup chopped green onion bottoms (white part)

2 tablespoons minced garlic

2 tablespoons minced peeled fresh ginger

3 cups cooked, chilled long-grain brown rice

1 large egg

3 tablespoons mirin (sweet rice wine)

3 tablespoons lower-sodium soy sauce

1 teaspoon dark sesame oil

¼ teaspoon freshly ground black pepper

2 cups fresh bean sprouts

¼ cup canned diced water chestnuts, rinsed and drained

1 cup sliced green onion tops

1. Heat a large skillet over medium-high heat. Add 1 tablespoon peanut oil to pan; swirl to coat. Sprinkle ⅛ teaspoon salt over pork. Add pork

Try Twists on the Classics

MAKING WHOLE GRAINS a regular part of your cooking routine can be easy and delicious. Many dishes require only simple swaps like subbing whole-wheat breadcrumbs for regular or brown rice for white. You—and your family—will never notice the difference.

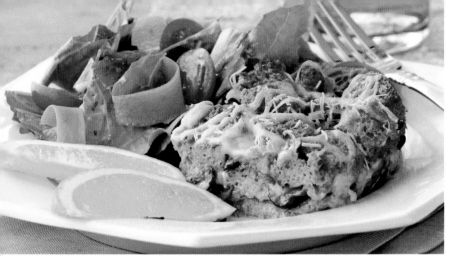

to pan; sauté 2 minutes or until browned on all sides. Remove pork from pan. Add carrot and celery to pan; sauté 2 minutes or until lightly browned, stirring frequently. Add carrot mixture to pork.

2. Add remaining 1 tablespoon peanut oil to pan; swirl to coat. Add green onion bottoms, garlic, and ginger; cook 15 seconds, stirring constantly. Add rice, stirring well to coat rice with oil; cook, without stirring, 2 minutes or until edges begin to brown. Stir rice mixture, and cook, without stirring, 2 minutes or until edges begin to brown. Make a well in center of rice mixture. Add egg; stir-fry 30 seconds or until soft-scrambled, stirring constantly.

3. Return pork mixture to pan. Stir in mirin, and cook 1 minute or until mirin is absorbed. Stir in remaining ⅜ teaspoon salt, soy sauce, sesame oil, and pepper. Remove from heat, and stir in bean sprouts and water chestnuts. Sprinkle with green onion tops. Serves 4 (serving size: about 2 cups).

CALORIES 408; FAT 12.4g (sat 2.6g, mono 5.4g, poly 3.6g); PROTEIN 21g; CARB 49.3g; FIBER 6.5g; CHOL 82mg; IRON 2.4mg; SODIUM 627mg; CALC 79mg

Fontina and Parmesan Mushroom Bread Pudding

6 cups (1-inch) cubed sturdy 100% whole-wheat bread (about 12 ounces)
Cooking spray
1 teaspoon olive oil
⅓ cup chopped shallots
2 (8-ounce) packages presliced cremini mushrooms
2 tablespoons chopped fresh parsley
1 tablespoon chopped fresh thyme
¼ teaspoon salt
¼ teaspoon freshly ground black pepper
1 cup (4 ounces) shredded fontina cheese
2 tablespoons grated fresh Parmesan cheese
1½ cups 1% low-fat milk
½ cup fat-free, lower-sodium chicken broth
3 large eggs, lightly beaten

1. Preheat oven to 350°.
2. Place bread cubes on a jelly-roll pan; coat with cooking spray. Bake at 350° for 20 minutes or until lightly toasted, turning twice. Remove from oven; cool. Heat a large nonstick skillet over medium-high heat. Add oil to pan; swirl to coat. Add shallots and mushrooms; sauté 12 minutes or until lightly browned and moisture evaporates. Remove from heat; stir in parsley, thyme, salt, and pepper.

3. Place half of bread cubes in an 11 x 7–inch glass or ceramic baking dish coated with cooking spray. Arrange mushroom mixture evenly over bread cubes; sprinkle with ½ cup fontina and 1 tablespoon Parmesan. Top with remaining bread cubes. Combine milk, broth, and eggs, stirring with a whisk; pour over bread mixture. Gently press with back of a spoon; let stand 30 minutes. Top with remaining ½ cup fontina and remaining 1 tablespoon Parmesan.

4. Bake at 350° for 45 minutes or until set. Let stand 10 minutes. Cut into 6 squares. Serves 6 (serving size: 1 square).

CALORIES 316; FAT 12.1g (sat 5.1g, mono 3.4g, poly 0.8g); PROTEIN 18.9g; CARB 36.7g; FIBER 4.8g; CHOL 131mg; IRON 2.6mg; SODIUM 696mg; CALC 228mg

READER TIP:
Change Your Method

"Brown rice was not a favorite with my kids until I changed how I cooked it. Now I combine 1 cup brown rice with 2½ cups chicken broth, 1 tablespoon oil, and seasonings like lemon rind and rosemary. I cover and bake this at 350° for 1 hour. I get the most delicious, perfect rice every time!"

—*Michelle Arndt*

Incorporate Whole-Wheat Pastas

PERHAPS YOU THINK WHOLE-WHEAT PASTA TASTES LIKE THE BOX it's sold in. If so, give it another shot. The quality and taste of whole-grain pastas have improved significantly since their debut. The dark color lightens considerably when cooked, and the texture is smoother than you may think. Check out various brands until you find one you like, or try mixing half whole-grain and half refined pasta when making your favorite dishes.

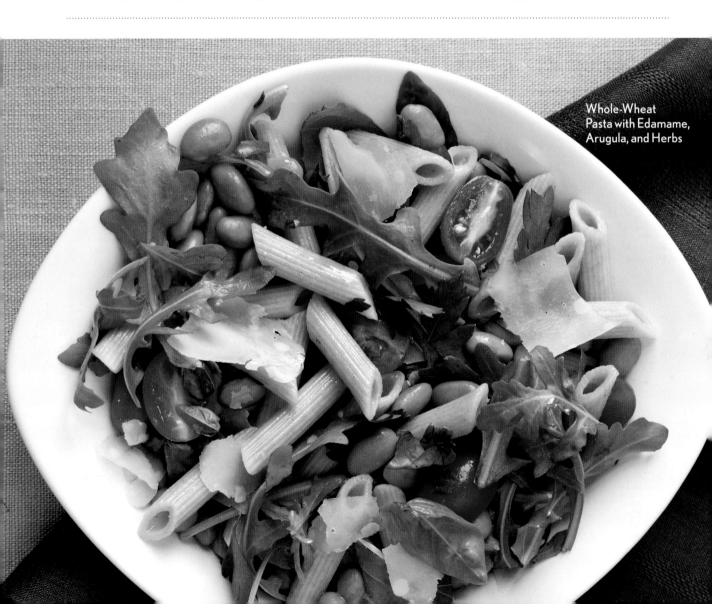

Whole-Wheat Pasta with Edamame, Arugula, and Herbs

Whole-Wheat Pasta with Edamame, Arugula, and Herbs

8 ounces uncooked whole-wheat penne
2 tablespoons olive oil
1 tablespoon butter
2 cups frozen shelled edamame (green soybeans), thawed
2 cups loosely packed baby arugula
1 cup grape tomatoes, halved
1/4 cup chopped fresh flat-leaf parsley
1/4 cup fresh lemon juice
3 tablespoons chopped fresh basil
1 tablespoon chopped fresh thyme
1/2 teaspoon kosher salt
2 ounces fresh Parmigiano-Reggiano cheese, shaved

1. Cook pasta according to package directions, omitting salt and fat. Drain. Heat oil and butter in a large skillet over medium heat. Add edamame to pan; cook 2 minutes or until edamame is thoroughly heated, stirring occasionally. Combine pasta and edamame in a large bowl. Stir in arugula and next 6 ingredients, tossing well. Sprinkle each serving with cheese. Serves 4 (serving size: about 1¾ cups pasta mixture and ½ ounce cheese).

CALORIES 477; FAT 21.6g (sat 5.4g, mono 7.8g, poly 6.1g); PROTEIN 25.6g; CARB 56.6g; FIBER 13.1g; CHOL 18mg; IRON 2.8mg; SODIUM 521mg; CALC 264mg

Sesame Noodles with Broccoli

This meatless main dish uses whole-wheat spaghetti and incorporates sesame seeds in two forms: tahini (sesame seed paste) in the sauce and toasted seeds as a garnish. Tumbles on CookingLight.com said she uses half peanut butter and half tahini for the sauce, and Dlk1217 incorporates even more veggies and dials up the chile paste for more heat.

Sauce:

2 tablespoons tahini (sesame seed paste)
2 tablespoons water
2 tablespoons rice wine vinegar
2 tablespoons lower-sodium soy sauce
1½ tablespoons dark sesame oil
2 teaspoons honey
1/2 teaspoon salt
1/2 teaspoon grated peeled fresh ginger
1/2 teaspoon chile paste with garlic (such as sambal oelek)
2 garlic cloves, minced

Noodles:

8 ounces uncooked whole-wheat spaghetti
5 cups broccoli florets
2 cups matchstick-cut carrots
3/4 cup thinly sliced green onions
1/3 cup chopped fresh cilantro
3 tablespoons sesame seeds, toasted
1/4 teaspoon salt

1. To prepare sauce, combine first 10 ingredients in a small bowl; stir with a whisk.
2. To prepare noodles, cook pasta in a large pot of boiling water 5 minutes, omitting salt and fat. Add broccoli to pan, and cook 1 minute. Add carrots to pan; cook 1 minute. Drain; place in a large bowl. Sprinkle with onions and remaining ingredients. Drizzle with sauce; toss well. Serve immediately. Serves 4 (serving size: 2 cups).

CALORIES 401; FAT 13.7g (sat 2g, mono 4.9g, poly 5.9g); PROTEIN 14.9g; CARB 62.7g; FIBER 13.6g; CHOL 0mg; IRON 4.1mg; SODIUM 798mg; CALC 119mg

EXPERT TIP: *Preventing Whole-Grain Boredom*

"If you're bored with whole-wheat pasta, and not ready to make the leap to millet and quinoa, try whole-grain Asian noodles instead. Japanese soba is made with buckwheat flour, and some varieties of chewy udon noodles are made with Kamut berries and spelt. You can also find brown rice Chinese vermicelli."

—*Gloria Tsang, RD, blogger, HealthCastle*

Eggplant Bolognese

2 tablespoons olive oil
2¼ cups chopped onion
¾ teaspoon kosher salt, divided
½ teaspoon freshly ground black
    pepper, divided
½ pound ground sirloin
8 cups chopped eggplant
    (about 1½ pounds)
1 tablespoon minced garlic
1 tablespoon tomato paste
½ cup red wine
1 (28-ounce) can whole tomatoes,
    undrained
1 tablespoon red wine vinegar
10 ounces uncooked whole-wheat
    fettuccine
1 tablespoon kosher salt
¼ cup small fresh basil leaves

1. Heat a Dutch oven over medium-high heat. Add oil to pan; swirl to coat. Add onion, ¼ teaspoon salt, ¼ teaspoon pepper, and beef, and cook 10 minutes or until beef is browned, stirring to crumble beef. Add eggplant, garlic, ¼ teaspoon salt, and remaining ¼ teaspoon pepper, and cook 20 minutes or until eggplant is very tender, stirring occasionally. Add tomato paste; cook 2 minutes, stirring constantly. Add wine; cook 1 minute, scraping pan to loosen browned bits. Add tomatoes, and bring to a boil. Reduce heat; simmer 10 minutes, stirring occasionally and breaking up tomatoes as necessary. Add remaining ¼ teaspoon salt and red wine vinegar.

2. Cook pasta according to package directions, adding 1 tablespoon kosher salt to cooking water. Drain. Toss pasta with sauce; sprinkle with basil leaves. Serves 6 (serving size: 1 cup sauce, about ¾ cup pasta, and 2 teaspoons basil).

CALORIES 323; **FAT** 7.3g (sat 1.5g, mono 4.1g, poly 1.1g); **PROTEIN** 17.3g; **CARB** 53.1g; **FIBER** 12.3g; **CHOL** 20mg; **IRON** 3.9mg; **SODIUM** 553mg; **CALC** 92mg

Pasta with Fresh Tomato Sauce and Clams

Inspired by salsa cruda, or "raw sauce," this dish features a simple and delicious combination of tomatoes, chives, garlic, and balsamic vinegar.

5 cups chopped tomato (about 4 large)
6½ tablespoons chopped fresh
    chives, divided
2½ tablespoons minced garlic,
    divided
1 tablespoon balsamic vinegar
¾ teaspoon kosher salt
½ teaspoon black pepper
2 quarts water
1 tablespoon kosher salt
8 ounces uncooked whole-wheat
    spaghetti or linguine
1 tablespoon butter
1 tablespoon olive oil
16 littleneck clams

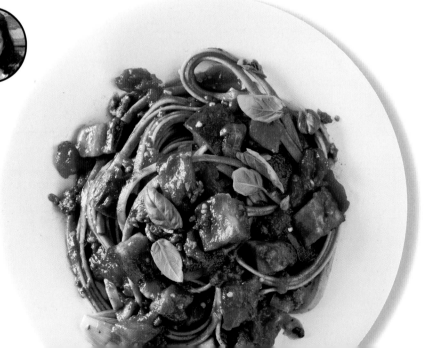

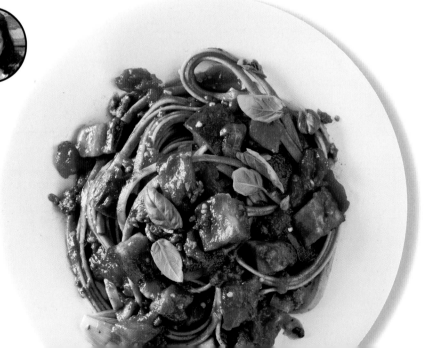

> **BLOGGER TIP:**
> *Whole-Grain Meal Ideas*
>
> "I make a lot of whole-grain pastas at home. If you use the right sauce you seriously can't tell. If I have extra pasta on hand, I like to make a quick salad and throw some in. It's a great way to add healthy carbs and feel full."
>
> —*Nisha Singh, blogger,*
> *Honey What's Cooking*

1. Combine tomato, ⅓ cup chives, 1 tablespoon garlic, vinegar, ¾ teaspoon salt, and pepper in a large bowl; let stand 15 minutes. Drain mixture in a colander over a bowl, reserving liquid.

2. While tomato stands, bring 2 quarts water to a boil in a large saucepan. Add 1 tablespoon salt and pasta. Cook pasta 10 minutes or until al dente, and drain.

3. Heat butter, olive oil, and remaining 1½ tablespoons garlic in a large skillet over low heat; cook 4 minutes or until fragrant. Increase heat to medium-high. Add reserved tomato liquid, and bring to a boil; cook until reduced to ½ cup (about 6 minutes). Add clams; cover and cook 4 minutes or until shells open. Remove clams from pan, and discard any unopened shells. Add reserved tomato mixture and pasta to pan; cook 2 minutes or until thoroughly heated. Top with remaining chives. Serves 4 (serving size: about 2 cups pasta mixture, 4 clams, and about 1 teaspoon chives).

CALORIES 332; **FAT** 7.9g (sat 2.6g, mono 3.4g, poly 1.1g); **PROTEIN** 15.4g; **CARB** 55g; **FIBER** 10.2g; **CHOL** 20mg; **IRON** 8mg; **SODIUM** 563mg; **CALC** 79mg

If you've got delicious ripe tomatoes, you don't need to bother seeding or peeling them. Just core them and roughly chop.

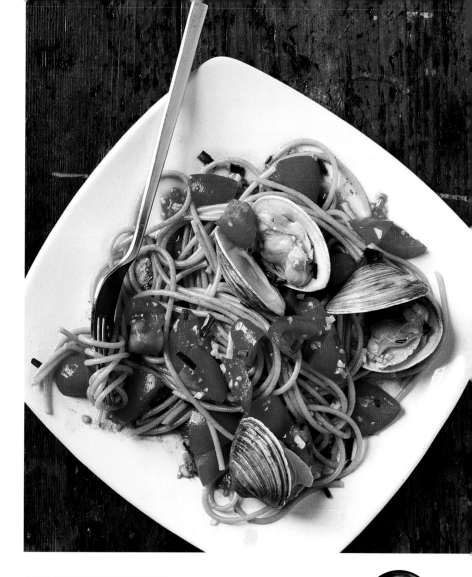

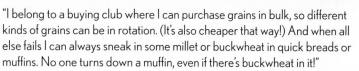

BLOGGER TIP: *Consider a Buying Club*

"I belong to a buying club where I can purchase grains in bulk, so different kinds of grains can be in rotation. (It's also cheaper that way!) And when all else fails I can always sneak in some millet or buckwheat in quick breads or muffins. No one turns down a muffin, even if there's buckwheat in it!"

—*Julia Sforza, blogger,*
What Julia Ate

Make Risottos Whole Grain

MANY WHOLE GRAINS CAN BE COOKED RISOTTO-STYLE for a delicious, comforting main dish. You won't get quite the same silken creaminess as traditional rice risotto, but the nutty flavor and enhanced nutrition will make up for that. Try barley, farro, spelt, wheat berries, or even steel-cut oats.

Farro Risotto with Mushrooms

1 cup dried wild mushroom blend (about 1 ounce)
5½ cups Mushroom Stock (recipe on page 101)
2 tablespoons extra-virgin olive oil
1½ cups uncooked farro
½ cup finely chopped onion
2 garlic cloves, minced
6 cups sliced cremini mushrooms (about 1 pound)
¾ teaspoon salt, divided
½ cup dry white wine
1 teaspoon chopped fresh thyme
¼ cup (1 ounce) grated fresh Parmigiano-Reggiano cheese
¼ cup chopped fresh flat-leaf parsley
½ teaspoon freshly ground black pepper

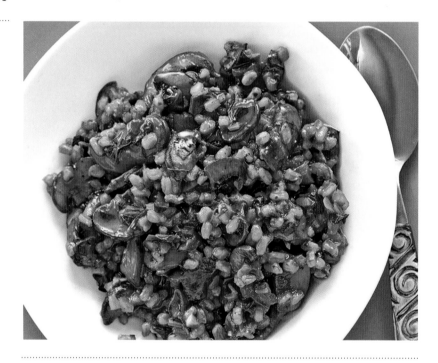

1. Place dried mushrooms in a bowl; cover with boiling water. Let stand 30 minutes or until tender; drain. Coarsely chop mushrooms.
2. Bring Mushroom Stock to a simmer in a small saucepan (do not boil). Keep stock warm over low heat.
3. Heat a Dutch oven over medium heat. Add oil to pan; swirl to coat. Add farro and onion; cook 5 minutes, stirring occasionally. Add garlic; cook 1 minute, stirring constantly. Add rehydrated mushrooms, cremini mushrooms, and ½ teaspoon salt; sauté 5 minutes or until cremini mushrooms are tender, stirring occasionally. Add wine and thyme; cook until liquid almost evaporates.
4. Add ½ cup stock to farro mixture; cook over medium heat 4 minutes or until liquid is nearly absorbed, stirring occasionally. Add 4½ cups stock, ½ cup at a time, stirring occasionally until each portion of stock is absorbed before adding the next (about 40 minutes total).
5. Add remaining ¼ teaspoon salt, remaining ½ cup stock, cheese, parsley, and pepper; stir until cheese melts. Serves 6 (serving size: 1 cup).

CALORIES 271; FAT 7.1g (sat 1.7g, mono 3.9g, poly 1g); PROTEIN 12.2g; CARB 43.4g; FIBER 8.5g; CHOL 4mg; IRON 1.8mg; SODIUM 378mg; CALC 71mg

Mushroom Stock

2 cups boiling water
1/2 cup dried porcini mushrooms
    (about 1/2 ounce)
1 whole garlic head
1 tablespoon extra-virgin olive oil
2 cups (1-inch-thick) slices onion
2 cups (1-inch-thick) slices leek
1 pound cremini mushrooms,
    quartered
10 black peppercorns
4 parsley sprigs
4 thyme sprigs
1 bay leaf
1/4 cup dry white wine
6 1/2 cups water

1. Combine 2 cups boiling water and porcini mushrooms in a bowl. Cover and let stand 30 minutes or until tender. Strain through a fine sieve over a bowl; reserve 1 1/2 cups liquid and mushrooms.
2. Cut off and discard pointed end of garlic just to expose cloves; set garlic head aside.
3. Heat a Dutch oven over medium-high heat. Add oil to pan; swirl to coat. Add onion and leek to pan, and sauté 5 minutes or until tender, stirring occasionally. Add porcini mushrooms, garlic, cremini mushrooms, and next 4 ingredients; sauté 10 minutes or until cremini mushrooms are tender, stirring occasionally. Add wine; cook until liquid evaporates (about 2 minutes). Add reserved 1 1/2 cups mushroom liquid and 6 1/2 cups water; bring to a boil. Reduce heat, and simmer 50 minutes. Strain through fine sieve over a bowl; discard solids. Store in an airtight container in refrigerator up to 1 week. Serves 6 (serving size: 1 cup).

CALORIES 28; FAT 2.4g (sat 0.3g, mono 1.7g, poly 0.3g); PROTEIN 0.5g; CARB 1.6g; FIBER 0.3g; CHOL 0mg; IRON 0.2mg; SODIUM 3mg; CALC 5mg

Mushroom—Brown Rice Risotto

1 1/2 teaspoons kosher salt, divided
1 cup short-grain brown rice
1/2 cup dried porcini mushrooms
    (about 1/2 ounce)
3 cups hot water
2 tablespoons olive oil, divided
1 pound button or cremini mushrooms,
    sliced
3 cups (1-inch) cut green beans
1/2 teaspoon black pepper, divided
1/2 cup chopped shallots
1/2 cup white wine
2 ounces Parmigiano-Reggiano
    cheese, grated (about 1/2 cup)
1/4 cup chopped fresh flat-leaf parsley
2 tablespoons chopped fresh thyme

1. Bring a saucepan of water to a boil; add 1 teaspoon salt. Stir in rice; reduce heat, and simmer 15 minutes (rice will not be done). Drain. Set aside.
2. Place porcini in a medium bowl; add 3 cups hot water. Let stand 15 minutes. Drain through a sieve over a bowl; reserve liquid. Chop porcini.
3. Heat a large skillet over medium-high heat. Add 1 tablespoon oil to pan; swirl to coat. Add sliced fresh mushrooms; sauté 8 minutes or until moisture evaporates and mushrooms begin to brown, stirring occasionally. Stir in reserved porcini, green beans, 1/4 teaspoon salt, and 1/4 teaspoon black

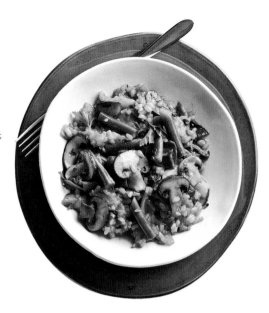

pepper; cook 2 minutes or until green beans are crisp-tender. Place mushroom mixture in a bowl; keep warm.
4. Return pan to medium-high heat. Add remaining 1 tablespoon oil to pan; swirl to coat. Add shallots; sauté 4 minutes or until tender. Add rice; cook 2 minutes, stirring occasionally. Stir in remaining 1/4 teaspoon salt and 1/4 teaspoon black pepper. Stir in wine; cook 2 minutes or until wine evaporates, stirring constantly. Add 1/2 cup reserved mushroom liquid to rice mixture; cook 3 minutes or until liquid is nearly absorbed, stirring constantly. Stir in remaining mushroom liquid, 1/2 cup at a time, stirring constantly until each portion is absorbed before adding the next (about 30 minutes total). Stir in mushroom mixture, cheese, and parsley; sprinkle with thyme. Serve immediately. Serves 4 (serving size: about 1 3/4 cups).

CALORIES 434; FAT 11.8g (sat 2.8g, mono 6.1g, poly 1.3g); PROTEIN 19.1g; CARB 60.6g; FIBER 9.1g; CHOL 9mg; IRON 6.6mg; SODIUM 534mg; CALC 180mg

Amp Up Soups and Stews

BOLSTER YOUR SOUPS and stews with whole grains, including barley, brown and wild rice, and whole-grain noodles. Don't forget that corn is considered a vegetable *and* a whole grain, so make a corn chowder or drop corn kernels into vegetable soups. Thick stews are delicious poured over a bowl of cooked brown rice, whole-wheat couscous, or wheat berries.

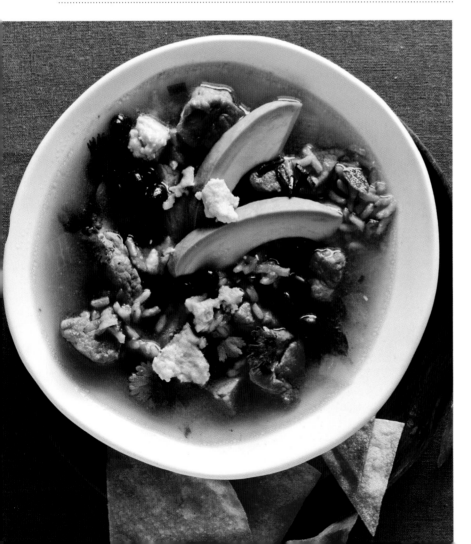

Pork and Wild Rice Soup

1 tablespoon extra-virgin olive oil, divided
1 (1-pound) pork tenderloin, trimmed and cut into ½-inch pieces
⅓ cup brown and wild rice blend
¼ cup finely chopped onion
3 garlic cloves, minced
2 serrano chiles, seeded and minced
1 cup water
1 teaspoon chopped fresh oregano
1 (32-ounce) carton fat-free, lower-sodium chicken broth
1 (15-ounce) can black beans, rinsed and drained
¼ cup chopped fresh cilantro
2½ tablespoons fresh lime juice
¼ teaspoon kosher salt
¼ teaspoon freshly ground black pepper
1 sliced peeled avocado
3 tablespoons crumbled queso fresco
24 baked tortilla chips

Switching from refined grains to whole grains may seem like a major change, but you'll discover that whole grains have an appealing chewy texture and help you feel satisfied and full for longer.

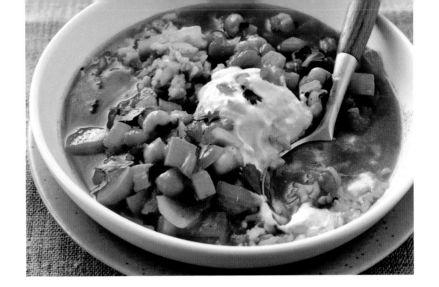

1. Heat a Dutch oven over medium-high heat. Add 1½ teaspoons oil to pan; swirl to coat. Add pork to pan; brown pork on all sides. Remove from pan.

2. Heat remaining 1½ teaspoons oil in pan, scraping pan to loosen browned bits. Add rice, onion, garlic, and chiles; sauté 3 minutes or until onion is tender. Add pork, 1 cup water, oregano, broth, and beans; bring to a boil. Cover, reduce heat, and simmer 15 minutes or until rice is tender. Stir in cilantro, juice, salt, and pepper; simmer 2 minutes.

3. Top each serving with cheese, avocado, and chips. Serves 6 (serving size: 1⅓ cups soup, about 2 avocado slices, 1½ teaspoons cheese, and 4 chips).

CALORIES 282; FAT 12.1g (sat 2.7g, mono 6.7g, poly 1.7g); PROTEIN 21.6g; CARB 24.6g; FIBER 5.1g; CHOL 52mg; IRON 2.3mg; SODIUM 638mg; CALC 61mg

Curried Chickpea Stew with Brown Rice Pilaf

This curry hails from the Indian region of Punjab. The cardamom pods puff up to almost twice their size and float to the top, so they're easy to find and discard before serving.

Pilaf:
1 tablespoon canola oil
1 cup finely chopped onion
1 cup uncooked brown rice
½ teaspoon ground turmeric
3 cardamom pods, crushed
1 (3-inch) cinnamon stick
1 garlic clove, minced
1⅔ cups water
1 bay leaf

Stew:
1 tablespoon canola oil
2 cups chopped onion
1 tablespoon grated peeled fresh ginger
1 teaspoon ground cumin
1 teaspoon ground coriander
¾ teaspoon ground turmeric
¼ teaspoon ground red pepper
4 garlic cloves, minced
3 cardamom pods, crushed
1 (3-inch) cinnamon stick
2½ cups water
1 cup diced carrot
¼ teaspoon kosher salt
1 (15-ounce) can chickpeas (garbanzo beans), rinsed and drained
1 (14.5-ounce) can fire-roasted crushed tomatoes, undrained
½ cup plain fat-free yogurt
¼ cup chopped fresh cilantro

1. To prepare pilaf, heat a large nonstick skillet over medium heat. Add 1 tablespoon oil to pan; swirl to coat. Add 1 cup onion; cook 6 minutes or until golden, stirring frequently. Add rice and next 4 ingredients, and cook 1 minute, stirring constantly. Add 1⅔ cups water and bay leaf; bring to a boil. Cover, reduce heat, and simmer 45 minutes. Let stand 5 minutes. Discard cardamom, cinnamon, and bay leaf. Keep warm.

2. To prepare stew, heat a large Dutch oven over medium-high heat. Add 1 tablespoon oil; swirl to coat. Add 2 cups onion; sauté 6 minutes or until golden. Add ginger and next 7 ingredients; cook 1 minute, stirring constantly. Add 2½ cups water, carrot, ¼ teaspoon salt, chickpeas, and tomatoes; bring to a boil. Cover, reduce heat, and simmer 20 minutes or until carrots are tender and sauce is slightly thick. Discard cardamom and cinnamon stick.

3. Place 1 cup rice mixture into each of 4 bowls; spoon 1¼ cups chickpea mixture over rice. Top each serving with 2 tablespoons yogurt and 1 tablespoon cilantro. Serves 4.

CALORIES 431; FAT 9.6g (sat 1g, mono 5.1g, poly 2.9g); PROTEIN 11.9g; CARB 77.9g; FIBER 9.6g; CHOL 1mg; IRON 3.1mg; SODIUM 626mg; CALC 121mg

Add Whole Grains on the Side

LOOK FOR WAYS TO SERVE a whole grain at every meal. Try rotating in some of these grain-based side dishes several nights a week instead of other starches, such as potatoes, white rice, or noodles. You can start off by mixing half white rice and half brown rice (or other whole grains) to make the transition easier.

Multigrain Pilaf with Sunflower Seeds

This recipe calls for long-cooking barley and brown rice, but if you're in a hurry, substitute instant brown rice and quick-cooking barley. Just be sure to adjust cooking times according to package directions.

4 teaspoons canola oil, divided
1/3 cup sunflower seed kernels
1/2 teaspoon salt, divided
2 teaspoons butter
1 cup thinly sliced leek (about 1 large)
2 1/2 cups water
1 1/2 cups fat-free, lower-sodium chicken broth
1/2 cup uncooked pearl barley
1/2 cup brown rice blend or brown rice
1/2 cup dried currants
1/4 cup uncooked bulgur
1/4 cup chopped fresh parsley
1/4 teaspoon freshly ground black pepper

1. Heat a Dutch oven over medium-high heat. Add 2 teaspoons oil, sunflower seeds, and 1/4 teaspoon salt; sauté 2 minutes or until lightly browned. Remove from pan; set aside.
2. Heat pan over medium heat; add remaining 2 teaspoons oil and butter.

Add leek; cook 4 minutes or until tender, stirring frequently. Add 2 1/2 cups water and next 3 ingredients; bring to a boil. Cover, reduce heat, and simmer 35 minutes. Stir in currants and bulgur; cover and simmer 10 minutes or until grains are tender. Remove from heat; stir in remaining 1/4 teaspoon salt, sunflower seeds, parsley, and pepper. Serve immediately. Serves 8 (serving size: 1/2 cup).

CALORIES 198; FAT 6.6g (sat 1.1g, mono 2.2g, poly 2.6g); PROTEIN 5g; CARB 32.7g; FIBER 4.9g; CHOL 3mg; IRON 1.5mg; SODIUM 266mg; CALC 26mg

Bulgur with Dried Cranberries

1 cup coarse-ground bulgur
2 cups boiling water
2 cups (1/4-inch) cubed peeled English cucumber
1 cup dried cranberries
1 cup finely chopped fresh flat-leaf parsley
1/3 cup thinly sliced green onions
1 teaspoon grated lemon rind
1/3 cup fresh lemon juice
1/3 cup extra-virgin olive oil
3/4 teaspoon kosher salt
3/4 teaspoon freshly ground black pepper

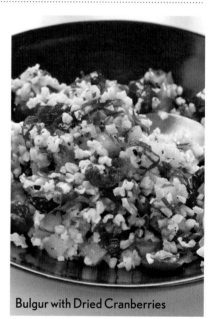

Bulgur with Dried Cranberries

1. Place bulgur in a large bowl; cover with 2 cups boiling water. Cover; let stand 30 minutes or until liquid is absorbed. Fluff with a fork. Add cucumber and remaining ingredients; toss gently to combine. Serves 8 (serving size: 1 cup).

CALORIES 197; FAT 9.6g (sat 1.3g, mono 6.7g, poly 1.2g); PROTEIN 2.7g; CARB 28.2g; FIBER 4.7g; CHOL 0mg; IRON 1.2mg; SODIUM 186mg; CALC 27mg

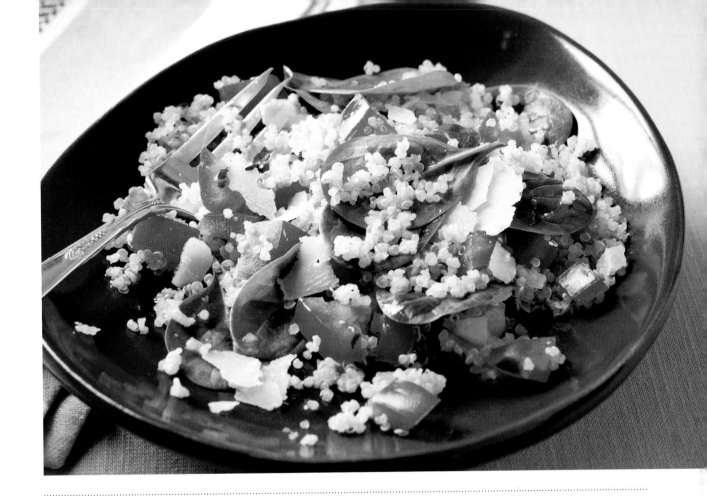

Quinoa with Roasted Garlic, Tomato, and Spinach

1 whole garlic head
1 tablespoon olive oil
1 tablespoon finely chopped shallots
¼ teaspoon crushed red pepper
½ cup uncooked quinoa, rinsed and drained
1 tablespoon dry white wine
1 cup fat-free, lower-sodium chicken broth
½ cup fresh baby spinach leaves
⅓ cup chopped seeded tomato (1 small)
1 tablespoon shaved fresh Parmesan cheese
¼ teaspoon salt

1. Preheat oven to 350°.
2. Remove papery skin from garlic head. Cut garlic head in half crosswise, breaking apart to separate whole cloves. Wrap half of head in foil; reserve remaining garlic for another use. Bake at 350° for 1 hour; cool 10 minutes. Separate cloves; squeeze to extract garlic pulp. Discard skins.
3. Heat a saucepan over medium heat. Add oil to pan; swirl to coat. Add shallots and red pepper to pan, and cook 1 minute. Add quinoa to pan; cook 2 minutes, stirring constantly. Add wine; cook until liquid is absorbed, stirring constantly. Add broth; bring to a boil. Cover, reduce heat, and simmer 15 minutes or until liquid is absorbed. Remove from heat; stir in garlic pulp, spinach, tomato, cheese, and salt. Serve immediately. Serves 4 (serving size: ½ cup).

CALORIES 130; FAT 5g (sat 0.7g, mono 3.1g, poly 1g); PROTEIN 4.1g; CARB 16.6g; FIBER 1.8g; CHOL 1mg; IRON 1.7mg; SODIUM 305mg; CALC 49mg

Boost Your Salads

WITH A NUTTY TASTE, mild flavor, and chewy texture, whole grains are a fitting canvas for salads because they harmonize with bright, fresh flavors. You can make whole-grain salads in advance, chill, and enjoy for easy lunches and dinners.

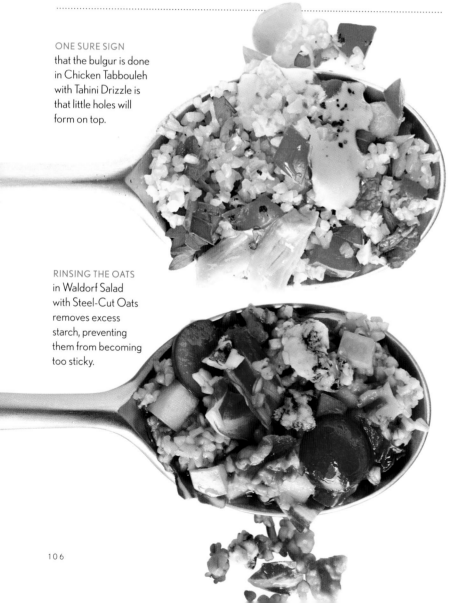

ONE SURE SIGN that the bulgur is done in Chicken Tabbouleh with Tahini Drizzle is that little holes will form on top.

RINSING THE OATS in Waldorf Salad with Steel-Cut Oats removes excess starch, preventing them from becoming too sticky.

Chicken Tabbouleh with Tahini Drizzle

1¼ cups water
1 cup uncooked bulgur, rinsed and drained
2 tablespoons olive oil, divided
1 teaspoon kosher salt, divided
½ pound skinless, boneless chicken thighs
½ teaspoon freshly ground black pepper
3 cups chopped tomato
1 cup chopped fresh parsley
1 cup chopped fresh mint
1 cup chopped green onions
1 teaspoon minced garlic
¼ cup tahini (roasted sesame seed paste)
¼ cup plain 2% reduced-fat Greek yogurt
3 tablespoons fresh lemon juice
1 tablespoon water

1. Combine 1¼ cups water, 1 cup bulgur, 1 tablespoon olive oil, and ½ teaspoon salt in a medium saucepan; bring to a boil. Reduce heat; simmer 10 minutes (do not stir) or until liquid almost evaporates. Remove from heat; fluff with a fork. Place bulgur in a medium bowl; let stand 10 minutes.
2. Heat a large nonstick skillet over medium-high heat. Add remaining 1 tablespoon oil to pan; swirl to coat. Add chicken to pan; sprinkle with ¼ teaspoon salt and black pepper. Sauté 4 minutes on each side or until done; shred chicken. Combine bulgur, chicken, tomato,

and next 4 ingredients in a large bowl; toss gently.

3. Combine remaining ¼ teaspoon salt, tahini, and remaining ingredients in a small bowl, stirring with a whisk. Drizzle over salad. Serves 4 (serving size: about 1½ cups).

CALORIES 395; FAT 18.2g (sat 3g, mono 8.8g, poly 5.1g); PROTEIN 21.5g; CARB 41g; FIBER 10.9g; CHOL 48mg; IRON 4.2mg; SODIUM 573mg; CALC 127mg

Waldorf Salad with Steel-Cut Oats

1 cup steel-cut oats, rinsed and drained
1 cup water
1 teaspoon kosher salt, divided
⅔ cup coarsely chopped walnuts
1½ teaspoons honey
⅛ teaspoon ground red pepper
3 tablespoons extra-virgin olive oil
2 tablespoons sherry vinegar
½ teaspoon freshly ground black pepper
1½ cups diced Granny Smith apple (about 1 large)
1½ cups torn radicchio
1½ cups seedless red grapes, halved
½ cup (2 ounces) crumbled blue cheese

1. Combine oats, 1 cup water, and ½ teaspoon salt in a medium saucepan; bring to a boil. Reduce heat, and simmer 7 minutes (do not stir) or until liquid almost evaporates. Remove from heat; fluff with a fork. Place oats in a medium bowl, and let stand 10 minutes.
2. Combine walnuts, honey, and red pepper in a small nonstick skillet over medium heat; cook 4 minutes or until nuts are fragrant and honey is slightly caramelized, stirring occasionally.

3. Combine remaining ½ teaspoon salt, olive oil, vinegar, and black pepper in a small bowl, stirring with a whisk. Add dressing, apple, radicchio, and grapes to oats; toss well. Place 1½ cups oat mixture on each of 4 plates, and top each serving with about 3 tablespoons walnut mixture and 2 tablespoons blue cheese. Serves 4 (serving size: 1 salad).

CALORIES 410; FAT 26.5g (sat 5.4g, mono 10.5g, poly 9.6g); PROTEIN 9g; CARB 37.9g; FIBER 5.1g; CHOL 11mg; IRON 2mg; SODIUM 683mg; CALC 106mg

Wheat Berry Salad with Raisins and Pistachios

1 cup uncooked wheat berries
¾ teaspoon salt, divided
3 tablespoons shelled pistachios
2 tablespoons olive oil
2 tablespoons fresh lemon juice
2 teaspoons honey
½ teaspoon ground coriander
½ teaspoon grated peeled fresh ginger
½ cup golden raisins
¼ cup thinly sliced green onions
2 tablespoons chopped fresh cilantro
½ cup (2 ounces) crumbled goat cheese

1. Place wheat berries and ½ teaspoon salt in a medium saucepan. Cover with water to 2 inches above wheat berries, and bring to a boil. Cover, reduce heat to medium-low, and simmer 1 hour or until tender. Drain.
2. Preheat oven to 350°.
3. Place pistachios on a baking sheet. Bake at 350° for 8 minutes, stirring once. Cool slightly, and chop.

4. Combine oil, juice, honey, coriander, ginger, and remaining ¼ teaspoon salt in a large bowl, stirring with a whisk. Add hot wheat berries and raisins; stir well to combine. Let stand 20 minutes or until cooled to room temperature.
5. Add nuts, ¼ cup green onions, and cilantro to wheat berry mixture. Transfer to a serving bowl, and sprinkle with goat cheese. Serves 6 (serving size: about ½ cup).

CALORIES 240; FAT 8.9g (sat 2.3g, mono 4.8g, poly 1.3g); PROTEIN 7.2g; CARB 36.8g; FIBER 5g; CHOL 4mg; IRON 0.7mg; SODIUM 284mg; CALC 28mg

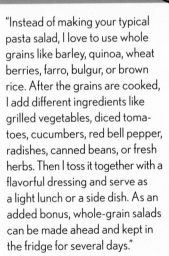

BLOGGER TIP:
Make a Grain Salad

"Instead of making your typical pasta salad, I love to use whole grains like barley, quinoa, wheat berries, farro, bulgur, or brown rice. After the grains are cooked, I add different ingredients like grilled vegetables, diced tomatoes, cucumbers, red bell pepper, radishes, canned beans, or fresh herbs. Then I toss it together with a flavorful dressing and serve as a light lunch or a side dish. As an added bonus, whole-grain salads can be made ahead and kept in the fridge for several days."

—Kalyn Denny, blogger, Kalyn's Kitchen

Toasted Millet and Confetti Vegetable Salad with Sesame and Soy Dressing

Toasting the millet helps bring out the nutty taste of this ancient grain. Use bulgur, whole-wheat couscous, or wheat berries if you can't find millet.

Dressing:
3 tablespoons rice vinegar
1 tablespoon cold water
1 tablespoon lower-sodium soy sauce
1 teaspoon canola oil
½ teaspoon dark sesame oil
1 teaspoon grated peeled fresh ginger
½ teaspoon salt
1 garlic clove, minced

Salad:
1 cup uncooked millet
2 cups water
3 tablespoons chopped walnuts
1 tablespoon lower-sodium soy sauce
1 cup diced carrot
1 cup chopped fresh cilantro
½ cup finely chopped red bell pepper
½ cup finely chopped green bell pepper
½ cup thinly sliced green onions
1 tablespoon finely chopped seeded jalapeño pepper

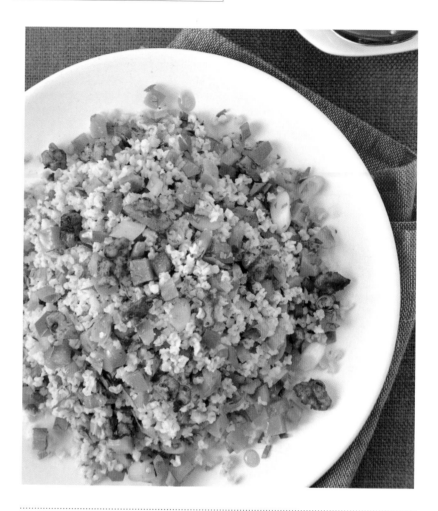

1. To prepare dressing, combine first 8 ingredients in a small bowl.
2. To prepare salad, heat a medium saucepan over medium-high heat. Add millet to pan; cook 5 minutes or until golden, stirring often. Add 2 cups water; bring to a boil. Cover, reduce heat, and simmer 20 minutes. Remove from heat; let stand, covered, 10 minutes. Fluff with a fork. Cool completely.
3. Heat a small saucepan over medium-high heat. Add nuts; cook 3 minutes or until lightly toasted, stirring occasionally. Add 1 tablespoon soy sauce; cook 30 seconds, stirring constantly.
4. Cook carrot in boiling water 3 minutes or until tender. Drain, and rinse with cold water. Drain. Combine millet, carrot, cilantro, bell peppers, onions, and jalapeño in a large bowl. Drizzle dressing over millet mixture, and toss well. Top with walnuts. Serves 4 (serving size: 1¾ cups salad and about 2 teaspoons nuts).

CALORIES 238; FAT 7.3g (sat 0.8g, mono 1.7g, poly 3.9g); PROTEIN 7.3g; CARB 42.1g; FIBER 5.6g; CHOL 0mg; IRON 4.5mg; SODIUM 587mg; CALC 35mg

Grains can be cooked in advance and kept in the refrigerator for several days or frozen in zip-top plastic freezer bags. Simply reheat in the microwave or on the stovetop with a little extra liquid.

Quinoa and Parsley Salad

"Best quinoa recipe yet!" said Jugorji on CookingLight.com. "I've made this a few times now, and I always get requests for the recipe," said Katmandu.

1 cup water
½ cup uncooked quinoa
¾ cup fresh parsley leaves
½ cup thinly sliced celery
½ cup thinly sliced green onions
½ cup finely chopped dried apricots
3 tablespoons fresh lemon juice
1 tablespoon olive oil
1 tablespoon honey
¼ teaspoon salt
¼ teaspoon black pepper
¼ cup unsalted pumpkinseed
   kernels, toasted

1. Bring 1 cup water and quinoa to a boil in a medium saucepan. Cover, reduce heat, and simmer 20 minutes or until liquid is absorbed. Spoon into a bowl, and fluff with a fork. Add parsley, celery, onions, and apricots.
2. Combine lemon juice and next 4 ingredients in a small bowl, stirring with a whisk. Add to quinoa mixture, and toss well. Top with seeds. Serves 4 (serving size: about ⅔ cup).

CALORIES 238; FAT 8.6g (sat 1.3g, mono 4.3g, poly 2.8g); PROTEIN 5.9g; CARB 35.1g; FIBER 3.6g; CHOL 0mg; IRON 4.6mg; SODIUM 172mg; CALC 47mg

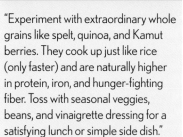

EXPERT TIP:
Step Outside Your Comfort Zone

"Experiment with extraordinary whole grains like spelt, quinoa, and Kamut berries. They cook up just like rice (only faster) and are naturally higher in protein, iron, and hunger-fighting fiber. Toss with seasonal veggies, beans, and vinaigrette dressing for a satisfying lunch or simple side dish."

—*Dana Angelo White, MS, RD, blogger, Healthy Eats*

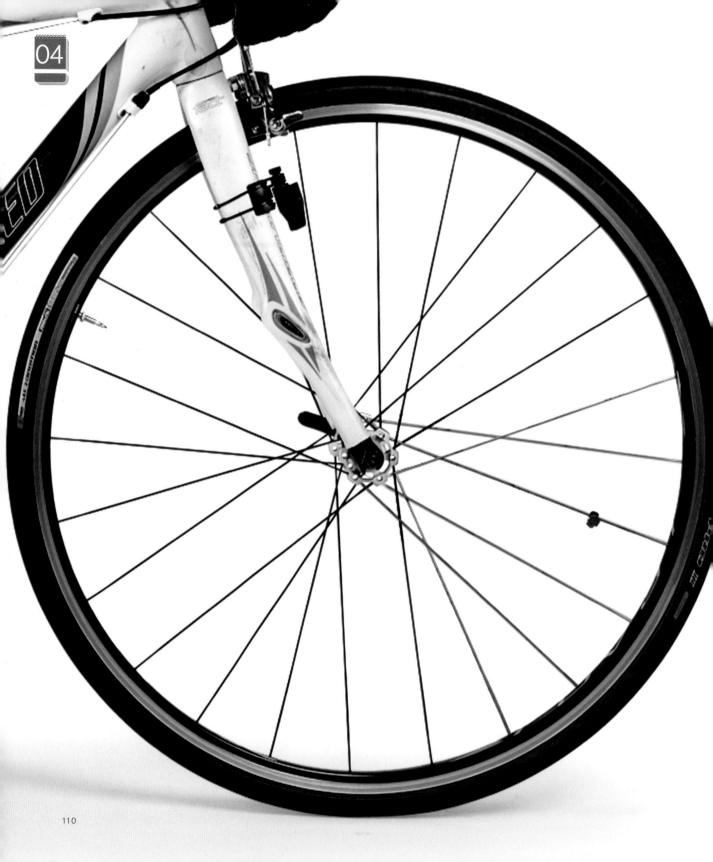

GET MOVING

SMALL DOSES DELIVER BIG PAYOFFS.

EXERCISE IS LIKELY already on your to-do list. And while it often seems impossible to squeeze such a good thing into a busy daily routine, it really is a crucial habit to adopt. Being active is what allows you to keep enjoying the wondrous pleasures of good food, and it gives you the energy to do the things you want to do, whether that's playing with your kids or running a marathon.

The vital thing to remember when incorporating more physical activity into your life is that you don't have to do it all at once. Breaking up exercise into 10- to 15-minute increments can yield health benefits and often makes getting 30 minutes a day more doable. And something is better than nothing. One study found that exercising for as little as 15 minutes a day can extend your life. When you're starting out, do what you can and work exercise in when you can.

The payoffs are immense. In addition to helping you lose extra pounds and maintain a healthy weight, exercise helps you sleep, improves your mood, relieves stress, strengthens your immune system, and decreases your risk of virtually every ailment—from heart disease and diabetes to osteoporosis and cancer.

The ideal fitness plan includes cardiovascular exercise as well as muscle-strengthening exercise (see page 248). This chapter is all about cardio—sustained, brisk physical activity that boosts your heart rate and accelerates your breathing.

Providing your body with the proper fuel before and after exercise is key. The right foods can keep you energized during your workout and help your muscles recover afterward.

If you're not exercising much (or at all), your goal here is to be active for 30 minutes, three times a week—or the equivalent. If you're at that level now, bump it up to five times per week or increase your intensity. Wherever you're starting out, be sure to discuss your plans with your physician first.

YOUR GOAL

Be active for 30 minutes a day, three times a week.

The 12 Healthy Habits

| · 01 · GET COOKING | · 02 · BREAKFAST DAILY | · 03 · WHOLE GRAINS | · 04 · GET MOVING | · 05 · VEGGIE UP | · 06 · MORE SEAFOOD | · 07 · HEALTHY FATS | · 08 · GO MEATLESS | · 09 · GET STRONGER | · 10 · LESS SALT | · 11 · BE PORTION-AWARE | · 12 · EAT MINDFULLY |

Begin with the Basics

WANT TO START AN EXERCISE ROUTINE but don't know where to begin? You don't need expensive exercise equipment for a super cardio workout. Here, the three ingredients that can get you started:

HEART RATE MONITOR

Use a heart rate monitor to keep track of exercise intensity. Our pick: Sportline's DUO 1060 heart rate monitor ($119.99; sportline.com). The best heart rate monitors require you to wear a belt around your chest, but the DUO 1060 gives you the option of just placing your finger on the watch for an equally precise readout. What we really love is that it gives you that information in three beats or less, making it the fastest, most accurate contact heart-rate measuring device on the market.

FOOTWEAR

Invest in a pair of comfortable running shoes and reserve them just for exercise, like Asic's GEL-Uptempo and GEL-Upshot ($85 each; asics.com). To be able to tackle any type of exercise, you need a training shoe that offers your feet stability from any angle, shock absorption from heel to toe, and a breathable mesh upper that lets your feet air out as you work out. Both the Uptempo and Upshot offer a superior mix of cushioning, traction, and support, all in a lightweight pair of shoes with a sock-like fit that almost makes you forget you're wearing them.

HYDRATION

If you do more than an hour of cardio, you're losing fluid and sweating out electrolytes like sodium and potassium. You don't need to spend money on expensive, calorie-laden sports drinks. Water can do the trick, or try one of these five choices instead:

- **Low-fat chocolate milk:** Provides an ideal mix of carbs and proteins that tired muscles need for recovery.
- **Iced green tea:** Contains catechins that may help reduce muscle damage caused by exercise.
- **Tart cherry juice:** Full of anthocyanins that help decrease inflammation, oxidative stress, and muscle pain after exercise.
- **Coconut water:** Rich in potassium and helps rehydrate the body as effectively as a sports drink, although it's lower in sodium.
- **Tomato juice:** Contains potassium and sodium to help replenish stores after sweating.

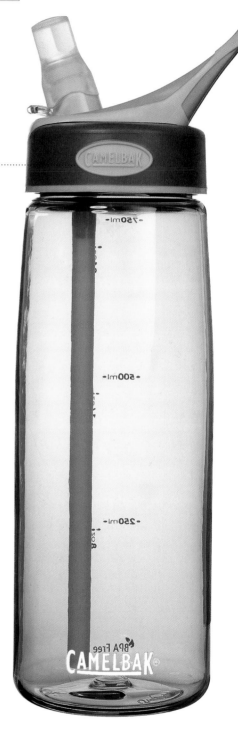

The Injured Athlete

"I want to exercise— but injuries plague me."

PHOEBE WU
Cooking Light *Assistant Editor*

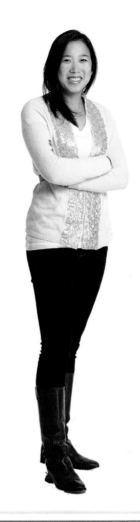

➤ **GET MOVING CHALLENGE:** Even though she's a spring chicken, Phoebe is thwarted by ankle aches and pains that come from a lifetime of playing sports like soccer and field hockey. "I've always done cardio, but lately the problem is that it hurts when I walk. If I do nothing, it will go away for a while, but as soon as I do something like running, it comes back immediately."

OUR ADVICE

■ **Consult a sports medicine physician.** While a lot of people have a pain or injury that prevents them from exercising, ironically that pain can often be rectified—by exercise. In Phoebe's case, she may just need a few sessions of physical therapy to give her ankle a boost.

■ **Mix up your cardio every few days.** Each type of aerobic exercise trains different groups of muscles. If you keep exercising the same way every day, you can cause muscular imbalances that can pull your knees, lower back, and hips out of alignment (and create more unnecessary pain for yourself). Trying a new type of cardio at least every week (or even every time you exercise) will ensure you'll hit every muscle group evenly.

■ **Consider a water workout.** In the water, your body weighs 10% of what it does on land, which helps reduce the stress on your joints. If you can't swim a stroke, simply tread water for one minute, rest for one minute, then repeat this cycle 8 to 10 times to start for a full-body cardio minus the aches and pains.

■ **Don't be a weekend warrior.** When you don't have time to fit in a full workout during the week, it's tempting to go double the distance on Saturday and Sunday. But don't: You'll most likely overdo it and reinjure yourself. Stick to a reasonable routine and try to sneak in an extra exercise session or two during the week if possible.

EXPERT TIP: *Stay Hydrated*

"Dehydration is one of the most common causes of fatigue during exercise. Hydrate before, during, and after workouts—the more you sweat, the more you need to drink. Choose sports drinks for hot conditions and endurance activities; otherwise, stick to plain old H_2O. Water flavored with thin slices of fresh citrus, cucumber, or melon is extra refreshing."

—*Dana Angelo White, MS, RD, certified athletic trainer and blogger, Healthy Eats*

Get Equipped

THERE'S NO NEED TO SPLURGE on an expensive gym membership; you can get in shape at home. These five pieces of equipment can be the basis of great workouts.

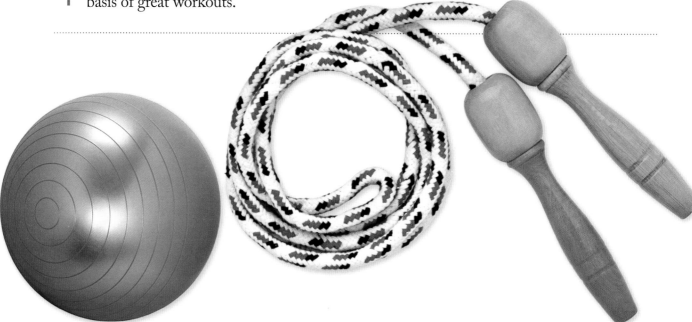

What is the one thing that would help you the most to be more active? Here's what the *Cooking Light* community had to say.

42% Exercising with friends
29% More motivation
19% Time
7% Other (confidence, instruction, support from family)
3% Decreased pain

JUMP ROPE

Hop to it! Jumping rope is a great form of cardio that works virtually all your main muscles while improving your balance. If you haven't tried it since elementary school, start with a two- to three-minute jumping session, then gradually add in extra minutes as you build up your stamina. A fifteen-minute skipping session will burn just over 200 calories.

HULA HOOP

It was all the rage in the 1950s, and now it's making a comeback. A recent study sponsored by the American Council on Exercise found that 30 minutes of hooping burned around 210 calories—similar to the results you'd get in a kickboxing or step aerobics class.

STABILITY BALL

Instead of using a chair to watch TV, sit at your desk, or eat dinner with the family, try sitting on a stability ball. Researchers at the University of Buffalo found that people sitting on an exercise ball burned 4.1 calories more per hour (a 6% boost) compared to sitting in a regular office chair. Even though your body isn't technically moving as you sit, using a ball forces your muscles to actively work—and burn calories—just to keep you balanced.

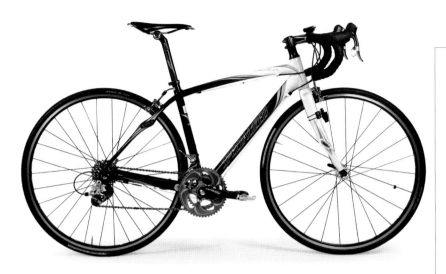

THE BASICS

Cardio doesn't just mean running. Walking, playing with your kids, or even cleaning the house count, too. And don't underestimate the workout you can get from your staircase—walk continuously up and down for 15 minutes, and you'll be feeling the burn.

The American College of Sports Medicine and the American Heart Association recommend moderate intensity cardiovascular exercise for 30 minutes, five days a week. Any of these activities count toward your quota (the calorie count is what a 150-pound person would burn in a half hour).

Cleaning the house	122
Walking the dog	148
Mowing the lawn	162
Gardening	162
Biking with your family	220
Kicking a soccer ball with the kids	234
Playing football with the kids	275

PEDOMETER

This device clips on your belt or waistband to count your steps or mileage. Just by wearing one you'll end up more active—studies have shown that people who regularly wear a pedometer walk about a mile more each day. Already a walker? Consider investing in one anyway to log your times and distances to track your training. You'll be inspired when you see improvements.

MP3 PLAYER

It's an easy way to energize any sort of at-home workout, whether you're running up and down your stairs or walking your favorite neighborhood route. Just make sure it's upbeat or you'll find yourself slowing down. And keep the volume low if you're outdoors; you need to be able to hear nearby traffic.

A Stanford University study found that people who regularly use a pedometer lose more weight, exercise more, and have lower blood pressure than those who do not.

EXPERT TIP:
Powering Through a Tough Workout

"Whether I'm exhausted or simply just bored, I always visualize the finish line of a race and push myself to keep going because I know that's always the hardest part."

–*Mary Creel, MS, RD*
Cooking Light *Special Publications Editor,*
who has run more than 50 marathons

Make It Natural

THE WORLD'S LONGEST-LIVING PEOPLE don't pump iron or hit the treadmill. Studies show that they live in environments that constantly nudge them into moving without thinking about it. Here, seven tips to help you add more activity into your day, no gym required:

MAKE EVERY DAY A LITTLE MORE CASUAL.

Researchers at the University of Wisconsin discovered that people who wore clothing that was more casual to work took an average of 491 extra steps a day and burned roughly 8% more calories compared to those who wore more restrictive outfits.

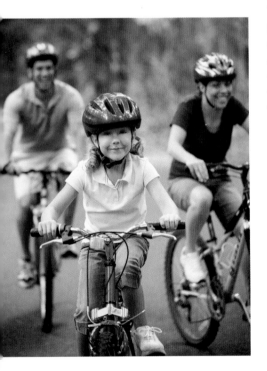

VOLUNTEER YOUR TIME.

Look for a volunteer group that will require you to do something physical—like weeding community gardens—to help out. Not only will you burn calories, but knowing you have others relying on you will hold you more accountable to stay the course—and stay active.

OFFER TO BABYSIT.

There's a reason why watching kids is exhausting—it's not just a chance to bond, it's an opportunity to burn calories. Once the play date is set, try to plan activities for them that you know will keep you up and active, like playing tag, hopscotch, skipping rope, or running around the park.

MAKE YOUR LIFE LESS CONVENIENT.

Intentionally park your car in the farthest spot possible, skip the elevator and use the stairs instead, use a basket when shopping instead of a cart, or simply leave the things you use every day—like your keys, phone, shoes, etc.—in places where you'll have to walk a little farther for them.

TAKE FIVE.

The moment you sit to do anything at home (surf the Internet, read, watch TV), limit yourself to 10 minutes, then make a point to get up and walk around for five minutes. Research from the American Cancer Society has found that women who sit for more than six hours a day are about 40% more likely to die prematurely than those who are on their duffs for less than three.

MIX WHAT YOU LIKE WITH WHAT YOU LOATHE.

Find that one activity you can't live without—such as talking on the phone, watching your favorite show, or shopping online—then only allow yourself to do it as you exercise or immediately afterward.

MAKE A FEW MICRO GOALS.

Try setting much smaller, less intimidating goals that are easier to achieve and may cause you to exercise more. For example, your goal could be "I will get up 15 minutes earlier to walk" or "I will run five more minutes." Small goals are easier to reach and usually lead to bigger success in the long run.

The Time-Pressed Professional

"I commute three and a half hours a day! How can I fit in exercise?"

JO-ANN MARTIN
Account Manager

➤ **GET MOVING CHALLENGE:** Jo-Ann has a doozy of an excuse not to exercise: a one-hour, 45-minute commute each way to work. She leaves her house by 7 a.m. and doesn't get home until 7 or 8. "After cooking dinner, the last thing I want to do is work out," she says.

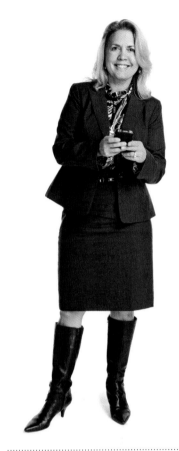

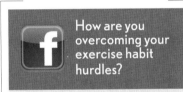
How are you overcoming your exercise habit hurdles?

"I now squeeze in all my workouts before work starts. It feels great to be done before I've really started my day. Plus, it frees up my lunch hour to run errands, read, or take a short nap."

—*Amelia Nuss*

OUR ADVICE

■ **Map out every single workout.** A plan will play to Jo-Ann's work skills with schedules, deadlines, and goals. She should lay out a month's worth of workouts as a list of to-dos in the exact same way she plans to call clients.

■ **Make a commitment to exercise on the busiest day of the week.** Once you've done that, it becomes much harder to convince yourself you have no time to work out the rest of the week. And weekends are critical.

■ **Get a partner involved.** Research has shown that having an exercise partner can increase your chances of getting in shape faster than trying to go it alone.

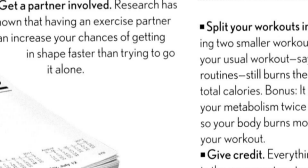

■ **Split your workouts in half.** Performing two smaller workouts that add up to your usual workout—say, two 15-minute routines—still burns the same amount of total calories. Bonus: It temporarily revs your metabolism twice instead of once, so your body burns more calories after your workout.

■ **Give credit.** Everything from walking in the grocery store to carrying your child through the mall is exercise, so add up those minutes on days when you're actively busy, so you can adjust your workouts accordingly.

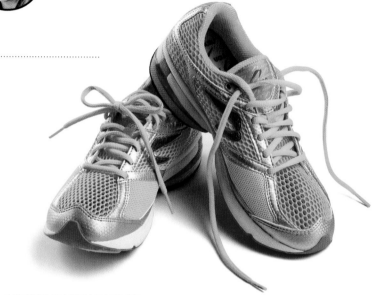

COACHING SESSION
with JANET HELM, MS, RD

"YES, YOU CAN DO IT!"

If you're new to working out, you'll be amazed at what you can do if you start slowly. I learned that in a big way recently when I became a runner for the first time in my life. Before joining a marathon training group, I couldn't even run three blocks. I signed up for a run-walk training program to help novices like me learn to run.

We started out by running three minutes, then walking two minutes. Mile by mile, we kept up those intervals of walk, run, walk, run, and each week we increased our distance. I could barely get out of bed the next morning after our first group run, but after a few weeks I felt myself getting stronger. Finishing the marathon was a huge accomplishment for me. Before, I never even imagined that this was possible, but I did it. I wasn't fast, and I certainly wasn't elegant, but I finished. Often starting is the hardest part of all, but there's something incredibly powerful about setting a goal and seeing it through.

A FEW THINGS I LEARNED ALONG THE WAY

- **Going outside helps.** I never really enjoyed being on a treadmill. I think I was so focused on the magazine I had propped up on the rack or the time left on the clock. Running outside is an entirely different experience.
- **Make a commitment.** Signing up for a group training program helped me be more accountable. Explore local races in your area (although I'd recommend starting with a 5K), then share your intentions with your family, announce it at work, or post it on Facebook—whatever helps you stick with your goal.
- **Run your own race.** Don't compare yourself to others. I was often the slowest in our training group, but I was OK with that. Focus on your own improvements.
- **Cherish the time.** The minutes you've carved out to run or walk are all about you. Enjoy this time alone to focus on yourself, make plans in your head, and think positive thoughts without any distractions.

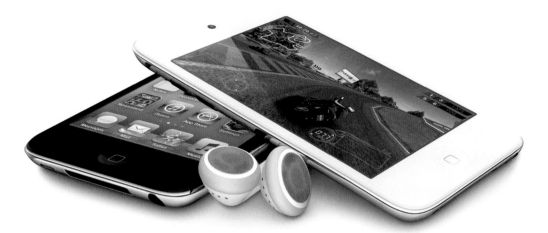

A FEW THINGS THAT HELPED

These three items helped keep me motivated to tackle my workouts:

- **My iPod.** I could never have gotten through my long runs without it. I put together a specific playlist for my training: upbeat, motivating music such as U2's "It's a Beautiful Day," Rascal Flatts' "Unstoppable," and Bruce Springsteen's "Born to Run."
- **My Starbucks coffee.** We had gear drop-off right by Starbucks, so the group would always gather for a quick coffee afterwards. It was great to connect with so many people who were all in the same boat as me—first-time runners who had never dreamt they could train for a marathon before. We commiserated about aches and pains and shared tips.
- **My running shoes.** This was the first time I ever got fitted for workout shoes— before, I'd always buy them based on looks. Having the right shoes and socks really made a huge difference. I was not only more comfortable, I had such a positive mindset I knew I'd finish, no matter how long it took me.

Being active will likely help you live longer. A now-classic study that followed 7,000 people in California for 35 years found that daily exercise was one of seven habits that predicted how long people will live and how healthy they'll be during their lifetime. The people in the study exercised 30 minutes at a time, several times a week; walking vigorously was their top exercise choice.

BLOGGER TIP: *Let Go of "All or Nothing."*

"I thought, 'Someday I'm going to start that really intense exercise routine, and I will do it six days a week.' Allison Fishman [the 12HH coach] told me to start with the goal of three and see what happened. It was the nudge I needed. To my surprise, when I relaxed and said, 'Let's see if I can do it three times a week,' three became four, then five."

—Shauna James Ahern, blogger,
Gluten-Free Girl and the Chef, and Healthy Habits graduate

COACHING SESSION
with MYATT MURPHY, CSCS

CARDIO BLAST WORKOUT

NO TREADMILL? NO PROBLEM. These five moves will get your heart pumping—anywhere, any time. This cardio plan busts boredom by mixing up the moves and working your body from head to toe while elevating your heart rate. Better still, it can be done indoors or out, morning or night—no equipment necessary.

GAME PLAN

- Do each exercise for one minute; switch to the next move without resting.
- Make a 20-minute workout by repeating the sequence four times.
- Make a 30-minute workout by repeating the sequence six times.
- Perform the routine three times a week in the beginning, resting one day in between. When you're ready, try doing the workout four to five times a week.

1. SIDE SHUFFLES WITH KNEE RAISE

Step 1: Stand straight with your feet shoulder-width apart, knees unlocked. Quickly shuffle to your left for two seconds.
Step 2: Stop, then raise your right knee as high as you can toward your chest; lower your foot back to the floor. Quickly shuffle back to the right for two seconds, and raise your left knee toward your chest; lower your foot back to the floor.
Repeat: Continue the drill for one minute.

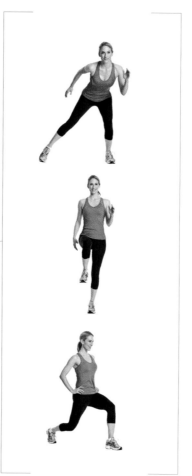

2. SQUAT THRUSTS

Step 1: Stand with your feet shoulder-width apart, arms at your sides. Squat down as low as you can, and place your palms flat on the floor, shoulder-width apart.
Step 2: Kick your legs out straight behind you (you should look like you're about to do a push-up).
Step 3: Quickly jump your feet back to squat position, knees at your chest, and immediately stand—or jump—up to standing as you raise your hands above your head.
Repeat: Continue the drill for one minute.

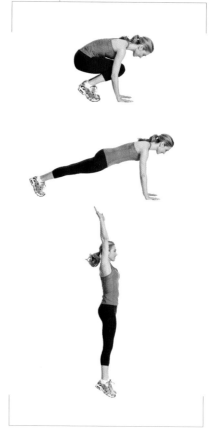

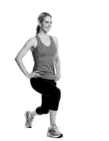
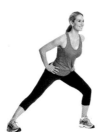
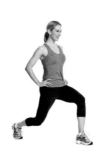
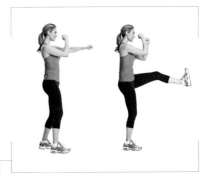
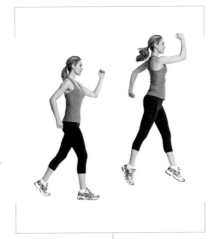

3. AROUND-THE-CLOCK LUNGES

Step 1: Stand straight with your feet and legs together, hands on your hips. Lunge forward with your left foot, then push back to standing.
Step 2: Perform a side lunge by planting your left foot out to your left side, then push back to standing.
Step 3: Extend your left leg behind you, and lower yourself into a reverse lunge, then push back to standing.
Repeat: Perform the drill with your right leg; continue alternating legs for one minute.

4. SCISSOR JUMPS

Step 1: Stand with your right foot in front of your left, spaced about 2 feet apart. Extend your right arm behind you and your left arm in front of you, elbows comfortably bent about 90 degrees.
Step 2: Quickly jump up and switch arm and leg positions while in the air, so that you land with your left foot in front of your right foot, your right arm in front of your body, and your left arm behind you.
Repeat: Continue jumping and alternating legs for one minute.

5. CROSS-PUNCH KICKS

Step 1: Stand with your feet about hip-width apart, right foot in front of left foot. Hold fisted hands in front of your face, palms facing each other. Quickly throw a left punch in front of your body at chest level, pull back, then throw a right punch and pull back.
Step 2: Next, kick your left leg forward about waist-high, then lower it back to the floor. Jump and switch your stance—left foot in front of right foot—and perform again, this time throwing a right punch, a left punch, then kicking forward with your right leg.
Repeat: Alternate for one minute.

EXPERT TIP: *Adopt Healthy Hobbies*

"Lots of hobbies can be physically active and not feel like typical exercise. You don't have to be a trained dancer to dance—you just dance! You can dance in your room alone or join a local drop-in class. In recent years, Bollywood and belly dancing have increased in popularity. Maybe you like nature. Pick up bird-watching or hiking."

—*Rebecca Scritchfield, MA, RD, blogger, Rebecca Thinks*

Choose Cardio-Friendly Foods

I F YOU'RE DOING CARDIO AT LEAST THREE TIMES A WEEK, you need enough daily carbs to fuel your workouts and replenish your energy stores. Remember: All carbs are not created equal, which means empty calories such as a candy bar won't cut it. The best carbs to choose are ones that contribute plenty of other nutrients such as protein, vitamins, fiber, and antioxidants, like these five below:

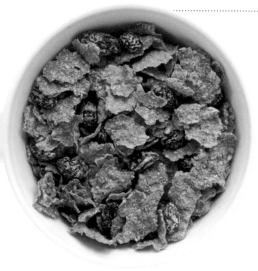

RAISIN AND ALMOND MIX

Raisins are rich in energy-boosting carbs as well as potassium, which maintains fluid balance and thus helps prevent dehydration as well as muscle cramps. Almonds are a top source of antioxidants, which protect against harmful free radicals your body produces during intense exercise. Cyclists who ate 60 almonds a day before meals for four weeks boosted their antioxidant capacity and increased their trial time distance, according to a study presented at the 2009 annual meeting of the American College of Sports Medicine.

LOW-FAT RICOTTA WITH HONEY

After a tough workout, your muscles are hungry for protein to help them repair and rebuild. Whey protein, used to make ricotta cheese, is a top pick. Whey is rich in B-lactoglobulin, a protein that's especially effective in stimulating muscle resynthesis, according to a 2010 *Nutrition & Metabolism* study. Adding some quickly digested carbs—like a drizzle of honey—to this post-exercise snack encourages your muscles to soak up that protein even faster.

GINGER SMOOTHIE

Does your workout leave you aching? Instead of heading to the medicine cabinet for a couple of aspirin, make a beeline to the kitchen for some ginger. According to a 2010 *Journal of Pain* study this potent anti-inflammatory root eases post-exercise muscle pain. It's also been shown to reduce joint stiffness and swelling, too. You can throw some fresh ginger into your favorite smoothie, or try the Carrot, Apple, and Ginger Refresher (recipe on page 125) as a post-workout snack.

WHOLE-GRAIN CEREAL AND MILK

It may sound boring, but it's anything but: In fact, a bowl of whole-grain cereal and milk was found to be just as good as a sports drink for recovery after exercise by researchers at the University of Texas at Austin.

ENERGY BAR

Nothing beats an energy bar for convenience. But set the "bar" high: Look for one with at least 3 grams of protein and fiber and less than 20 grams of sugar. We like Luna and Zing bars, which have 10 and 13 grams of protein, respectively, to give you a nice post-workout boost.

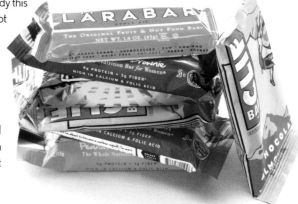

The Disinterested Exerciser

"Cardio is boring, so I just can't make myself do it."

PHILLIP RHODES
Cooking Light *Executive Managing Editor*

➤ **GET MOVING CHALLENGE:** Phillip doesn't have an exercise problem—he has a cardio problem: "I don't like getting on the treadmill or elliptical—you just go and go and go and nothing happens. I find it boring." He's a dedicated gym-goer, though, three to four times a week, focusing on weights. But Phillip wants to stop the pant-size progression, which means more cardio.

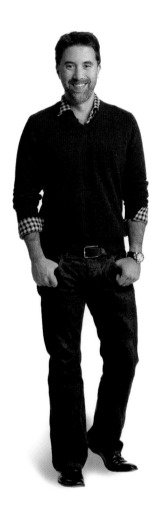

OUR ADVICE

■ **Mix it up.** A cardio program with some tricks—like intervals—will keep his muscles as intrigued as his brain, will intensify his workouts, and should help to evoke a more calorically intense response from his body. See our cardio blast workout on page 120 for more details.

■ **Set up workout dates.** If there's something that doesn't feel like work—say, tennis or racquetball, which introduce the buddy benefit—rein in a friend for a twice- or thrice-weekly game.

■ **Take it outdoors.** As an Alabama resident, Phillip has many months of outdoor-fitness weather.

One of the biggest reasons most people prefer to exercise outdoors is that it always feels different.

■ **Count the seconds.** Researchers at the University of New South Wales found that people who exercised at a high intensity for 8 seconds, then at a low intensity for 12 seconds, lost three times more fat in 20 minutes than exercisers who worked out at a constant pace for 40 minutes. It's hard to do this for a full 20 minutes, but boy, does it focus the brain.

If you're easily bored, sign up for a short-term cardio activity that lasts three months or less, like a 12-week spin class or training to run a 5K.

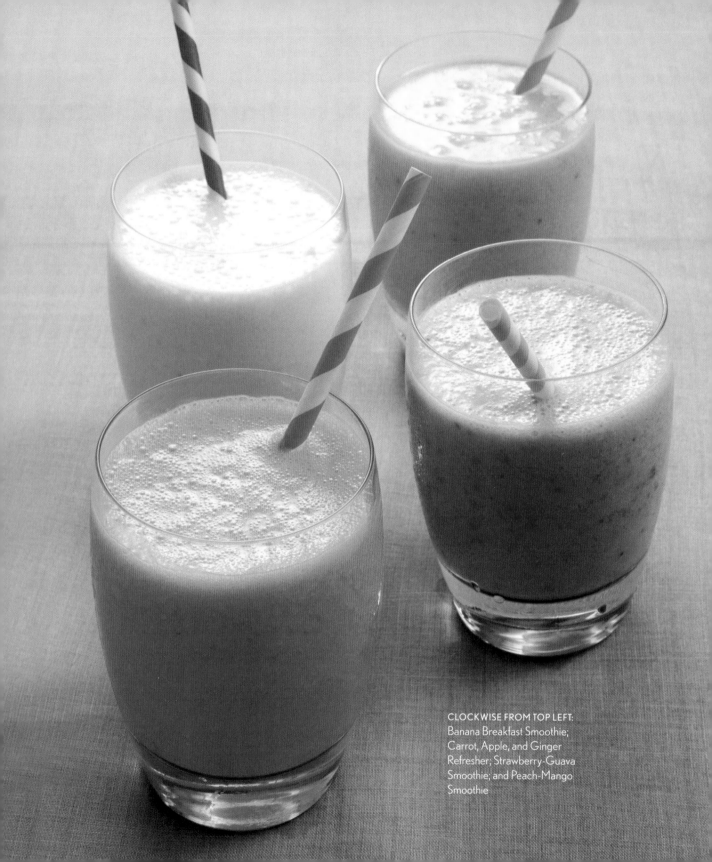

CLOCKWISE FROM TOP LEFT:
Banana Breakfast Smoothie;
Carrot, Apple, and Ginger
Refresher; Strawberry-Guava
Smoothie; and Peach-Mango
Smoothie

Prepare a Pre-Workout Smoothie

WHEN IT COMES TO A PRE- OR POST-WORKOUT SNACK, smoothies are a hands-down winner. Yogurt or milk adds protein and some calcium, while fruit contributes natural sweetness and vitamin C for tired, sore muscles. Drink these smoothies about an hour before a cardio session to fuel your workout, or within the ideal recovery window—between 30 and 60 minutes after exercise—when your body is best able to repair itself and replenish the energy you've spent.

Banana Breakfast Smoothie

½ cup 1% low-fat milk
½ cup crushed ice
1 tablespoon honey
⅛ teaspoon ground nutmeg
1 large sliced ripe banana, frozen
1 cup plain 2% reduced-fat Greek yogurt

1. Place first 5 ingredients in a blender; process 2 minutes or until smooth. Add yogurt; process just until blended. Serve immediately. Serves 2 (serving size: 1 cup).

CALORIES 212; FAT 3.6g (sat 2.5g, mono 0.2g, poly 0.1g); PROTEIN 14.2g; CARB 34.2g; FIBER 2g; CHOL 9mg; IRON 0.3mg; SODIUM 75mg; CALC 200mg

Strawberry-Guava Smoothie

1 cup quartered strawberries (about 5 ounces)
½ cup guava nectar
1 (6-ounce) carton organic strawberry fat-free yogurt
1 small sliced ripe banana, frozen
5 ice cubes (about 2 ounces)

1. Place all ingredients in a blender; process 2 minutes or until smooth. Serve immediately. Serves 2 (serving size: about 1¼ cups).

CALORIES 156; FAT 0.5g (sat 0.1g, mono 0.1g, poly 0.2g); PROTEIN 4.2g; CARB 36.2g; FIBER 3.6g; CHOL 2mg; IRON 0.5mg; SODIUM 49mg; CALC 116mg

Peach-Mango Smoothie

⅔ cup frozen sliced peaches
⅔ cup frozen mango pieces
⅔ cup peach nectar
1 tablespoon honey
1 (6-ounce) carton organic peach fat-free yogurt

1. Place all ingredients in a blender; process 2 minutes or until smooth. Serve immediately. Serves 2 (serving size: 1 cup).

CALORIES 184; FAT 0.3g (sat 0.1g, mono 0.1g, poly 0.1g); PROTEIN 4.1g; CARB 44g; FIBER 2.4g; CHOL 2mg; IRON 0.4mg; SODIUM 50mg; CALC 107mg

Carrot, Apple, and Ginger Refresher

½ cup 100% carrot juice, chilled
½ cup unsweetened applesauce
½ cup organic vanilla fat-free yogurt
1 teaspoon fresh lemon juice
½ teaspoon grated peeled fresh ginger
1 sliced ripe banana, frozen
5 ice cubes (about 2 ounces)

1. Place all ingredients in a blender; process 2 minutes or until smooth. Serve immediately. Serves 2 (serving size: about 1¼ cups).

CALORIES 138; FAT 0.1g (sat 0g; mono 0g; poly 0.1g); PROTEIN 4.3g; CARB 32.7g; FIBER 2.3g; CHOL 2mg; IRON 0.3mg; SODIUM 79mg; CALC 126mg

A 2010 *Journal of Pain* study found that ginger, a potent anti-inflammatory, eases post-exercise muscle pain.

Power Up with Pasta

PASTA IS A HEARTY MEAL that provides easy-to-digest carbs that can power you through your next race or workout. Add in some lean protein like shrimp or pork if you're looking to help repair muscles and refuel your tank after exercise. Toss in your favorite fresh vegetables for texture, color, extra vitamins, and fiber.

Mini Farfalle with Roasted Peppers, Onions, Feta, and Mint

8 ounces uncooked mini farfalle (bow tie pasta)
¼ cup pine nuts
1 tablespoon extra-virgin olive oil
1 cup prechopped onion
¼ cup golden raisins
1 tablespoon minced garlic
1 cup sliced bottled roasted red bell peppers, rinsed and drained
1 cup (4 ounces) crumbled feta cheese
2 tablespoons chopped fresh mint
2 tablespoons chopped fresh basil
¼ teaspoon black pepper

1. Cook pasta according to package directions, omitting salt and fat. Drain pasta over a bowl; reserve ½ cup cooking liquid.
2. While pasta cooks, heat a small nonstick skillet over medium heat. Add nuts; cook 4 minutes or until golden brown, stirring frequently.
3. Heat a large skillet over medium heat. Add oil; swirl to coat. Add onion, raisins, and garlic; cook 8 minutes or until onion begins to brown, stirring frequently. Add bell peppers; cook 4 minutes or until heated, stirring occasionally. Add

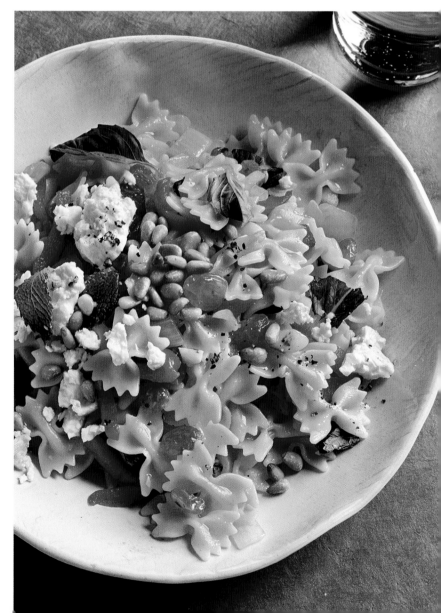

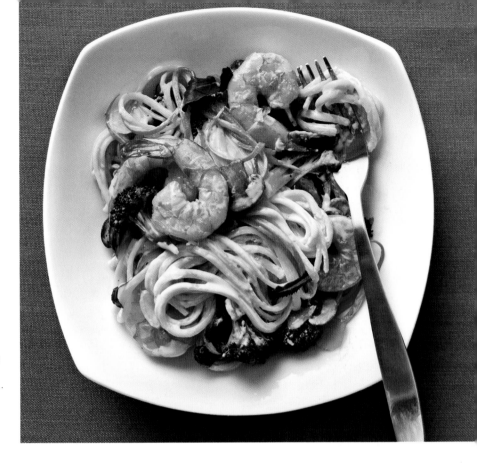

pasta and ½ cup reserved cooking liquid; cook 1 minute, stirring to combine. Remove from heat; stir in feta, mint, basil, and black pepper. Sprinkle with nuts. Serves 4 (serving size: about 1½ cups pasta and 1 tablespoon nuts).

CALORIES 453; FAT 17.4g (sat 5.1g; mono 4.1g; poly 3.3g); PROTEIN 16.6g; CARB 59.7g; FIBER 4.2g; CHOL 25mg; IRON 3.5mg; SODIUM 558mg; CALC 131mg

Creamy Linguine with Shrimp and Veggies

6 quarts water
1 teaspoon salt, divided
8 ounces uncooked linguine
3 cups small broccoli florets
1½ tablespoons butter
1 cup chopped onion
8 ounces sliced mushrooms
2 garlic cloves, minced
12 ounces peeled and deveined medium shrimp
1 julienne-cut carrot
¾ cup (6 ounces) ⅓-less-fat cream cheese
¼ teaspoon ground black pepper

1. Bring 6 quarts water to a boil in a saucepan. Add ½ teaspoon salt and pasta; cook 5 minutes. Add broccoli; cook 3 minutes or until pasta is al dente. Drain through a sieve over a bowl, reserving ½ cup pasta water.

2. Melt butter in a Dutch oven over medium-high heat. Add onion and mushrooms to pan; sauté 5 minutes, stirring occasionally. Add garlic; sauté 1 minute, stirring constantly. Add remaining ½ teaspoon salt, shrimp, and carrot; sauté 3 minutes, stirring occasionally. Add pasta mixture, ½ cup reserved pasta water, cream cheese, and pepper to pan; cook 3 minutes or until cheese melts and shrimp are done, stirring occasionally. Serves 4 (serving size: 2 cups).

CALORIES 501; FAT 16.3g (sat 9.4g, mono 3.9g, poly 1.2g); PROTEIN 32.2g; CARB 57g; FIBER 5.6g; CHOL 171mg; IRON 4.8mg; SODIUM 691mg; CALC 136mg

HOW TO COOK PASTA

To make great pasta, cook it *al dente,* or "to the tooth." That means the pasta will be tender and not raw-tasting, but you'll get a slight resistance when you bite. With long pastas like spaghetti and linguine, you can tell that it has been cooked al dente if there is a dot of white at the center. For tube-shaped pasta, such as penne and ziti, look for a faint but clear ring of white around the center of the pasta. If you're going to simmer cooked pasta with a sauce, cook the pasta slightly less than al dente—it will finish cooking in the sauce.

Pack Salads with Protein

I F YOU'RE SQUEEZING FITNESS into your lunch hour, nothing beats a salad topped with lean protein for a post-workout meal. Studies show that a protein-carb combo enhances muscle recovery after exercise more effectively than carbs alone. It'll also keep you full, so you're less tempted to snack later.

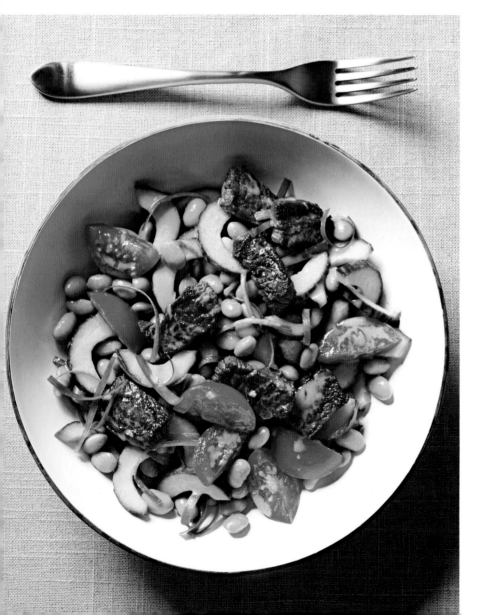

Edamame Salad with Crisp Steak Bits

3 cups frozen shelled edamame (green soybeans)
2 tablespoons lower-sodium soy sauce
1 tablespoon minced peeled fresh ginger
1 tablespoon mayonnaise
1 tablespoon Dijon mustard
2 teaspoons rice wine vinegar
1 teaspoon dark sesame oil
1 pint cherry tomatoes, quartered
1½ cups sliced seeded English cucumber (about 1)
4 green onions, chopped
1 tablespoon olive oil
8 ounces flank steak, cut into small pieces
¼ teaspoon kosher salt
¼ teaspoon freshly ground black pepper

1. Cook edamame according to package directions; drain. Rinse with cold water; drain.
2. Combine soy sauce and next 5 ingredients in a large bowl, stirring with a whisk. Add edamame, tomatoes, cucumber, and onions; toss to coat.
3. Heat a medium cast-iron skillet over high heat. Add olive oil to pan; swirl to coat. Sprinkle steak with

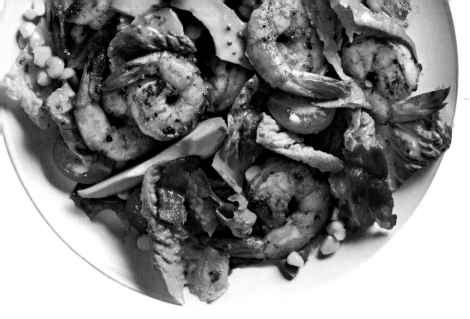

Studies show that people are more likely to make exercise a habit if they choose a simple cue or trigger to get them started, such as lacing up their shoes before breakfast or running as soon as they get home from work.

salt and pepper. Add to pan; cook 5 minutes or until well browned and crisp, stirring frequently. Spoon 1½ cups edamame mixture onto each of 4 plates; top evenly with steak. Serves 4.

CALORIES 277; FAT 14.8g (sat 2.7g, mono 6.7g, poly 2.8g); PROTEIN 23.1g; CARB 14.6g; FIBER 6.1g; CHOL 20mg; IRON 3.5mg; SODIUM 540mg; CALC 97mg

Shrimp Cobb Salad

4 center-cut bacon slices
1 pound large shrimp, peeled and
    deveined
½ teaspoon paprika
¼ teaspoon black pepper
Cooking spray
¼ teaspoon salt, divided
2½ tablespoons fresh lemon juice
1½ tablespoons extra-virgin olive oil
½ teaspoon whole-grain Dijon mustard
1 (10-ounce) package romaine salad
2 cups cherry tomatoes, quartered
1 cup shredded carrot (about 2 carrots)
1 cup frozen whole-kernel corn, thawed
1 ripe peeled avocado, cut into 8 wedges

1. Cook bacon in a large skillet over medium heat until crisp. Remove bacon from pan; cut in half crosswise. Wipe pan clean with paper towels. Increase heat to medium-high. Sprinkle shrimp with paprika and pepper. Coat pan with cooking spray. Add shrimp to pan; cook 2 minutes on each side or until done. Sprinkle with ⅛ teaspoon salt; toss to coat.
2. While shrimp cooks, combine remaining ⅛ teaspoon salt, juice, oil, and mustard in a large bowl, stirring with a whisk. Add lettuce; toss to coat.
3. Arrange about 1½ cups lettuce mixture on each of 4 plates. Top each serving with about 6 shrimp, ½ cup tomatoes, ¼ cup carrot, ¼ cup corn, 2 avocado wedges, and 2 bacon pieces. Serves 4.

CALORIES 332; FAT 15.2g (sat 2.9g, mono 8g, poly 2.6g); PROTEIN 30g; CARB 21.8g; FIBER 7.5g; CHOL 181mg; IRON 4.3mg; SODIUM 551mg; CALC 110mg

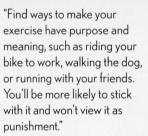

EXPERT TIP:
Give Exercise Meaning

"Find ways to make your exercise have purpose and meaning, such as riding your bike to work, walking the dog, or running with your friends. You'll be more likely to stick with it and won't view it as punishment."
—*Nancy Clark, MS, RD sports nutritionist, author of* Nancy Clark's Sports Nutrition Guidebook

Refuel with Sandwiches

YOU CAN'T GO WRONG with a sandwich after a workout—it's got everything in a hand-held package and provides just the right balance of protein and carbs. Throw in some antioxidant-rich fresh veggies such as lettuce and tomatoes to further help your muscles repair. You can easily use 100% whole-wheat bread to boost fiber content and get a whole-grain serving (another 12HH challenge).

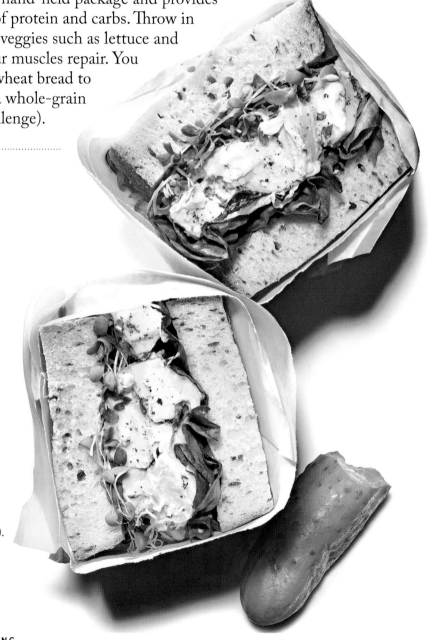

Herbed Chicken Salad Sandwiches

3 tablespoons canola mayonnaise
3 tablespoons plain 2% reduced-fat
 Greek yogurt
1 tablespoon finely chopped fresh
 tarragon
1 tablespoon fresh lemon juice
⅛ teaspoon kosher salt
2 cups chopped skinless, boneless
 rotisserie chicken breast
¼ cup minced sweet onion
8 (1½-ounce) slices rye sandwich
 bread
4 red leaf lettuce leaves
1 cup microgreens or arugula

1. Combine first 5 ingredients in a large bowl. Stir in chicken and onion. Top each of 4 bread slices with 1 lettuce leaf, about ½ packed cup chicken salad, ¼ cup microgreens, and 1 bread slice. Serves 4 (serving size: 1 sandwich).

CALORIES 382; **FAT** 9g (sat 1.4g, mono 3.9g, poly 2.4g); **PROTEIN** 30.2g; **CARB** 42.9g; **FIBER** 5.1g; **CHOL** 60mg; **IRON** 3.2mg; **SODIUM** 745mg; **CALC** 89mg

The American College of Sports Medicine recommends refueling muscles with 30 to 60 grams of carbohydrate in the first 30 minutes after an hour-long workout.

Tuscan Tuna Sandwiches

¼ cup finely chopped fennel bulb
¼ cup chopped red onion
¼ cup chopped fresh basil
2 tablespoons drained capers
2 tablespoons fresh lemon juice
2 tablespoons extra-virgin olive oil
¼ teaspoon black pepper
2 (6-ounce) cans solid white tuna in
    water, drained
1 (4-ounce) jar chopped roasted red
    bell peppers, drained
8 (1-ounce) slices 100% whole-wheat
    bread, toasted

1. Combine first 9 ingredients in a bowl, stirring well. Spoon ½ cup tuna mixture on each of 4 bread slices. Top each serving with 1 bread slice. Cut each sandwich in half. Serves 4 (serving size: 1 sandwich).

CALORIES 307; FAT 11.1g (sat 2g, mono 6.9g, poly 1.8g); PROTEIN 24.5g; CARB 26.5g; FIBER 4.4g; CHOL 30mg; IRON 2.3mg; SODIUM 726mg; CALC 83mg

Open-Faced Hummus Sandwiches

4 (1½-ounce) slices sourdough bread
1½ cups quartered grape
    tomatoes
⅓ cup chopped green onions
¼ cup sliced pitted kalamata
    olives
1 tablespoon olive oil
¼ teaspoon black pepper
⅛ teaspoon kosher salt
1 garlic clove, minced
1 (8-ounce) container plain hummus
½ cup (2 ounces) crumbled goat
    cheese

1. Preheat broiler.
2. Arrange bread on a baking sheet. Broil 1 minute or until toasted.
3. Combine tomatoes and next 6 ingredients. Spread about ¼ cup hummus over each bread slice. Divide tomato mixture evenly among servings. Top each serving with 2 tablespoons cheese. Serves 4 (serving size: 1 sandwich).

CALORIES 358; FAT 20.1g (sat 3.1g, mono 11.9g, poly 3.9g); PROTEIN 12.3g; CARB 36.5g; FIBER 4.3g; CHOL 7mg; IRON 3.5mg; SODIUM 811mg; CALC 100mg

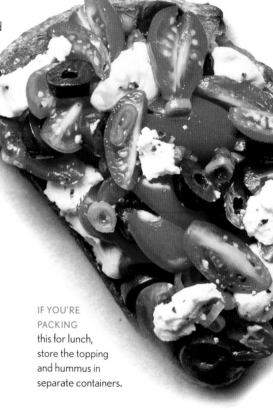

IF YOU'RE PACKING this for lunch, store the topping and hummus in separate containers.

 What are your tricks for staying active?

@Claire_Atwell: Going for a run before work in the morning! Get your cardio in before 9 a.m. and stay energized all day!

@ElizabethAFloyd: My healthy habits are walking or biking everywhere because I don't own a car! Well, or the bus! But I do go to the gym two times a week.

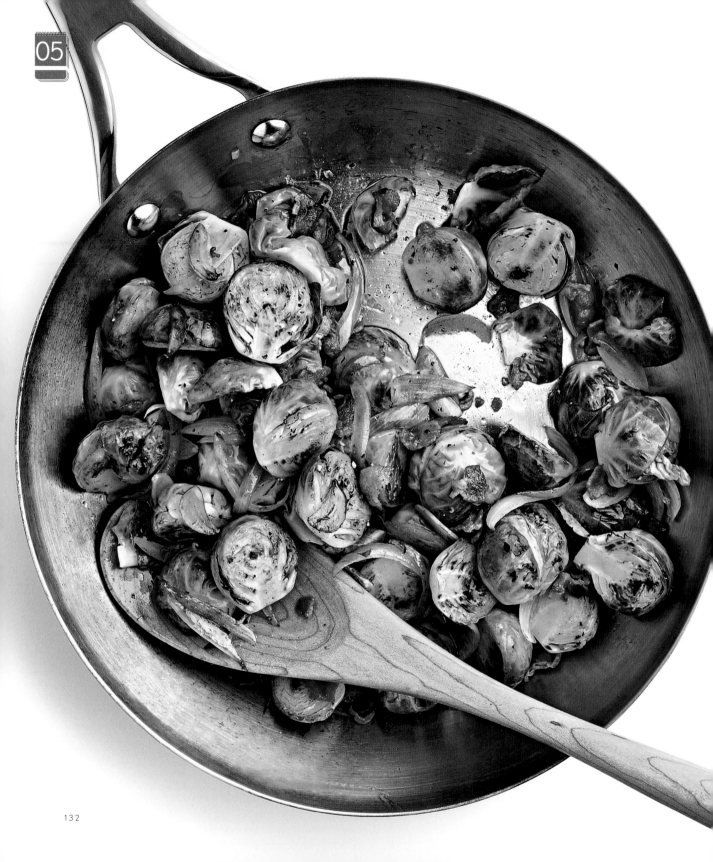

VEGGIE UP

CRANK UP COLOR, CROWD OUT CALORIES.

EAT YOUR VEGETABLES may be mom's original injunction, but she was right about this one. And now that you've grown up and (hopefully) stopped pushing peas around on your plate, it's time to give veggies the respect they deserve.

Sixty-three percent of our readers confess they don't eat the nine daily recommended servings of fruits and vegetables. But plants are the absolute foundation of a healthy diet, providing all sorts of nutrients and fiber that play a role in disease prevention. Eating more plants tends to displace higher-calorie foods, balancing your diet and controlling hunger. Countless studies have shown that people who load up on vegetables and fruits every day have a lower risk of heart disease, stroke, diabetes, and certain cancers. They also have lower blood pressure, tend to weigh less, and have higher-quality diets.

But it's not easy. Unlike fruits, which are sweeter and more convenient, it's harder to fit veggies in—they aren't exactly an ideal topping for your morning cereal. Spinach dip gets you nowhere, and pumpkin pie, tasty as it is, is not the ideal veggie delivery system. In supermarkets, especially during cold months, it's hard to find rich variety in great condition. Vegetables such as turnips and squash require prep and cooking time that you, like about one-fifth of our readers, might feel you don't have.

But upping your intake doesn't require a revolution. Just a few small and very simple substitutions to your everyday breakfasts, snacks, and suppers can help you get the 2½ to 3 cups of veggies the USDA recommends for most adults each day.

YOUR GOAL

Eat three more servings each day.

The 12 Healthy Habits

| · 01 ·
GET
COOKING | · 02 ·
BREAKFAST
DAILY | · 03 ·
WHOLE
GRAINS | · 04 ·
GET
MOVING | · 05 ·
VEGGIE
UP | · 06 ·
MORE
SEAFOOD | · 07 ·
HEALTHY
FATS | · 08 ·
GO
MEATLESS | · 09 ·
GET
STRONGER | · 10 ·
LESS
SALT | · 11 ·
BE PORTION-
AWARE | · 12 ·
EAT
MINDFULLY |

Boost Your Breakfast

ALMOST A FIFTH OF READERS admit the reason they don't consume enough veggies is because it simply seems to take too much time to prep them and add them in throughout the day. Breakfast can be particularly tricky because of the a.m. rush to get to work or school. The trouble is, missing out in the morning makes it that much harder to catch up by the end of the day. Chicago nutritionist David Grotto, RD, author of *101 Optimal Life Foods*, offers some tips:

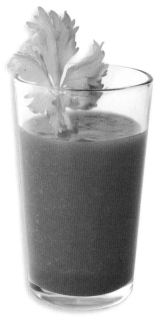

TRY A SWEET TOPPER
Spoon a couple tablespoons of mashed roasted sweet potato or pumpkin over your morning toast or oatmeal instead of your usual butter or sweetener.

BOOST YOUR BREAKFAST SANDWICH
Bolster that egg on a roll you order at your corner deli every morning by asking the cook to throw in a cup of cooked chopped veggies like peppers, tomatoes, mushrooms, or onions.

BUTTERNUT UP
Stir 1 cup of canned butternut squash into homemade pancake or waffle batter.

MUG IT UP
Take 2 eggs, 2 tablespoons of milk, and a couple handfuls of chopped veggies like peppers or tomatoes, and throw them into a microwave-safe coffee mug. Beat them until they're blended, microwave at HIGH 2 minutes, and voilà! You have an egg scramble you can take with you on the road. No time for pepper prep? No problem—add in tomato sauce instead.

MINCE SOME VEGGIES INTO YOUR MUFFINS
When you're baking your usual muffins or breakfast bread, add 1½ cups of grated carrots or zucchini to the batter. Your kids will never taste the difference.

GO FOR A VIRGIN MARY
Mix 1 cup of no-salt-added tomato juice, ½ tablespoon lemon juice, and a dash of Worcestershire sauce or hot pepper sauce (or both!), and pour over ice.

MAKE A PUMPKIN PARFAIT
Mix 1 cup of organic vanilla low-fat yogurt with 1 cup of canned pumpkin puree.

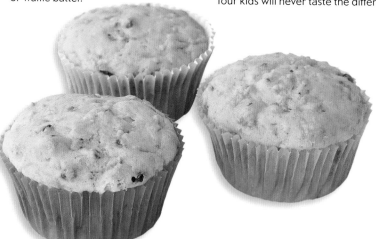

Only 27% of Americans eat vegetables three or more times per day.

MEET THE NEW PLATE

Who has time to measure out a cup of chopped broccoli or peppers or check the diameter of a sweet potato? Let's face it, most of us don't. Now, making sure you get enough veggies is simpler than ever, thanks to the U.S. Department of Agriculture's easy-to-understand MyPlate.

The recommendation? At each meal, simply fill half your plate with vegetables and fruits, one-fourth with grains like brown rice or whole-wheat bread, and one-fourth with a protein like chicken, eggs, fish, or a lean cut of beef or pork. The key is to build your meal around your fruits and veggies, rather than protein and a starchy side.

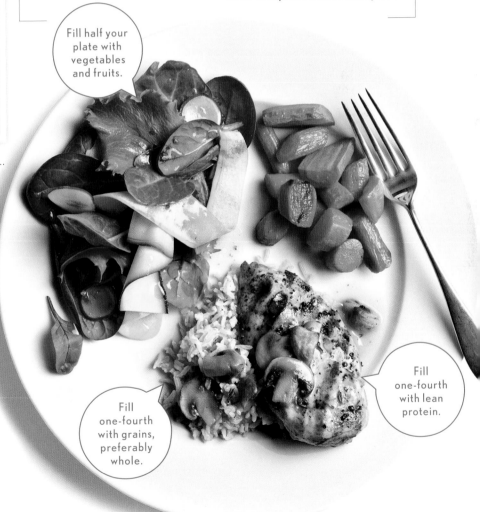

Fill half your plate with vegetables and fruits.

Fill one-fourth with grains, preferably whole.

Fill one-fourth with lean protein.

Double Your Vegetables

ABOUT A THIRD OF OUR READERS say finding new, tasty recipes containing veggies is a real challenge. But you don't need to reinvent the wheel to pump up your produce. Here, ways to sneak an extra serving (or two) into your family's favorite meal staples:

STIR EXTRA VEGGIES INTO SOUPS.

When it comes to something like soups, an overdose of chopped veggies won't ruin the recipe. Instead, they'll enhance the flavor, nutritional value, and your daily vegetable tally. Stirring in a few cups of chopped vegetables and dark leafy greens (which wilt down significantly in soup) is an easy way to amp up the veggie count.

CRAM THEM INTO CASSEROLES.

Cooking up a Mexican casserole? Add some extra peppers, mushrooms, and squash. Don't be shy when topping with tomato- and veggie-heavy salsa, either. Eggplant Parmesan? Double the eggplant. Chicken Pot Pie? Double those peas and carrots. You've got the idea.

PILE THEM ON PIZZA.

Don't hold back! Add extra veggies to a frozen pizza, order double veggies from delivery, or create your own where the sky is the limit.

Precook vegetables so they don't add too much moisture to the pizza.

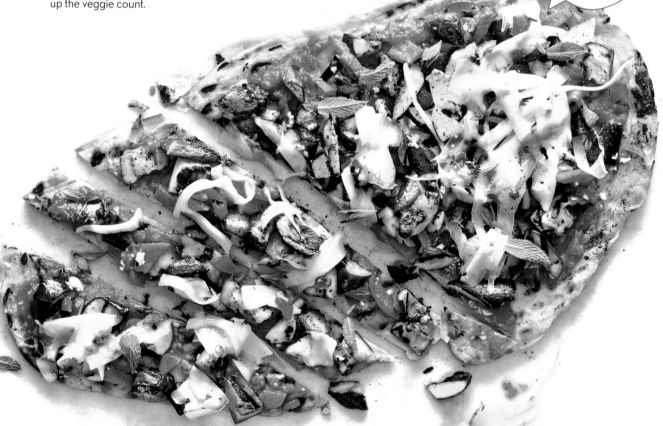

STUFF THEM INTO SANDWICHES.

A sandwich is another blank canvas just waiting to get stuffed with color. Take your routine turkey sandwich and jazz it up with sliced apples, cucumber, zucchini, sprouts, and spinach. A cup of this colorful combo just scored you another serving. Another tip: Pita bread and wraps are great for holding lots and lots of veggies.

GRATE YOUR WAY TO GOODNESS.

Shred or grate veggies and see how creative you can get with your favorite recipes. Grated zucchini and carrots do wonders for turkey burgers, meat loaf, and meatballs, adding both moisture and nutrients to the dish.

PREPARE SOME PUREES.

Veggies like cauliflower, winter squash, or red peppers can easily be pureed and stirred into sauces, mashed potatoes, pot pies, or that old kid staple, mac and cheese. See Creamy, Light Macaroni and Cheese on page 319.

COACHING SESSION
with ALLISON FISHMAN

SHARPEN YOUR KNIFE SKILLS

You can streamline veggie prep by sharpening up your knife skills, which will make chopping a breeze. Here, three quick tips from *Cooking Light* 12HH coach Allison Fishman:

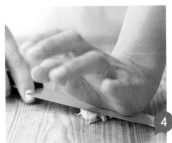

- **Onion.** To chop onion, (1) cut it in half and remove the papery skin. Place the onion flat side down, and hold the root end. (2) See those lines on the onion? Follow them. Cut two-thirds of the way through the onion without cutting the root end. (3) Once you've made those slices, cut across the onion in the opposite direction, directly perpendicular to where you were cutting.
- **Garlic.** Sure, you can buy chopped garlic in a jar, but that doesn't offer optimal flavor. You can make it less time consuming by (4) slicing off the root end, smashing the garlic to remove the papery skin, then slicing the semi-smushed piece of garlic.
- **Knives.** The best way to dull a knife is cleaning it in the dishwasher. Washing by hand takes less than 10 seconds. Ideally, you should get your knives professionally sharpened every six months.

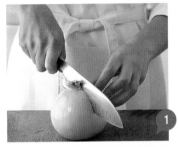

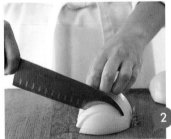

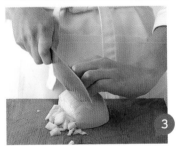

The Busy Mom

"I don't have time to deal with produce."

KRISTI HART
Human Resources Director

➤ **VEGGIE UP CHALLENGE:** As a working mom with two small children, Kristi is always rushing. She feels like she doesn't have time during the day to eat many vegetables herself, and she finds it hard to squeeze in dinnertime prep work.

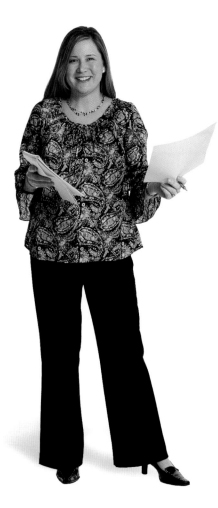

OUR ADVICE

■ **Make salad a staple.** Begin each dinner with one: Use no-prep bagged salad greens as a base, then load in other chopped veggies. This can add two servings.

■ **Fill up your freezer.** Frozen veggies are ideal for getting dinner on the table within minutes. You can steam them in the microwave for a quick cooking option or sauté with fresh herbs for an easy stovetop version.

■ **Pay a bit more for fresh precut veggies.** You can't beat the convenience factor—some are even designed to microwave-steam in the bag. You can also spread veggies on a baking sheet to roast.

■ **Augment lunch** with raw veggies and dip brought from home. (Hint: Get one of those little insulated lunch bags.) For variety, try snow peas, cauliflower, radishes, and cucumber paired with a store-bought tzatziki or hummus.

Instead of bread or tortillas, make your next sandwich or wrap inside a leafy green such as Bibb lettuce, romaine, or red lettuce.

The Restaurant-Goer

"How do I add in veggies when I'm always eating out?"

MARGARET BARNHART
Sales Manager

➤ **VEGGIE UP CHALLENGE:** A third of Margaret's meals are eaten out due to her hectic work schedule. "It's the lunches and dinners that get me," she says. "People say, 'Let's order some appetizers!'" And she's not talking crudités.

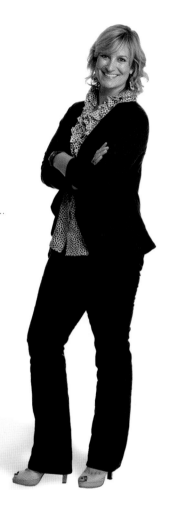

OUR ADVICE

■ **Customize your order.**
Don't hesitate to combine two or three appetizers or sides and skip the entrée to fit in your veggies. You can even ask if the kitchen will build a custom veggie plate with three sides.
■ **Opt for veggie-based entrées.**
Look for pasta topped with vegetables, chunky vegetable broth–based soups, veggie-loaded sandwiches, and vegetable pizzas—just ask them to hold half of the cheese.

■ **Entertain with ethnic.** If clients are willing to try them, Chinese, Thai, Indian, and Mexican eateries offer lots of vegetable-based entrées and side dishes. Even if the table is sharing apps, order a vegetable platter and savor it.
■ **Order entrée salads.** These salads can provide up to three servings of vegetables—just order dressings on the side so you can control how much you use and monitor rich, calorie-heavy toppings like blue cheese and bacon bits.

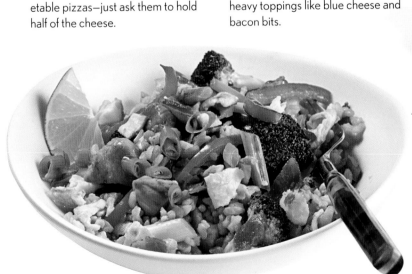

Oatmeal topped with fruit is an easy option for rushed morning meals or when you're grabbing breakfast from a fast-food restaurant.

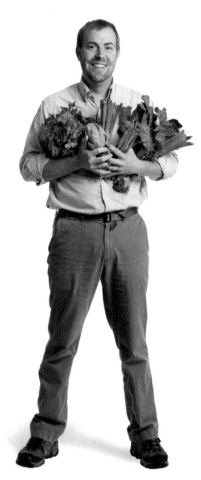

The Embattled Dad

"My kids won't eat their vegetables!"

ROBIN BASHINSKY
Cooking Light *Recipe Tester*

➤**VEGGIE UP CHALLENGE:** Robin cooks for a living, but when he gets home his kids turn up their noses at the vegetables he puts on their plates. To keep the peace, the kids get one meal and the grown-ups eat later. But by the time they've fed the kids and focused on their own meal, Robin and his wife Nan are so wiped out that they end up not eating many vegetables, either. Sound familiar?

OUR ADVICE

■ **Involve the kids in shopping.** Let each child pick an item for the family to try. Let them grab purple cauliflower or warty celeriac—if it's a veggie, it doesn't matter.

■ **Let your kids lend a hand.** Whether it's peeling carrots or simply pouring frozen peas into a bowl, if children feel a sense of pride from helping prepare a meal, they'll be more interested in eating it.

■ **Keep it crunchy.** How you prep veggies can make all the world of difference for picky kids. Dutch researchers found that children prefer vegetables that are steamed or boiled over mashed, grilled, stir-fried, and deep fried. Veggies that retained their original taste, color, and crunchiness were the most appealing. Noisy, crunchy veggies like raw carrots and bell peppers paired with one of the dips on pages 162-165 are sure crowd-pleasers.

■ **Please all palates with one dish.** Serve pan-grilled chicken breasts to kids along with sweet crisp veggies like cucumber sticks or blanched green beans. For the adults, slice and pile the chicken on top of a big bed of spinach or arugula tossed with the same veggies.

EXPERT TIP: *Be a Veggie Role Model*

"It's important to serve some type of vegetable on their plate every day so your kids realize it's simply part of the meal, and be sure they see you enjoying your own plate of vegetables. Don't underestimate your influence as a veggie role model."

—*Liz Weiss, MS, RD, and Janice Bissex, MS, RD, bloggers, Meal Makeover Moms' Kitchen*

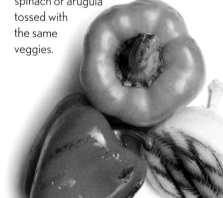

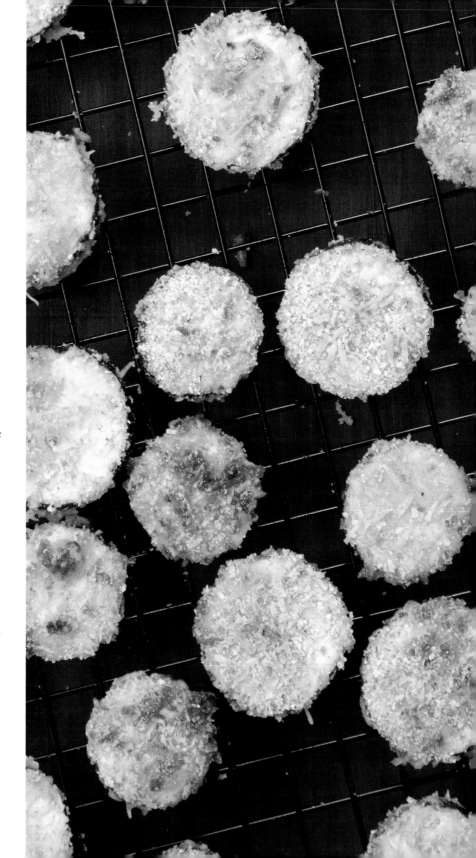

Quick Side

Zucchini Oven Chips

Preheat oven to 425°. Stir together ¼ cup dry breadcrumbs, ¼ cup grated fresh Parmesan cheese, ¼ teaspoon seasoned salt, and ⅛ teaspoon freshly ground pepper in a medium bowl. Pour 2 tablespoons fat-free milk in a shallow bowl. Dip ¼-inch-thick zucchini slices (about 2 small zucchini) in milk, and dredge in breadcrumb mixture. Place slices on an ovenproof wire rack coated with cooking spray; place rack on a baking sheet. Bake at 425° for 30 minutes, or until browned and crisp. Serve immediately. Serves 4 (serving size: about ¾ cup).

CALORIES 61; FAT 1.9g (sat 1g, mono 0.5g, poly 0.2g); PROTEIN 3.8g; CARB 7.6g; FIBER 1g; CHOL 5mg; IRON 0.6mg; SODIUM 231mg; CALC 87mg

Let your kids help prepare these tasty veggie chips. They can measure, mix, and dredge.

Purchase Produce in Season

IT'S TRICKY ENOUGH trying to squeeze in a few extra servings of veggies a day without worrying about how to find the freshest produce on the block. Robert Schueller, *Cooking Light*'s produce guru and director of public relations at Melissa's Produce, gives a few ideas on what to buy when:

FALL

Potatoes
They're cheaper in the fall and are the ultimate comfort food—great for thick soups or roasted for a holiday dinner.
Look for: Potatoes that are wrinkle free, without green tinges, sprouts, or cracks

Parsnips
When cooked they have the combined sweetness of a carrot with a taste of parsley and some subtle nuttiness.
Look for: Those that are firm and relatively smooth

Onions
They're great in fall stews or casseroles, or roasted with olive oil.
Look for: A firm bulb, without soft spots

WINTER

Leafy greens
Fresh greens are available year-round and are so versatile—you can add them to spaghetti, sauté them, or use them as a salad base.
User tip: Don't wash them until you're ready to use, since rinsing can break down the protective layer that extends their shelf life.

Winter squash
It brightens up this time of year with its array of colors, from green to yellow to orange, and makes a great add-in to soups and pasta.
Look for: Squash that seems heavy for its size, since it contains more edible flesh

Beets
They're great in winter soups, or served warm with butter.
User tip: It's much easier (and much less messy) to peel them when they're cooked.

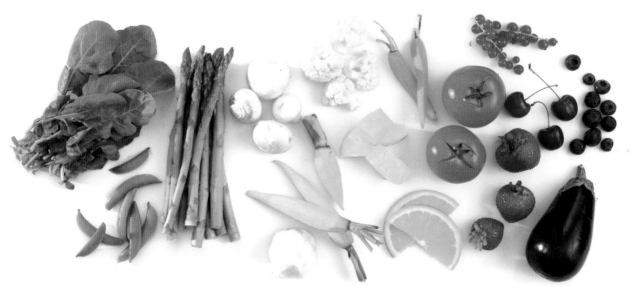

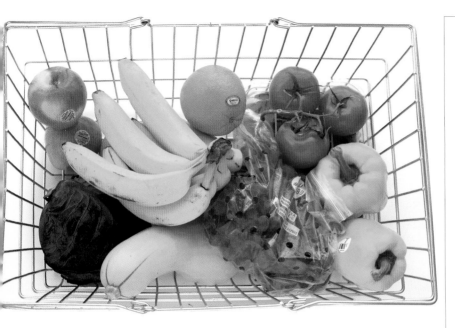

SPRING

Peas
They're great raw or cooked, or mashed and mixed with avocado to make guacamole.
Look for: Peas with bright green, glossy pods

Artichokes
March through May is peak season. They look tough, but cooking makes them buttery sweet.
Look for: Leaves that squeak when pressed together

Bell peppers
They're less expensive now, since you can get them domestically.
Look for: Firm peppers with shiny, wrinkle-free skins

SUMMER

Corn
You can't beat fresh corn in the summer, especially when it comes to its price!
User tip: Pull back portions of the husk to make sure the green silk is slightly sticky.

Tomatoes
They're a great addition to summer salads, as they pack a wallop of sweetness tinged with a bit of acidity.
Look for: Plump tomatoes that feel heavy for their size

Avocado
You can easily add it to salads or hamburgers at summer barbecues, or even serve up homemade guacamole.
User tip: Push the skin when buying—if it yields slightly, it's good for slicing or dicing, and if it leaves a small dent, it's ideal for mashing.

HOW TO BUY ORGANIC

The benefits of a fruit- and veggie-rich diet far outweigh the health risks of pesticide exposure. You can reduce your exposure by choosing organic when purchasing the fruits and vegetables that have the highest levels of pesticide residues—referred to as the Dirty Dozen™. The Clean 15™ includes items that are lowest in pesticide residues. Here's the list from the non-profit Environmental Working Group's Shopper's Guide to Pesticides in Produce:

THE DIRTY DOZEN
Apples
Celery
Sweet bell peppers
Peaches
Strawberries
Nectarines (imported)
Grapes
Spinach
Lettuce
Cucumbers
Blueberries (domestic)
Potatoes

THE CLEAN 15
Onions
Sweet corn
Pineapples
Avocado
Cabbage
Sweet peas
Asparagus
Mangoes
Eggplant
Kiwi
Cantaloupe (domestic)
Sweet potatoes
Grapefruit
Watermelon
Mushrooms

Eat More Greens

SALADS HAVE THE POTENTIAL to be a healthy habit goldmine, rich in fruits, vegetables, and nutritional value. But we're not talking about salads with a leaf of iceberg, and loads of bacon, cheese, and ranch. We're talking beds of dark, leafy greens with colorful, crunchy toppings to provide a wide array of phytonutrients.

Alternate your greens to keep things interesting—for a general rule of thumb, the darker the greens (like spinach, kale, or swiss chard) the more nutrient-rich they are. Pile on healthy toppings like chopped fruit and vegetables, and you can easily get half your daily recommended amount packed into one glorious salad. Don't cheat yourself on the dressing: A few splashes of a good, heart-healthy canola- or olive oil–based dressing can work wonders.

Honey Balsamic Arugula Salad

2 tablespoons balsamic vinegar
2 tablespoons olive oil
1 tablespoon minced shallots
1 tablespoon chopped fresh parsley
1 teaspoon Dijon mustard
1 teaspoon honey
¼ teaspoon salt
¼ teaspoon freshly ground
    black pepper
1 garlic clove, crushed
6 cups arugula
¼ cup sliced red onion
2 tablespoons chopped walnuts
1 ounce shaved fresh Parmesan cheese
    (about ¼ cup)

1. Combine first 9 ingredients in a large bowl; stir well with a whisk. Add arugula, onion, walnuts, and Parmesan; toss gently to coat. Serves 4.

CALORIES 139; FAT 11.2g (sat 2.4g, mono 5.8g, poly 2.6g); PROTEIN 4.1g; CARB 6.4g; FIBER 0.9g; CHOL 5mg; IRON 0.9mg; SODIUM 229mg; CALC 144mg

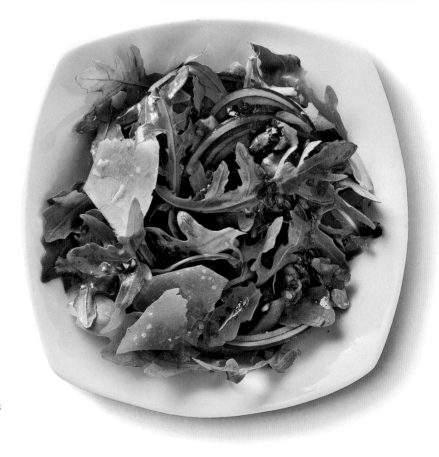

Shrimp, Avocado, and Grapefruit Salad

2½ tablespoons olive oil, divided
12 ounces peeled and deveined
    medium shrimp
½ teaspoon salt, divided
¼ teaspoon freshly ground black
    pepper, divided
1 grapefruit
2 tablespoons chopped fresh tarragon
2 teaspoons brown sugar
1 teaspoon chopped shallots
6 cups chopped romaine lettuce
1 peeled avocado, cut into 12 wedges

1. Heat a large skillet over medium-high heat. Add 1½ teaspoons oil to pan; swirl to coat. Sprinkle shrimp with ¼ teaspoon salt and ⅛ teaspoon pepper. Add shrimp to pan; cook 3 minutes or until shrimp are done, stirring frequently. Remove from pan; keep warm.
2. Peel and section grapefruit over a bowl, reserving 3 tablespoons juice. Combine grapefruit juice, remaining 2 tablespoons oil, remaining ¼ teaspoon salt, remaining ⅛ teaspoon pepper, tarragon, brown sugar, and shallots in a large bowl, stirring well with a whisk. Add lettuce; toss. Arrange 2 cups lettuce mixture on each of 4 plates. Top each serving with 3 avocado wedges; divide shrimp and grapefruit evenly among servings. Serves 4.

Sustainable Choice: Buy U.S. or Canadian wild or farmed shrimp.

CALORIES 291; FAT 17.7g (sat 2.6g, mono 11.3g, poly 2.5g); PROTEIN 19.9g; CARB 15.5g; FIBER 6g; CHOL 129mg; IRON 3.4mg; SODIUM 433mg; CALC 96mg

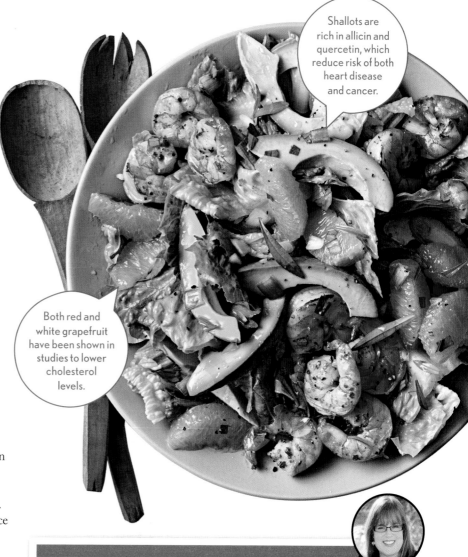

Shallots are rich in allicin and quercetin, which reduce risk of both heart disease and cancer.

Both red and white grapefruit have been shown in studies to lower cholesterol levels.

EXPERT TIP: *Open with Salad*

"Starting out the meal with a big bowl of greens is not just a way to grab onto nutrients. It's also a perfect way to put the skids on overeating. Penn State researchers find people who eat salad before a meal end up eating less."

—*Maureen Callahan, MS, RD, nutrition writer*

Shake Up Your Salads

T IRED OF THE SAME old boring lunchtime side salad? Here's a way to shake things up: Start with 2 cups of fresh mixed greens, add a tablespoon of your favorite vinaigrette, and then pile on one of these 100-calorie topping combinations.

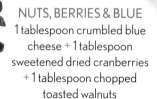

NUTS, BERRIES & BLUE
1 tablespoon crumbled blue cheese + 1 tablespoon sweetened dried cranberries + 1 tablespoon chopped toasted walnuts

PROTEIN-PACKED
2 tablespoons edamame + 1 tablespoon crunchy Chinese noodles + 2 tablespoons Mandarin orange segments + 1 tablespoon chopped roasted peanuts

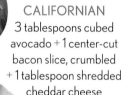

CALIFORNIAN
3 tablespoons cubed avocado + 1 center-cut bacon slice, crumbled + 1 tablespoon shredded cheddar cheese

SOUTHWESTERN
2 tablespoons rinsed and drained black beans + 2 tablespoons sweet yellow corn + 2 tablespoons crumbled queso fresco + 2 tablespoons cubed avocado

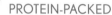
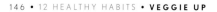

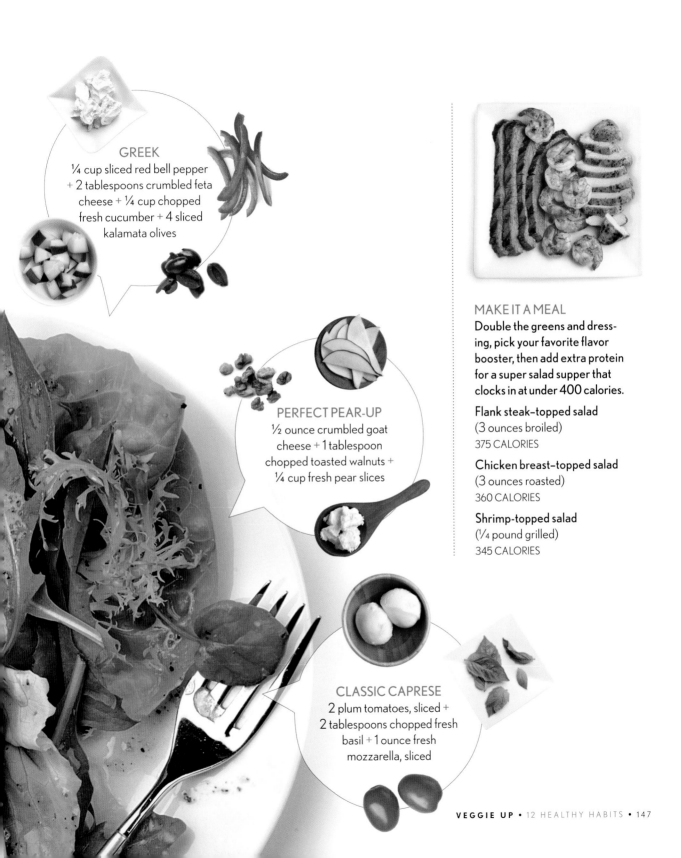

GREEK

¼ cup sliced red bell pepper
+ 2 tablespoons crumbled feta
cheese + ¼ cup chopped
fresh cucumber + 4 sliced
kalamata olives

PERFECT PEAR-UP

½ ounce crumbled goat
cheese + 1 tablespoon
chopped toasted walnuts +
¼ cup fresh pear slices

CLASSIC CAPRESE

2 plum tomatoes, sliced +
2 tablespoons chopped fresh
basil + 1 ounce fresh
mozzarella, sliced

MAKE IT A MEAL

Double the greens and dressing, pick your favorite flavor
booster, then add extra protein
for a super salad supper that
clocks in at under 400 calories.

Flank steak–topped salad
(3 ounces broiled)
375 CALORIES

Chicken breast–topped salad
(3 ounces roasted)
360 CALORIES

Shrimp-topped salad
(¼ pound grilled)
345 CALORIES

Roast to Build Flavor

ROASTING VEGGIES IS A SUREFIRE WAY to win over picky eaters. Unlike boiling, which can leave vegetables limp and soggy, roasting concentrates natural sugars, creating sweet vegetables bursting with flavor. It's ideal for dense veggies such as potatoes, carrots, and winter squash, as well as high-moisture ones like asparagus and summer squash. There's no better way to build big, intense flavors with so little effort.

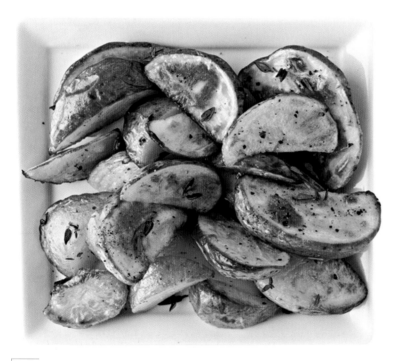

Quick Side
Roasted Potatoes with Thyme and Garlic
Preheat broiler. Combine 1 (20-ounce) package refrigerated potato wedges, 2 tablespoons olive oil, ¼ teaspoon kosher salt, and ¼ teaspoon freshly ground black pepper on a baking sheet. Broil 12 minutes, stirring after 6 minutes. Stir in 1 tablespoon minced garlic; broil 2 minutes or until potatoes are tender. Remove from oven; sprinkle with 2 teaspoons chopped fresh thyme. Serves 4 (serving size: about ¾ cup).

CALORIES 151; FAT 6.8g (sat 0.9g, mono 4.9g, poly 0.7g); PROTEIN 3.7g; CARB 18.4g; FIBER 3.6g; CHOL 0mg; IRON 0.8mg; SODIUM 269mg; CALC 6mg

ROAST 1-2-3

1. Cut the veggies into same-sized pieces so that they cook evenly.
2. Place the cut veggies on a baking sheet or roasting pan (for easy cleanup, line the pan with foil and coat with cooking spray), and toss them with a little olive or canola oil or spray with cooking spray. Then sprinkle with kosher salt, freshly ground black pepper, and any additional herbs of your choice. Just remember to spread the veggies in a single layer. If they're stacked on top of one another, the veggies on the bottom will steam rather than roast.

3. Stick the veggies in the oven and roast until browned. They usually need a moderate temperature near 375° so that the water inside the vegetables evaporates quickly to concentrate the flavor without the exterior browning too deeply or becoming too soft.

Roasting is an easy hands-off process that produces beautiful browned vegetables.

Roasted Asparagus with Browned Butter

1 pound asparagus spears, trimmed
1 tablespoon olive oil
½ teaspoon kosher salt
¼ teaspoon black pepper
1½ tablespoons butter
1½ tablespoons fresh Meyer lemon juice
1½ teaspoons chopped fresh thyme
1 teaspoon grated Meyer lemon rind

1. Preheat oven to 450°. Place asparagus in a roasting pan; drizzle with oil. Sprinkle evenly with salt and pepper. Bake at 450° for 8 minutes or until crisp-tender.
2. Melt butter in a small skillet over medium heat; cook 3 minutes or until lightly browned, shaking pan occasionally. Remove from heat; stir in juice. Drizzle butter mixture over asparagus; toss well to coat. Sprinkle thyme and rind over asparagus. Serves 4 (serving size: about 3 ounces).

CALORIES 82; FAT 7.8g (sat 3.2g, mono 3.6g, poly 0.6g); PROTEIN 1.4g; CARB 3.1g; FIBER 1.4g; CHOL 11mg; IRON 1.4mg; SODIUM 272mg; CALC 19mg

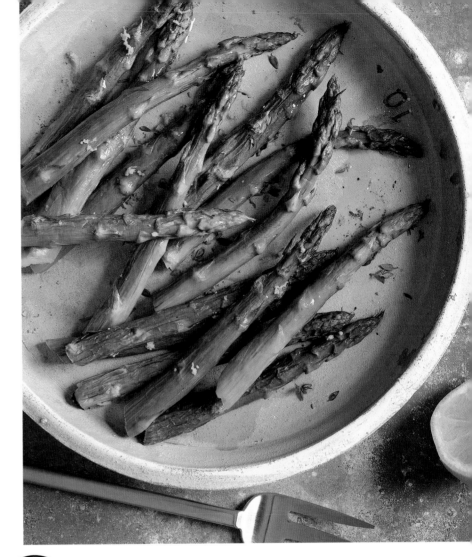

READER TIP: *Perfect Your Knife Skills*

"Learning to chop vegetables in different ways was huge. Now I can cut matchstick carrots and properly chop an onion. I'll do one big one and keep it in the fridge for several days. Having onions cut up makes a huge difference to me and cuts down on my prep time for meals. On a day when I was tired, that simple act would stop me from trying a recipe. Now I just pull it out of the fridge and go.

—*Mary Lynn Meyer, health-care consultant and Healthy Habits Graduate*

Steam to Preserve Flavor and Nutrients

OVERCOOKED VEGETABLES ARE A TURN-OFF. That's why steaming is ideal, because it cooks food more gently than almost any other method, which means the veggie retains its original texture. And unlike boiling, which leaches water-soluble nutrients from food, steaming keeps most of the nutrients—as well as the flavor and color—intact. Almost all veggies are good candidates, except for spongy ones like mushrooms or eggplant or tough ones like hearty greens. Best of all, you don't need to add much more than a tablespoon of olive or canola oil and your favorite fresh herbs to bring out the veggies' natural flavor.

STEAMING 1-2-3

Steaming requires little more than a pan with a well-fitting lid and a steamer to support the food over the liquid in the pan (most cookware sets come with one).

1. Fill the pan with a few inches of water, and bring to a boil.
2. Place the veggies in the metal steamer, and place in the pan (the boiling water shouldn't touch the vegetables).
3. Cover and steam until the vegetables are crisp-tender when pierced with a knife. Remember, creating a good seal with the lid is crucial for holding in steam. If the lid doesn't fit snugly, cover the pan with foil, and then cover it with the lid.

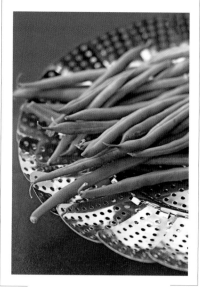

Simple Steamed Broccoli

4 cups broccoli florets
1 tablespoon butter
1/2 teaspoon grated lemon rind
1/8 teaspoon salt
1/8 teaspoon freshly ground black
    pepper

1. Steam broccoli 5 minutes or until crisp-tender. Place broccoli in a bowl. Add butter, rind, salt, and pepper; toss until butter melts. Serves 4 (serving size: 1 cup).

CALORIES 46; FAT 3.1g (sat 1.9g, mono 0.8g, poly 0.2g); PROTEIN 2.2g; CARB 3.8g; FIBER 2.2g; CHOL 8mg; IRON 0.7mg; SODIUM 113mg; CALC 36mg

Steamed Sugar Snap Peas

3 cups fresh sugar snap peas
1 tablespoon chopped fresh mint
    or tarragon
1 tablespoon butter
1/8 teaspoon salt
1/8 teaspoon freshly ground black
    pepper

1. Steam peas 5 minutes or until crisp-tender; drain. Combine peas, mint, butter, salt, and pepper; toss well. Serves 4 (serving size: 3/4 cup).

CALORIES 46; FAT 3g (sat 1.8g, mono 0.8g, poly 0.2g); PROTEIN 1.4g; CARB 3.7g; FIBER 1.3g; CHOL 8mg; IRON 1mg; SODIUM 96mg; CALC 22mg

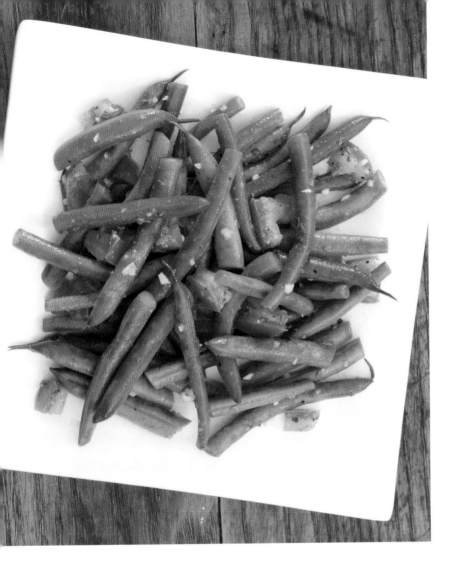

Use tongs or spatulas to remove food from the steamer. Steamed food often retains heat longer because the hot steam has permeated the food.

Steamed Green Beans with Tomato-Garlic Vinaigrette

1 tablespoon white wine vinegar
½ teaspoon Dijon mustard
¼ teaspoon salt
⅛ teaspoon freshly ground black
   pepper
2 garlic cloves, crushed and minced
1 tablespoon extra-virgin olive oil
½ cup seeded chopped tomato
2 teaspoons chopped fresh thyme
1 pound green beans, trimmed

1. Combine first 5 ingredients in a medium bowl; slowly add oil, whisking to combine. Stir in tomato and thyme; let stand 10 minutes.
2. Steam beans, covered, 7 minutes or until crisp-tender. Cut into 2-inch pieces; add to tomato mixture, tossing gently to coat. Serves 4 (serving size: ¾ cup).

CALORIES 73; FAT 3.6g (sat 0.5g, mono 2.5g, poly 0.5g); PROTEIN 2.4g; CARB 9.8g; FIBER 4.2g; CHOL 0mg; IRON 1.4mg; SODIUM 162mg; CALC 48mg

EXPERT TIP: *Add a Vinaigrette to Your Veggies*

"Vinaigrettes are not just for salads. Try adding them to cooked vegetables; it really sparkles them up. I also love to drizzle on roasted nut oils paired with a sprinkling of the same nut toasted and a finishing salt. The addition of these oils is a two-fer. The vegetables will not only taste better, so you'll want to eat more, but you'll enhance the bioavailability of some of the nutrients in the vegetables."

—*Mollie Katzen, best-selling cookbook author*

Sauté for Quick Results

PRESSED FOR TIME? You can streamline your vegetable cooking with a sauté. This method cooks food quickly over relatively high heat in a minimal amount of fat. The browning achieved lends richness to vegetables, and because the food cooks quickly, the flavor and texture remain intact. A good saucepan is all you need (along with some flavorful, heart-healthy olive oil or canola oil) to get delicious veggies on the table in a matter of minutes.

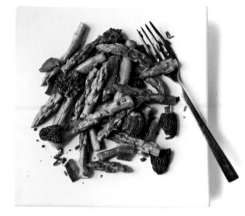

SAUTÉ 1-2-3

1. Cut vegetables to a uniform thickness and size to ensure they cook evenly. Veggies shouldn't be larger than bite-sized, or they run the risk of burning or forming a tough, overly browned outer crust.

2. Heat the pan over medium-high heat for a few minutes, since it needs to be quite hot to cook the food properly.

3. Once the pan is hot, add in the oil—ideally, one that has a high smoke point, such as olive oil (not extra-virgin) or canola oil. Let it heat for 10 to 30 seconds, then add in the veggies. You'll be done in about 3 minutes.

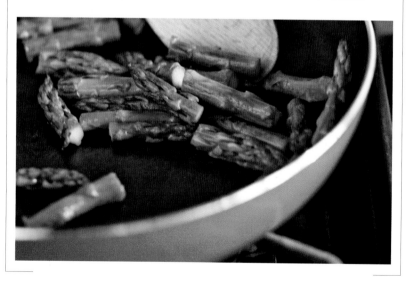

Quick Side
Smoky Asparagus and Mushroom Sauté

Cook 2 applewood-smoked bacon slices in a large skillet over medium heat until crisp. Remove bacon from pan; crumble. Add 1 tablespoon butter to drippings in pan; swirl to coat. Add 6 ounces quartered fresh morel mushrooms; sauté 4 minutes, stirring occasionally. Stir in 1 pound (1-inch) asparagus pieces, ¼ teaspoon freshly ground black pepper, and ⅛ teaspoon salt; sauté 5 minutes or until asparagus is crisp-tender, stirring occasionally. Remove from heat; sprinkle with bacon and 3 tablespoons chopped ramp greens or fresh chives. Serves 4 (serving size: about ⅔ cup).

CALORIES 107; FAT 7.5g (sat 3.6g, mono 1.7g, poly 0.4g); PROTEIN 5.4g; CARB 6.6g; FIBER 2.7g; CHOL 15mg; IRON 2.6mg; SODIUM 212mg; CALC 38mg

Broccoli Rabe with Onions and Pine Nuts

1½ pounds broccoli rabe (rapini)
1 tablespoon olive oil
1½ teaspoons butter
1 cup sliced onion
¼ teaspoon salt
2 tablespoons toasted pine nuts

1. Trim broccoli rabe; cut into 3-inch-long pieces. Cook in boiling water 1½ minutes; drain and rinse. Drain well. Heat olive oil and butter in a skillet over medium-high heat. Add onion; sauté 2 minutes or until lightly browned. Add broccoli rabe; sprinkle with salt, and toss to combine. Cook 1 minute. Sprinkle with pine nuts. Serves 4.

CALORIES 132; FAT 7.7g (sat 1.6g, mono 3.6g, poly 1.9g); PROTEIN 6.9g; CARB 11.2g; FIBER 0.6g; CHOL 4mg; IRON 1.8mg; SODIUM 207mg; CALC 88mg

Sautéed Snow Peas

1 tablespoon dark sesame oil
1 pound snow peas, trimmed
1½ tablespoons lower-sodium soy sauce
1 teaspoon sambal oelek (ground fresh chile paste; optional)

1. Heat a large skillet over medium-high heat. Add oil to pan; swirl to coat. Add peas; sauté 3 minutes or until crisp-tender. Remove from heat. Add soy sauce and sambal oelek, if desired. Toss to coat. Serves 4 (serving size: about 1 cup).

CALORIES 101; FAT 3.5g (sat 0.5g, mono 1.5g, poly 1.5g); PROTEIN 3g; CARB 8.6g; FIBER 2.7g; CHOL 0mg; IRON 1mg; SODIUM 160mg; CALC 54mg

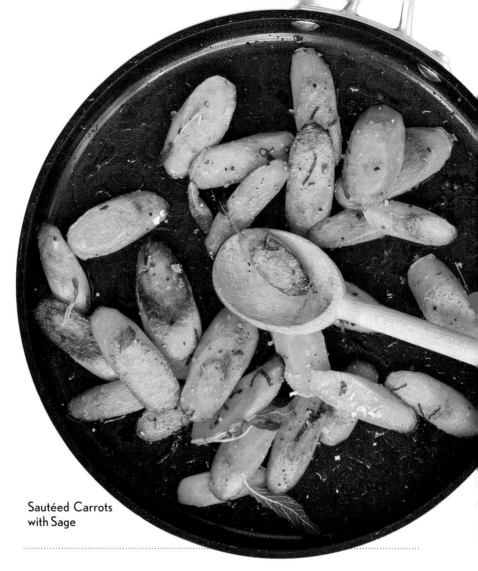

Sautéed Carrots with Sage

Sautéed Carrots with Sage

1 teaspoon butter
1 teaspoon olive oil
1½ cups diagonally sliced carrot
2 tablespoons water
⅛ teaspoon salt
⅛ teaspoon freshly ground black pepper
2 teaspoons small fresh sage leaves

1. Melt butter in a large nonstick skillet over medium heat. Add oil to pan; swirl to coat. Add carrot and 2 tablespoons water. Partially cover pan, and cook 10 minutes or until carrots are almost tender. Add salt and pepper to pan; increase heat to medium-high. Cook 4 minutes or until carrots are tender and lightly browned, stirring frequently. Sprinkle with sage. Serves 2 (serving size: ½ cup).

CALORIES 75; FAT 4.4g (sat 1.5g, mono 2.2g, poly 0.4g); PROTEIN 0.9g; CARB 9g; FIBER 2.6g; CHOL 5mg; IRON 0.3mg; SODIUM 224mg; CALC 35mg

Consider Cruciferous Vegetables

DON'T TURN UP YOUR NOSE at those Brussels sprouts—they contain several natural compounds called glucosinolates that may help lower the risk of cancer. These phytonutrients break down in the body to form isothiocynates, which may help block defective genes linked to tumor growth. Here's the catch: These disease-fighting compounds are the same sulfur-containing substances that give cruciferous veggies their strong smell and bitter taste. You can coax out their natural sweetness by roasting, or through a light steaming or a quick sauté.

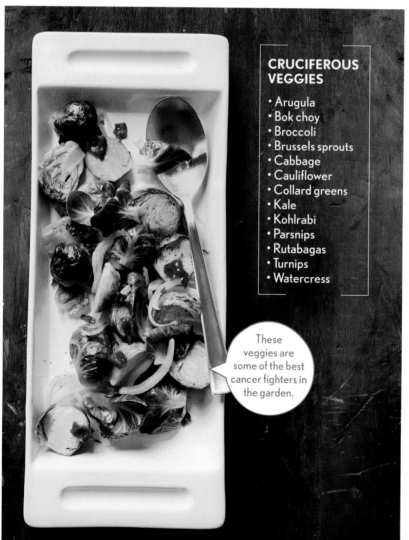

CRUCIFEROUS VEGGIES

- Arugula
- Bok choy
- Broccoli
- Brussels sprouts
- Cabbage
- Cauliflower
- Collard greens
- Kale
- Kohlrabi
- Parsnips
- Rutabagas
- Turnips
- Watercress

These veggies are some of the best cancer fighters in the garden.

Sautéed Brussels Sprouts with Bacon

3 center-cut bacon slices, finely chopped
1½ cups presliced onion
¼ teaspoon dried thyme
⅓ cup fat-free, lower-sodium chicken broth
1 pound Brussels sprouts, trimmed and halved

1. Heat a large skillet over medium-high heat. Add bacon; cook 7 minutes or until crisp. Remove bacon from pan with a slotted spoon; drain.
2. Add onion and thyme to pan; sauté 3 minutes. Add broth and Brussels sprouts; bring to a boil. Cover and simmer 6 minutes or until crisp-tender. Sprinkle with bacon. Serves 4 (serving size: about 1 cup).

CALORIES 81; FAT 1.5g (sat 0.5g, mono 0.1g, poly 0.2g); PROTEIN 6.1g; CARB 13.7g; FIBER 4.9g; CHOL 4mg; IRON 1.8mg; SODIUM 101mg; CALC 58mg

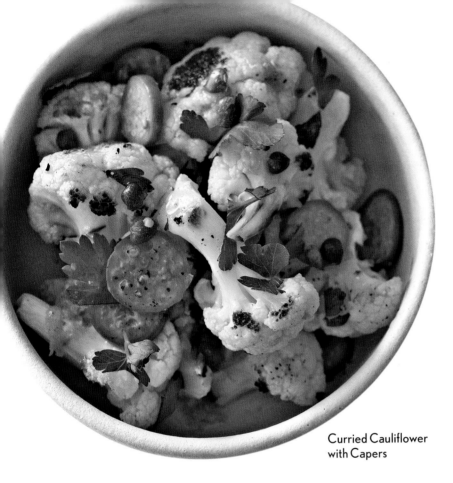

Curried Cauliflower
with Capers

In addition to their link to cancer prevention, cruciferous vegetables are also rich in fiber, vitamin C, and folate.

Steamed Baby Bok Choy with Soy-Ginger Drizzle

1 pound baby bok choy, cut in half lengthwise
1 tablespoon lower-sodium soy sauce
1 tablespoon fresh orange juice
1 teaspoon dark sesame oil
½ teaspoon grated peeled fresh ginger

1. Steam bok choy 5 minutes or until crisp-tender. Combine soy sauce, juice, oil, and ginger; drizzle over bok choy. Serves 4 (serving size: 4 ounces bok choy and about 1¾ teaspoons sauce).

CALORIES 27; FAT 1.4g (sat 0.2g, mono 0.5g, poly 0.6g); PROTEIN 2g; CARB 2.8g; FIBER 1.1g; CHOL 0mg; IRON 0.9mg; SODIUM 171mg; CALC 120mg

Curried Cauliflower with Capers

6 cups cauliflower florets (about 1 large head)
¼ cup extra-virgin olive oil, divided
2 teaspoons grated lemon rind
2 tablespoons fresh lemon juice
½ teaspoon curry powder
¼ teaspoon freshly ground black pepper
⅛ teaspoon salt
⅓ cup caperberries, thinly sliced
¼ cup chopped fresh flat-leaf parsley
¼ cup capers, drained

1. Preheat oven to 450°.
2. Combine cauliflower and 1 tablespoon oil on a jelly-roll pan, tossing to coat. Bake at 450° for 30 minutes or until browned, turning once.
3. Combine remaining 3 tablespoons oil, lemon rind, and next 4 ingredients in a large bowl; stir with a whisk. Add roasted cauliflower, caperberries, parsley, and capers to bowl; toss mixture well to combine. Serves 6 (serving size: about 1 cup).

CALORIES 107; FAT 9.5g (sat 1.3g, mono 6.6g, poly 1.2g); PROTEIN 2.1g; CARB 5.3g; FIBER 2.6g; CHOL 0mg; IRON 0.7mg; SODIUM 300mg; CALC 24mg

Choose Winter Squashes

IF ZUCCHINI AND YELLOW SUMMER SQUASH are the only members of the squash family that you're familiar with, it's time to get introduced to the rest of the brood. Maybe it's the hard, gnarled skin or the mysterious-sounding names (like kabocha) that are intimidating, but these winter squashes are worth getting to know. Their dark-colored flesh—usually yellow to deep orange—is packed with beta-carotene, a powerful antioxidant. Aim for at least three servings of orange-hued vegetables every week.

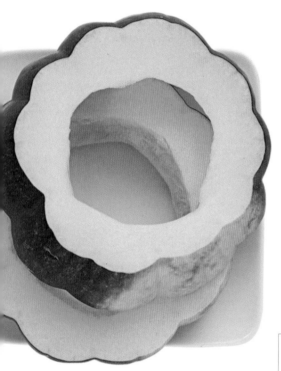

Acorn Squash Wedges with Maple-Harissa Glaze

Winter squash gets a little pizzazz with the addition of Moroccan chile paste, harissa. For a variation, replace the harissa with a couple teaspoons of minced canned chipotle chiles in adobo sauce and 1 teaspoon of the adobo sauce from the can.

2 medium acorn squash, each cut
   into 3 wedges and seeded
Cooking spray
½ teaspoon kosher salt
3 tablespoons maple syrup
1 tablespoon unsalted butter, melted
1 tablespoon water
1½ teaspoons harissa paste
4 teaspoons sesame seeds

1. Preheat oven to 400°. Arrange squash, cut sides up, on a parchment paper–lined baking sheet. Coat squash lightly with cooking spray; sprinkle evenly with salt. Combine syrup, butter, 1 tablespoon water, and harissa in a bowl, stirring well; drizzle evenly into each squash cavity. Bake at 400° for 30 minutes. Sprinkle squash evenly with sesame seeds; bake 20 minutes or until seeds are toasted and squash is tender. Serves 6 (serving size: 1 squash wedge).

CALORIES 113; FAT 3.1g (sat 1.4g, mono 0.9g, poly 0.6g); PROTEIN 1.5g; CARB 22.3g; FIBER 2.4g; CHOL 5mg; IRON 1.5mg; SODIUM 167mg; CALC 75mg

READER TIP: *Prepping Veggies*

"I prep my veggies as soon as possible after getting home from the store. I blanch green beans and freeze them. I cut the lettuce, and put it in zip-top bags, removing as much air as possible. I cut onions and tomatoes up to two days in advance. Same thing for zucchini and carrots. If you blanch them, they won't get bad as quickly."　　—*Sandrine Berger*

Roasted Butternut Squash Soup

1 (2½-pound) butternut squash
Cooking spray
1 tablespoon extra-virgin olive oil
1½ cups chopped onion
3 garlic cloves, minced
6 cups organic vegetable broth
2 cups coarsely chopped peeled
  Yukon gold potatoes
2 teaspoons chopped fresh sage
¼ teaspoon freshly ground black
  pepper
1 bay leaf
2 tablespoons chopped fresh
  parsley
2 teaspoons honey

1. Preheat oven to 400°.
2. Cut squash in half lengthwise; discard seeds. Place squash, cut sides down, on a foil-lined baking sheet coated with cooking spray. Bake at 400° for 30 minutes or until tender. Cool. Discard peel; mash pulp.
3. Heat a Dutch oven over medium-high heat. Add oil to pan; swirl to coat. Add onion; sauté 4 minutes, stirring occasionally. Add garlic; sauté 30 seconds, stirring constantly. Add squash, broth, and next 4 ingredients; bring to a boil. Reduce heat, and simmer 45 minutes or until potato is tender, stirring occasionally. Let stand 10 minutes. Discard bay leaf.
4. Place one-third of vegetable mixture in a blender. Remove center piece of blender lid (to allow steam to escape); secure blender lid on blender. Place a clean towel over opening in blender lid (to avoid splatters). Blend until smooth. Pour into a large bowl. Repeat procedure twice with remaining squash mixture. Return pureed mixture to pan; cook over medium heat 3 minutes or until thoroughly heated. Stir in parsley and honey. Serves 6 (serving size: about 1 cup).

CALORIES 166; FAT 2.7g (sat 0.4g, mono 1.8g, poly 0.3g); PROTEIN 2.9g; CARB 35.1g; FIBER 6.2g; CHOL 0mg; IRON 1.3mg; SODIUM 582mg; CALC 83mg

Quick Side
Goat Cheese Toasts

Preheat broiler. Place 6 (1-ounce) slices French bread baguette in a single layer on a baking sheet. Broil 2 minutes or until toasted. Sprinkle 2 ounces crumbled goat cheese (about ½ cup) evenly over slices; sprinkle evenly with 1 tablespoon finely chopped fresh chives. Serves 6 (serving size: 1 toast).

CALORIES 107; FAT 2.5g (sat 1.5g, mono 0.6g, poly 0.3g); PROTEIN 5.1g; CARB 16.1g; FIBER 0.7g; CHOL 4mg; IRON 1.2mg; SODIUM 219mg; CALC 26mg

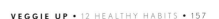

Roasted Pumpkin and Sweet Potato Pilaf

2 cups (½-inch) cubed peeled fresh pumpkin (about 12 ounces)
1½ cups (½-inch) cubed peeled sweet potato (about 1 medium)
Cooking spray
2 teaspoons olive oil
1 cup diced onion (1 small)
⅓ cup diced celery (about 1 stalk)
2 teaspoons minced garlic
4 cups fat-free, lower-sodium chicken broth
1 cup brown rice
2 teaspoons chopped fresh sage
½ teaspoon freshly ground black pepper
¼ teaspoon salt
1 bay leaf

1. Preheat oven to 400°.
2. Arrange pumpkin and sweet potato in an even layer on a jelly-roll pan coated with cooking spray. Bake at 400° for 35 minutes or until tender and vegetables just begin to brown, stirring after 18 minutes. Remove from oven, and set aside.
3. Heat a large saucepan over medium-high heat. Add oil to pan; swirl to coat. Add onion, celery, and garlic; sauté 3 minutes or until onion is tender. Add broth and remaining ingredients to onion mixture, stirring to combine; bring to a boil. Cover, reduce heat, and simmer 50 minutes or until rice is done and liquid is mostly absorbed. Remove from heat; discard bay leaf. Add pumpkin mixture; stir gently to combine. Serves 6 (serving size: about ¾ cup).

CALORIES 200; FAT 2.5g (sat 0.4g, mono 1.4g, poly 0.5g); PROTEIN 5.9g; CARB 38.8g; FIBER 3g; CHOL 0mg; IRON 1.3mg; SODIUM 428mg; CALC 45mg

Pumpkin and other winter squash are rich in beta-carotene, along with lutein and zeaxanthin, yellow-pigmented carotenoids that promote eye health.

HOW TO PREP PUMPKIN

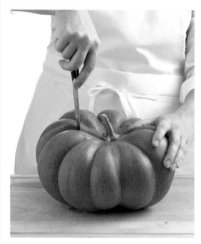

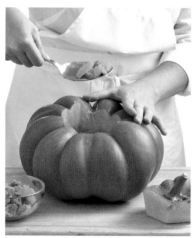

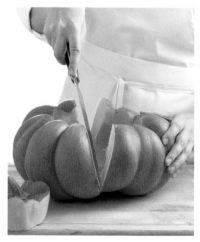

1. Place pumpkin on a steady surface, stem side up. Use a small knife to cut around the stem, about 2 inches out.

2. Scoop out stringy fibers and seeds; toss the fibers. Rinse and save the seeds to toast.

3. Cut the pumpkin in half using a heavy chef's knife. Scrape the flesh with a spoon to remove any remaining fibers.

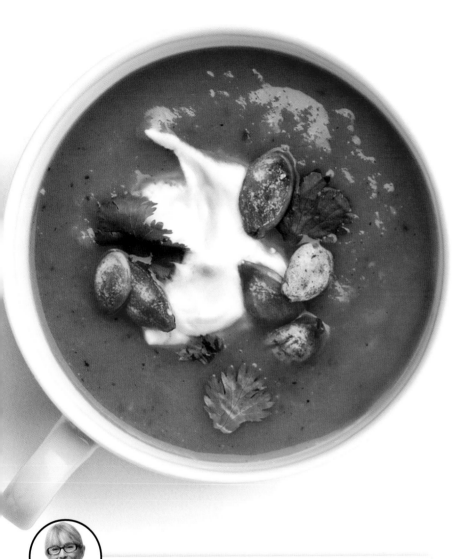

Indian-Spiced Roasted Squash Soup

1 cup chopped yellow onion
8 ounces carrot, chopped
4 garlic cloves, peeled
1 (1-pound) butternut squash, peeled and cut into ½-inch cubes
1 (8-ounce) acorn squash, quartered
1 tablespoon olive oil
½ teaspoon black pepper
2 cups water
1 teaspoon Madras curry powder
½ teaspoon garam masala
¼ teaspoon ground red pepper
2 (14-ounce) cans fat-free, lower sodium chicken broth
¼ teaspoon kosher salt
6 tablespoons Greek yogurt
6 teaspoons honey

1. Preheat oven to 500°.
2. Arrange first 5 ingredients on a jelly-roll pan. Drizzle with oil; sprinkle with pepper. Toss. Roast at 500° for 30 minutes or until vegetables are tender, turning once. Cool 10 minutes. Peel acorn squash; discard skin.
3. Place vegetable mixture, 2 cups water, curry powder, garam masala, and red pepper in a food processor; pulse to desired consistency. Scrape mixture into a large saucepan over medium heat. Stir in broth; bring to a boil. Cook 10 minutes, stirring occasionally, and stir in salt. Combine yogurt and honey, stirring well. Serve with soup. Serves 6 (serving size: 1 cup soup and 4 teaspoons yogurt mixture).

CALORIES 143; FAT 3.1g (sat 0.7g, mono 1.8g, poly 0.4g); PROTEIN 4.8g; CARB 27g; FIBER 4.4g; CHOL 1mg; IRON 1.5mg; SODIUM 343mg; CALC 98mg

EXPERT TIP: *Put Some Soup On*

"Soups are among the easiest, most inexpensive, and quickest dishes to make, especially with the bounty of winter vegetables—winter squash, Jerusalem artichokes, potatoes, carrots, parsnips, and mixtures of all those vegetables. They're healthy, inexpensive, and filling. Plus, you can make a big batch and have leftovers. Soups are always better reheated."

—*Deborah Madison, chef and author of multiple cookbooks, including* Vegetarian Cooking for Everyone

Add In More Beans

BEANS HELP REDUCE THE RISK OF HEART DISEASE, help keep blood sugar in check, and even lower the risk of certain cancers. Best of all, they're not only veggies, but they're packed with protein, fiber, and folate and can serve as a satisfying stand-in for meat. They're quick additions to salads, soups, and entrées, and can even be the spotlight of their own meal. Is there anything they can't do?

Zesty Three-Bean and Roasted Corn Salad

2½ cups (1-inch) cut green beans (about 1 pound)
¾ cup fresh corn kernels (about 2 medium ears)
¾ cup diced red bell pepper
½ cup minced red onion
¼ cup chopped fresh cilantro
1 tablespoon minced seeded jalapeño
1 (16-ounce) can cannellini beans or other white beans, rinsed and drained
1 (15-ounce) can black beans, rinsed and drained
¼ cup fresh lime juice
¼ cup red wine vinegar
1 tablespoon minced garlic
1 tablespoon olive oil
2 teaspoons ground cumin
1 teaspoon chili powder
½ teaspoon salt
¼ teaspoon red chile sauce
Dash of ground red pepper
1 cup diced seeded tomato (about 2 medium)
1 cup diced avocado

1. Heat a large nonstick skillet over medium-high heat. Add green beans and corn to pan; sauté 3 minutes or until lightly browned. Transfer green bean mixture to a large bowl. Add bell pepper and next 5 ingredients to bowl; toss well. Combine juice, vinegar, and next 7 ingredients in a small bowl; stir with a whisk. Add juice mixture to bean mixture; toss well. Cover and chill 30 minutes. Gently stir in tomato and avocado. Serve immediately. Serves 10 (serving size: about 1 cup).

CALORIES 146; FAT 5.3g (sat 0.6g, mono 3g, poly 0.7g); PROTEIN 6.6g; CARB 23.1g; FIBER 6.9g; CHOL 0mg; IRON 1.7mg; SODIUM 233mg; CALC 64mg

TOP-NOTCH BEANS

Best in Fiber:
Navy Beans
You'll get 9.6g of filling fiber in just half a cup, which is a third of the 25 to 30g you need daily. Navy beans edge out black beans (7.5g) and pintos (7.7g) for the high-fiber honor.

Best in Iron:
Soybeans
They have almost twice the iron of other beans (4.5mg per half cup, a quarter of the amount women ages 19 to 50 need) and are one of the few complete proteins the plant world has to offer.

Best in Folate:
Lentils
All legumes have folate, but lentils take the top prize at 179mcg (micrograms) per half cup. That's close to half of the 400mcg of naturally occurring folate you're supposed to eat every day.

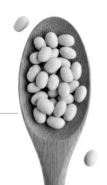
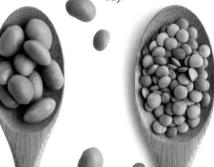

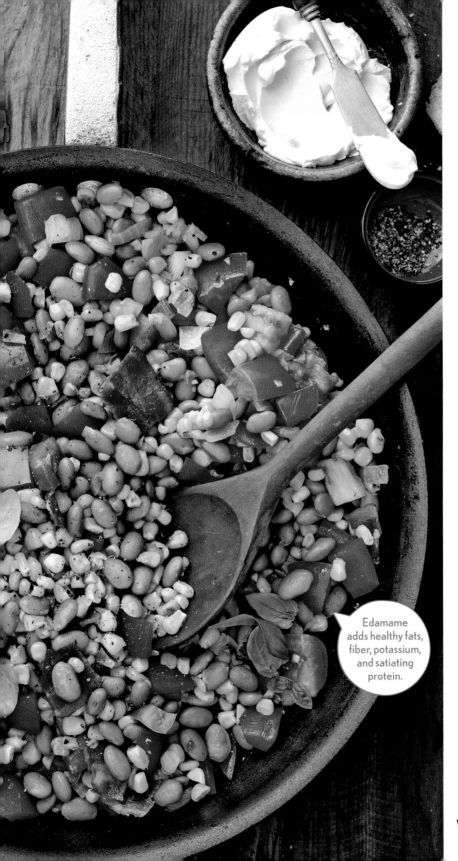

Edamame
adds healthy fats,
fiber, potassium,
and satiating
protein.

Edamame Succotash

1 center-cut bacon slice
1 tablespoon butter
2 cups chopped sweet onion
2 cups fresh corn kernels
    (about 3 ears)
1 (16-ounce) bag frozen shelled
    edamame, thawed
2 tablespoons red wine vinegar
½ teaspoon salt
½ teaspoon freshly ground
    black pepper
½ teaspoon sugar
3 plum tomatoes, coarsely chopped
1 red bell pepper, seeded and
    coarsely chopped
3 tablespoons torn basil

1. Cook bacon in a nonstick skillet
over medium heat until crisp.
Remove bacon from pan, reserving
2 teaspoons drippings in pan;
coarsely chop bacon.
2. Increase heat to medium-high.
Melt butter in drippings in pan.
Add onion; sauté 3 minutes, stirring
occasionally. Add corn kernels; sauté
3 minutes or until lightly charred.
Add edamame, and sauté 3 minutes,
stirring occasionally. Stir in vinegar
and next 5 ingredients; cook 30
seconds, stirring occasionally. Sprinkle
with bacon and basil. Serves 4 (serving size: 1¼ cups).

CALORIES 300; FAT 12.1g (sat 3.3g, mono 3.3g, poly 3.6g);
PROTEIN 17.9g; CARB 37.2g; FIBER 10g; CHOL 10mg;
IRON 0.9mg; SODIUM 386mg; CALC 28mg

Re-do Your Dips

DON'T LET FAT- and calorie-laden sour cream– and mayonnaise-based dips overpower your beautifully arranged vegetable tray. Instead, sub in healthy plant-based dips such as hummus, salsa, and black bean. You're not only helping your heart and waistline, but you're also getting an extra serving of veggies.

Traditional Hummus

Prepare and refrigerate a day ahead; let it stand at room temperature 30 minutes before serving.

2 (15.5-ounce) cans no-salt-added chickpeas (garbanzo beans), rinsed and drained
2 garlic cloves, crushed
½ cup water
¼ cup tahini (sesame seed paste)
3 tablespoons fresh lemon juice
2 tablespoons extra-virgin olive oil
¾ teaspoon salt
¼ teaspoon black pepper
Lemon wedge (optional)

1. Place beans and garlic in a food processor; pulse 5 times or until chopped. Add ½ cup water and remaining ingredients; pulse until smooth, scraping down sides as needed. Garnish with lemon wedge, if desired. Serves 26 (serving size: 2 tablespoons).

CALORIES 44; FAT 2.5g (sat 0.3g, mono 1.2g, poly 0.7g); PROTEIN 1.5g; CARB 4.4g; FIBER 0.9g; CHOL 0mg; IRON 0.3mg; SODIUM 74mg; CALC 12mg

Feta-Baked Hummus variation:

Preheat oven to 400°. Combine Traditional Hummus, 2 ounces crumbled feta cheese (about ½ cup), ¼ cup chopped fresh parsley, and ½ teaspoon ground cumin. Transfer mixture to an 8-inch square glass or ceramic baking dish coated with cooking spray. Sprinkle with 2 ounces crumbled feta cheese (about ½ cup). Bake for 25 minutes or until lightly browned. Garnish with small oregano leaves and, if desired, additional feta. Serves 32 (serving size: about 2 tablespoons).

CALORIES 46; FAT 2.8g (sat 0.8g, mono 1.2g, poly 0.6g); PROTEIN 1.8g; CARB 3.8g; FIBER 0.8g; CHOL 3mg; IRON 0.3mg; SODIUM 100mg; CALC 28mg

White Bean and Roasted Garlic Hummus variation:

Since this version calls for roasted garlic, you can just omit the raw crushed garlic cloves from the Traditional Hummus. Preheat oven to 350°. Remove white papery skin from 2 whole garlic heads (do not peel or separate the cloves). Wrap each head separately in foil. Bake for 1 hour; cool 10 minutes. Separate cloves; squeeze to extract garlic pulp. Discard skins. Place garlic pulp, Traditional Hummus, and 1 (15-ounce) can rinsed and drained cannellini beans (or other white beans) in a food processor; pulse 5 times or until chopped. Add ¼ cup water; process until smooth, scraping down sides as needed. Stir in ¾ teaspoon chopped fresh rosemary. Garnish with additional chopped rosemary, if desired. Serves 32 (serving size: about 2½ tablespoons).

CALORIES 45; FAT 2g (sat 0.3g, mono 1g, poly 0.6g); PROTEIN 1.8g; CARB 5.3g; FIBER 1.2g; CHOL 0mg; IRON 0.4mg; SODIUM 81mg; CALC 16mg

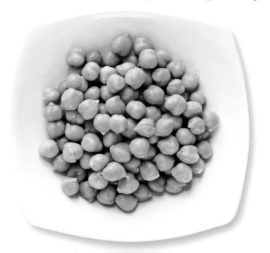

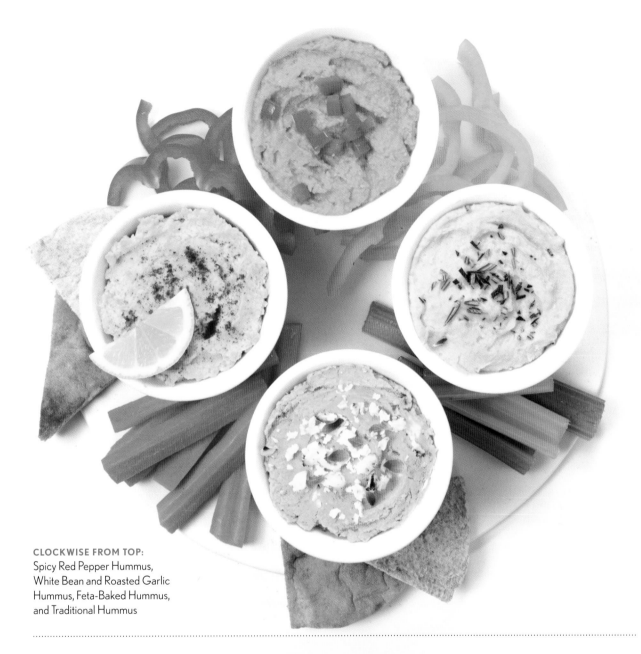

CLOCKWISE FROM TOP:
Spicy Red Pepper Hummus,
White Bean and Roasted Garlic
Hummus, Feta-Baked Hummus,
and Traditional Hummus

Spicy Red Pepper Hummus variation:

Preheat broiler. Cut 2 red bell peppers in half lengthwise; discard seeds and membranes. Place pepper halves, skin sides up, on a foil-lined baking sheet; flatten with hand. Broil 15 minutes or until blackened. Place in a paper bag, and fold to close tightly. Let stand 15 minutes. Peel and cut into strips. Place bell peppers, 2 teaspoons sambal oelek (ground fresh chile paste), ½ teaspoon paprika, and ⅛ teaspoon ground red pepper in a food processor; pulse until smooth. Transfer pepper mixture to a serving bowl; stir in Traditional Hummus. Garnish with chopped red bell pepper, if desired. Serves 32 (serving size: about 2 tablespoons).

CALORIES 39; FAT 2g (sat 0.3g, mono 1g, poly 0.6g); PROTEIN 1.4g; CARB 4.3g; FIBER 1g; CHOL 0mg; IRON 0.3mg; SODIUM 74mg; CALC 11mg

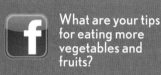
"If I buy melon, I cut it up and put it in plastic containers in the fridge. My family always eats more of fruit that's ready than fruit that needs preparing. If we're hanging around waiting for dinner to be ready, I'll put out celery sticks, baby carrots, fennel, and any other cut vegetables to munch on while we're waiting so that we don't go into the cheese and crackers routine."

—*Virginia Rotella*

Salsa Verde

2 poblano peppers
½ cup fat-free, lower-sodium chicken broth
1 pound tomatillos
2 tablespoons fresh lime juice
2 garlic cloves
⅔ cup chopped white onion
⅓ cup chopped fresh cilantro
½ teaspoon kosher salt
1 fresh serrano chile, finely chopped

1. Preheat broiler.
2. Broil poblano peppers 5 minutes per side or until blackened. Place in a paper bag; fold to close tightly. Let stand 10 minutes; peel and chop. Bring broth and tomatillos to a boil in a saucepan over medium heat. Cover and simmer 8 minutes. Remove from heat; let stand 20 minutes. Pour into a blender. Add lime juice and garlic; process until smooth. Pour into a bowl; stir in poblanos, onion, cilantro, salt, and serrano chile. Chill. Serves 8 (serving size: ¼ cup).

CALORIES 34; FAT 0.7g (sat 0.1g, mono 0.1g, poly 0.3g); PROTEIN 1.3g; CARB 7g; FIBER 1.7g; CHOL 0mg; IRON 0.4mg; SODIUM 146mg; CALC 10mg

Black-Eyed Pea and Tomato Salsa

1 cup chopped tomatoes
¼ cup prechopped red onion
3 tablespoons chopped poblano chile
2 tablespoons chopped fresh cilantro
2 ½ tablespoons fresh lime juice
¼ teaspoon minced fresh garlic
⅛ teaspoon salt
⅛ teaspoon ground cumin
⅛ teaspoon freshly ground black pepper
1 (15.8-ounce) can black-eyed peas, rinsed and drained

1. Place all ingredients in a large bowl, and toss to combine. Serves 8 (serving size: about ⅓ cup).

CALORIES 35; FAT 0.3g (sat 0.1g, mono 0g, poly 0.1g); PROTEIN 1.9g; CARB 6.6g; FIBER 1.5g; CHOL 0mg; IRON 0.4mg; SODIUM 139mg; CALC 11mg

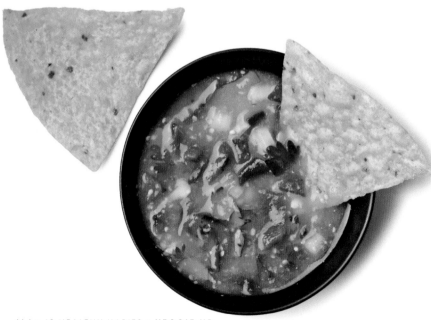

Artichoke, Spinach, and White Bean Dip

¼ cup (1 ounce) grated fresh
  pecorino Romano cheese
¼ cup canola mayonnaise
1 teaspoon fresh lemon juice
¼ teaspoon salt
¼ teaspoon freshly ground
  black pepper
⅛ teaspoon ground red pepper
2 garlic cloves, minced
1 (15-ounce) can organic white
  beans, rinsed and drained
1 (14-ounce) can baby artichoke
  hearts, drained and quartered
1 (9-ounce) package frozen chopped
  spinach, thawed, drained, and
  squeezed dry
Cooking spray
½ cup (2 ounces) shredded part-skim
  mozzarella cheese

1. Preheat oven to 350°.
2. Place first 8 ingredients in a food processor, and process until smooth. Spoon into a medium bowl. Stir in artichokes and spinach. Spoon mixture into a 1-quart glass or ceramic baking dish coated with cooking spray. Sprinkle with ½ cup mozzarella. Bake at 350° for 20 minutes or until bubbly and brown. Serves 12 (serving size: ¼ cup).

CALORIES 87; FAT 5.4g (sat 1.4g, mono 2.3g, poly 1g); PROTEIN 3.7g; CARB 4.9g; FIBER 1g; CHOL 6mg; IRON 0.7mg; SODIUM 232mg; CALC 91mg

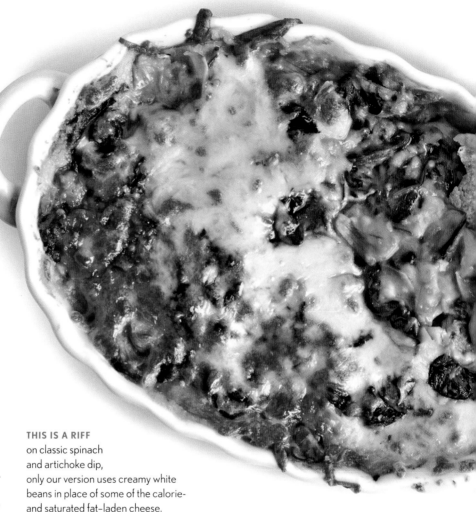

THIS IS A RIFF
on classic spinach
and artichoke dip,
only our version uses creamy white
beans in place of some of the calorie-
and saturated fat–laden cheese.

READER TIP: *Consider Canned*

"Canned vegetables can be healthy additions to stews and soups all winter long. Of course, you have to be careful of the sodium and sugar content."

—*Terrie Hull Moeny*

Finesse with Fruit

FRUITS ARE OFTEN RELEGATED TO BREAKFAST or dessert, but this juicy produce has greater potential. Chop some for your lunchtime salad, create a fruit salsa, roast some for a deliciously simple side, or throw into a veggie-based dish like cole slaw as a surprise add-in.

Quick Side
Pomegranate-Orange Salsa

Combine 1 cup chopped orange sections, ⅔ cup pomegranate seeds (about 2 pomegranates), ⅓ cup fresh pomegranate juice, ¼ cup minced shallots, 2 tablespoons minced jalapeño pepper, 1 tablespoon chopped fresh cilantro, 1 tablespoon fresh lime juice, ¼ teaspoon kosher salt, and ¼ teaspoon freshly ground black pepper. Serves 6 (serving size: ¼ cup).

CALORIES 46; FAT 0g (sat 0g, mono 0g, poly 0g); PROTEIN 0.6g; CARB 11.4g; FIBER 0.8g; CHOL 0mg; IRON 0.2mg; SODIUM 83mg; CALC 18mg

Quick Side
Green Apple Slaw

Combine 2 tablespoons cider vinegar, 1 tablespoon extra-virgin olive oil, 1½ teaspoons sugar, ¼ teaspoon kosher salt, and ¼ teaspoon freshly ground black pepper in a medium bowl; stir until sugar dissolves. Add 3 cups thinly sliced fennel bulb (about 1 large), 2 cups thinly sliced Granny Smith apple (1 large), ¼ cup fresh flat-leaf parsley leaves, and ¼ cup slivered red onion; toss to coat. Serves 4 (serving size: about 1 cup).

CALORIES 91; FAT 3.6g (sat 0.5g, mono 2.5g, poly 0.4g); PROTEIN 1.2g; CARB 14.9g; FIBER 3.6g; CHOL 0mg; IRON 0.9mg; SODIUM 155mg; CALC 43mg

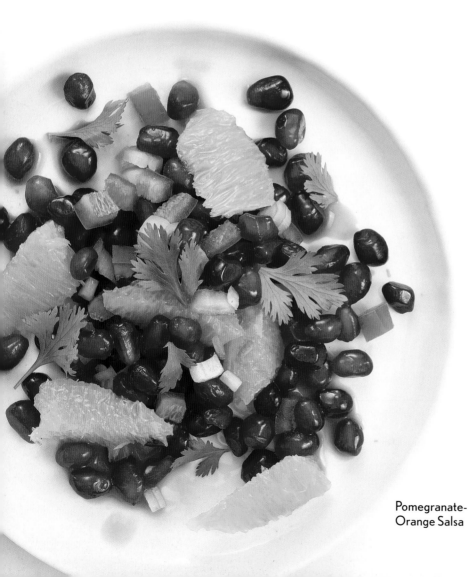

Pomegranate-Orange Salsa

Asian Caramelized Pineapple

1½ teaspoons canola oil
1½ tablespoons minced red onion
1 large garlic clove, minced
2 cups diced fresh pineapple
1 tablespoon lower-sodium soy sauce
1½ teaspoons chopped seeded
　red jalapeño pepper
1½ teaspoons fresh lime juice
1 teaspoon chopped peeled fresh ginger
1½ teaspoons chopped fresh cilantro

1. Heat a large nonstick skillet over medium heat. Add oil to pan; swirl to coat. Add onion and garlic to pan; cook 2 minutes. Add pineapple; cook 5 minutes or until lightly browned. Add soy sauce, pepper, juice, and ginger; cook 2 minutes. Remove from heat; stir in cilantro. Serves 4 (serving size: about ½ cup).

CALORIES 61; FAT 1.9g (sat 0.1g, mono 1.1g, poly 0.6g); PROTEIN 0.9g; CARB 11.6g; FIBER 1.3g; CHOL 0mg; IRON 0.4mg; SODIUM 135mg; CALC 15mg

Spinach-Strawberry Salad

1½ cups quartered strawberries
¼ cup Easy Herb Vinaigrette
　(page 223)
1 tablespoon finely chopped fresh mint
1 (6-ounce) package fresh baby
　spinach
2 tablespoons sliced almonds, toasted
¼ teaspoon black pepper

1. Combine first 4 ingredients in a large bowl; toss gently to coat. Sprinkle with almonds and pepper; serve immediately. Serves 4 (serving size: 2 cups).

CALORIES 136; FAT 10.3g (sat 0.7g, mono 6g, poly 3g); PROTEIN 2.1g; CARB 11g; FIBER 3.6g; CHOL 0mg; IRON 1.7mg; SODIUM 113mg; CALC 50mg

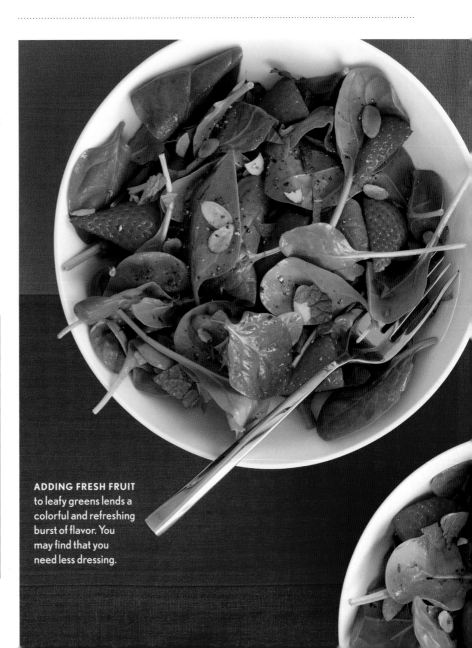

ADDING FRESH FRUIT to leafy greens lends a colorful and refreshing burst of flavor. You may find that you need less dressing.

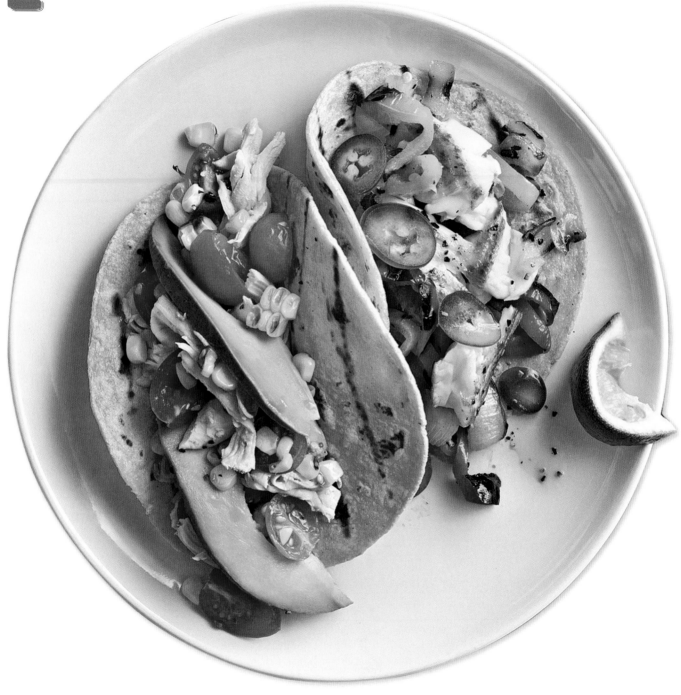

EAT MORE FISH

EXPAND YOUR SEAFOOD HORIZONS.

SOME PEOPLE HAVE A LOVE-HATE relationship with seafood. And then there are those who enjoy seafood in restaurants, but are intimidated by the prospect of buying it and preparing it at home. Regardless of which camp you fall into, increasing the amount of seafood you eat can have a good effect on your health.

When scientists compare diets around the globe, the healthiest have one thing in common: lots of seafood. For example, people in Iceland and Japan, where people live the longest—81 years on average—have the world's highest per capita consumption of seafood. Fish isn't the only reason behind this longevity, but it helps.

What makes seafood so healthy? First, it's a lean protein, with very little saturated fat. Also, the fat it does contain is mostly good-for-you omega-3 fatty acids, a type of poly-unsaturated fat that has been shown to protect against heart disease, stroke, and some forms of cancer; reduce blood pressure; and control inflammation. In the U.S., we barely eat 16 pounds of seafood, on average, each year (our average life expectancy is 78 years). That's one reason why the Dietary Guidelines for Americans recommend two 4-ounce servings per week in place of beef, pork, or poultry. Most Americans eat only about half of that.

This chapter is full of tips and strategies to help you overcome your habit hurdles. You'll find budget-conscious and family-friendly fish meals and simple cooking techniques for seafood novices. If you already eat fish twice a week, focus on trying new, sustainable species. If you're a vegetarian, you'll find other ways to get your omega-3s.

YOUR GOAL

Make seafood the centerpiece of two meals a week.

The 12 Healthy Habits

| · 01 · GET COOKING | · 02 · BREAKFAST DAILY | · 03 · WHOLE GRAINS | · 04 · GET MOVING | · 05 · VEGGIE UP | · 06 · MORE SEAFOOD | · 07 · HEALTHY FATS | · 08 · GO MEATLESS | · 09 · GET STRONGER | · 10 · LESS SALT | · 11 · BE PORTION-AWARE | · 12 · EAT MINDFULLY |

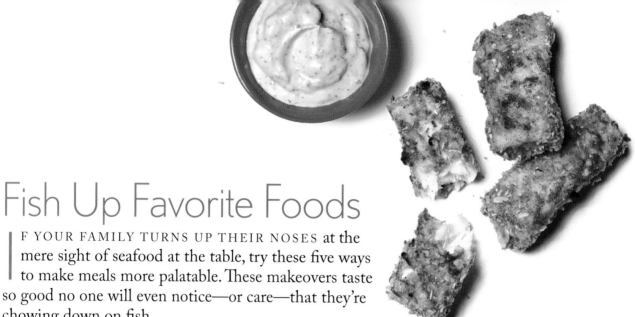

Fish Up Favorite Foods

I F YOUR FAMILY TURNS UP THEIR NOSES at the mere sight of seafood at the table, try these five ways to make meals more palatable. These makeovers taste so good no one will even notice—or care—that they're chowing down on fish.

SEAFOOD PASTA

If you already make pasta several nights a week, try adding in some grilled or canned fish. One good option for picky eaters: shrimp. It's sweet, succulent, and

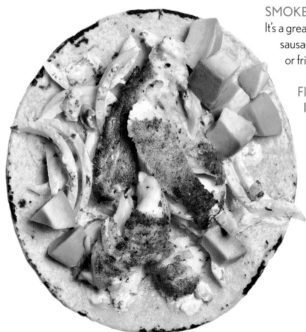

incredibly versatile: It cooks quickly using a variety of cooking techniques and can be served hot or cold. Try a few shrimp recipes like Peppery Pasta with Arugula and Shrimp on page 192.

SMOKED SALMON

It's a great sub for ham, bacon, or sausage in your morning omelet or frittata or dinnertime quiche.

FISH TACOS

Instead of using ground beef, take taco night to the ocean with tilapia, halibut, or other mild fish fillets. Try the Blackened Tilapia Baja Tacos or the Chimichurri Halibut Tacos on page 190 to get started.

TUNA OR SALMON BURGERS

Our Salmon Burger on page 188, for example, has only 372 calories (that's including the bun) and 16 grams of fat, most of which is the heart-healthy poly- and monounsaturated kinds. If you're using tuna, pair it with ginger to bring out its natural flavor.

FISH STICKS

They're usually a big hit due to their real crunch appeal, but your basic fried fish stick dunked in tangy tartar sauce can add up to half a day's sodium and saturated fat allowances. Try our makeover instead, which features strips of meaty halibut seasoned and breaded in a panko-pumpkinseed coating—the seeds add extra crunch and heart-healthy fat—on page 41.

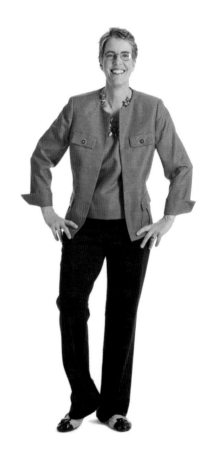

No Way, No How, No Fish!

"I have a visceral reaction to seafood. Eww!"

ANDREA STILLWELL
Postal Clerk

➤ **FISH CHALLENGE:** Andrea's dislike for fish started at a young age. "I grew up near the ocean and saw what washes up. I didn't want to eat anything out of there!" Add to that the fact that Andrea's early culinary exposure to seafood consisted of her mom's tuna casserole and "stinky" tuna sandwiches, and it's no wonder she skips half the recipes in her *Cooking Light* cookbook collection because of the fish.

OUR ADVICE

■ **Steer clear of "fishy" fish.** Arctic char looks like salmon, but it's less oily, so there's less fishy taste. Flounder and catfish are also mild and readily available, as are rainbow trout and haddock. Tilapia is the boneless, skinless chicken breast of the sea—it has an almost neutral flavor. All of these, with varying levels of omega-3s, are great to experiment with in recipes.

■ **Pack seafood dishes with other flavors.** Andrea loves curry, soups, and stews—all foods with robust flavors—and seafood versions will likely be enjoyable for her, too. Try Saffron Fish Stew with White Beans on page 194—it's chock-full of spices sure to please any palate.

■ **Cook outside.** Grilling gives seafood great smoky flavor, and cooking outdoors means the fishy smell doesn't get in your house. (Just be sure to thoroughly oil the grates first, or risk leaving delicate fish stuck to the grill.)

■ **Go for shrimp.** This sweet, succulent shellfish is available peeled and deveined, which helps lessen the eww factor. Once you've mastered a few shrimp recipes, you're ready to move on to scallops and mussels, two other seafood options with a naturally sweet flavor.

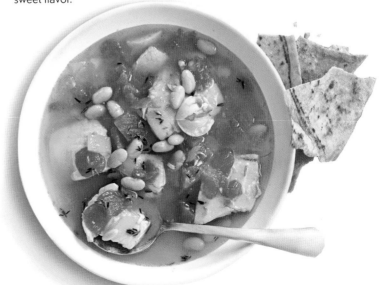

COACHING SESSION
with ALLISON FISHMAN

GAIN FISH-COOKING CONFIDENCE

If you're not in the habit of preparing fish at home, you might lack seafood-cooking confidence. Here's how to overcome your fear of fish:

■ **Grill it.** While you can get a special fish basket for the grill, you don't need one as long as you use the proper technique. First, preheat your grill and make sure the grate is clean and dry. Then oil the grate and your fish. When the fish is done cooking, it will release when gingerly nudged by your spatula. If it does not release from a clean, well-oiled grill, then it's simply not ready! Give it a little more time; the fish will release easily when done.

■ **Sauté it.** A nonstick skillet will allow you to get a crispy, golden brown sear on your fish. Yes, you'll still need a spritz of oil, but nothing beats a nonstick skillet when it comes to cooking fish on the stovetop.

■ **Broil it.** All you need to do is coat a sheet pan with nonstick cooking spray, place your fish on top, season, and broil. It's quick, easy, and leaves no scent behind. The rule of thumb for cooking fish is 8 to 10 minutes for every inch of thickness.

■ **Get the right tools.** Let's face it, fish has a different texture from other proteins, which is part of its appeal, but that's why it may be a bit challenging in the kitchen. I'm not one for unnecessary gadgets, but a fish spatula is a good investment. It's extra flexible, which means you can really get under that fish when you turn it.

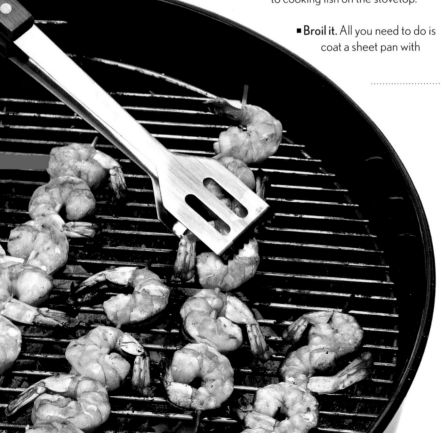

One study of 85,000 women found that those who ate five or more servings of fish per week had a 30% lower risk of heart failure, but only if the fish was broiled or baked. Eating just one serving of fried fish per week was linked to a 48% *higher* risk of heart failure.

Menu Navigator

Fish may start out as a wonder protein, but it can undergo a drastic transformation when it hits a commercial kitchen. Seafood restaurants have a long history of serving heaping baskets of heavily battered, deep-fried fish paired with even more deep-fried accompaniments. Here, our guide to the dishes at your local seafood restaurant:

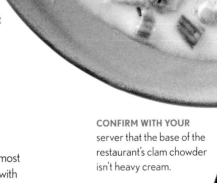

SPLURGE ONLY

Fish and Chips
943 calories
A thick batter and oil that's slightly too cool will cause whatever's being fried to soak up oil—and fat and calories—like a sponge. Split one order among a group.

Fish and Shellfish Platters
1,194 calories
In addition to thickly coated, deep-fried seafood, you're getting fried starches, slaw, sauce, melted butter, and maybe a biscuit or two. Go for grilled instead.

ASK YOUR SERVER

Mixed Grill
667 calories
Mixed grills generally offer several types of grilled seafood; the calorie and fat savings help mitigate the cup of slaw and fries.

Crab Cakes
492 calories
These may be a lower-calorie choice, but there's probably more saturated fat from the mayo in the filling and butter in which they're cooked than you need.

HEALTHY CHOICE

Cup of Clam Chowder
262 calories
Contrary to popular belief, most restaurants make chowder with milk and flour, not cream.

Blackened (or Grilled) Fish
367 calories
Blackened fish is usually cooked with very little, if any, fat. If spicy heat doesn't light your fire, go for the grilled version.

CONFIRM WITH YOUR server that the base of the restaurant's clam chowder isn't heavy cream.

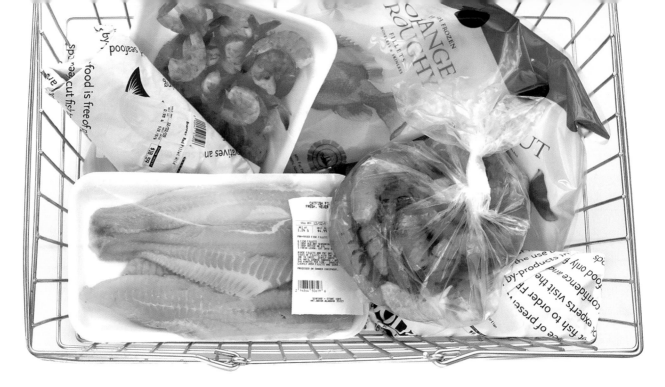

Be a Savvy Seafood Shopper

DON'T BE INTIMIDATED BY THE SEAFOOD COUNTER at your grocery store. You can find fresh and frozen options that fit your budget. Here's what to look for:

WHOLE FRESH FISH
- Look for shiny skin; tightly adhering scales; bright, clear eyes; firm, taut flesh that springs back when pressed; and a moist, flat tail.
- Gills should be cherry-red, not brownish.
- Saltwater fish should smell briny; freshwater fish should smell like a clean pond.

FRESH FILLETS AND STEAKS
- When buying white-fleshed fish, choose translucent-looking fillets with a pinkish tint.

- When buying any color fish, the flesh should appear dense without any gaps between layers.
- If the fish is wrapped in plastic, the package should contain little to no liquid.
- Ask the fishmonger to remove any pin bones, which run crosswise to the backbone.

FROZEN FISH
- Look for shiny, rock-hard frozen fish with no white freezer-burn spots, frost, or ice crystals.

- Choose well-sealed packages from the bottom of the freezer case that are at most three months old.

HANDLE WITH CARE
When shopping, ask for your fish to be packed with a separate bag of crushed ice to keep it cold. Refrigerate whole fish up to two days; fillets and steaks one to two days. Place the fish in a plastic bag, then top with a zip-top plastic bag filled with ice. Thaw frozen fish in the refrigerator.

The Fish-on-a-Budget Challenge

"We're sticklers about money, and seafood can be expensive."

JOSH RUTLEDGE
Cooking Light *Assistant Production Editor*

➤ **FISH CHALLENGE:** Like many young couples, Josh and his wife Meredith work hard to maximize their food dollars, and when Josh sees fish, he sees dollar signs. The couple's weekly grocery budget is just $50. At checkout, that translates to bulk quantities of skinless, boneless chicken breasts and less-expensive cuts of red meat. And though Josh will occasionally pick up tilapia or shrimp if it's on sale, fish comes to the family plate at most once a week. "I love salmon, but it's quite a bit more money than a chicken breast."

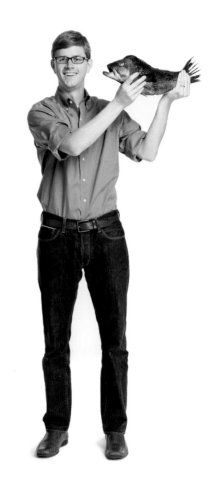

OUR ADVICE

■ **Look for bargains.** Grocery stores sell large packs of individually wrapped, frozen fish fillets, usually at a rate dramatically discounted from fresh varieties. In-season, fresh varieties are also a good buy; you can enjoy them now or freeze them for later.

■ **Use a little, save a lot.** Look for recipes that use less-expensive varieties or smaller amounts of pricier seafood in multiple servings. Peppery Pasta with Arugula and Shrimp on page 192 uses half a pound of shrimp in four servings.

■ **Break open a can.** Canned or jarred seafood is an easy, often inexpensive way to incorporate fish into your meals when fresh selections are limited or too pricey. For example, use just two 5-ounce cans of solid white tuna (at about $2 a can) for the Tuna and White Bean Salad on page 201. While you're comparing prices, check the labels, too. Unlike fresh, canned fish often comes packed with added salt (200mg to 300mg sodium in 2 ounces), so choose the low-sodium or unsalted variety, if available, or give it a good rinse before mixing it in.

■ **Try whole fish.** If you're adventurous, look for meaty heads, tails, and trimmings of larger fish like salmon, cod, and halibut, which are often sold at bargain prices. Simmer or steam, pick off the meat, and add to chowders and casseroles.

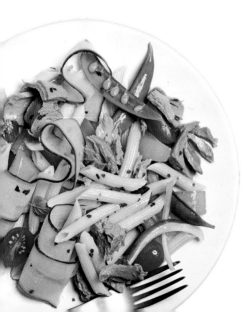

Know Your Omega-3s

A LL THOSE ABBREVIATIONS and technical-sounding terms linked to omega-3s can be confusing. But the basics are this: Not all omega-3s are created equal.

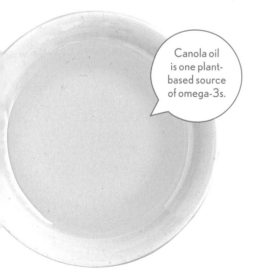

Two tablespoons of walnuts contain 1.3 grams of omega-3s.

WHAT THEY ARE

There are three major types of omega-3 fatty acids. The two most important ones are found mostly in cold-water fish and are eicosapentaenoic acid (EPA) and docosahexaenoic acid (DHA). The third type of omega-3 is alpha-linolenic acid (ALA), which is found in plant sources, including canola and soybean oils, walnuts, and flaxseeds.

THE HEALTH BENEFITS

Unlike the fat in a porterhouse or French fries, omega-3 fatty acids are polyunsaturated, so they don't cause the plaque build-up in arteries that can lead to heart disease. In fact, when substituted for saturated or trans fat, polyunsaturated fats raise "good" high-density lipoprotein (HDL) cholesterol, helping to lower the risk of cardiovascular disease. Studies suggest they may also help with rheumatoid arthritis and depression.

HOW MUCH YOU NEED

The Dietary Guidelines of Americans recommend 8 ounces of fish a week to help supply at least 250mg per day of EPA and DHA, or 1.75g each week. The American Heart Association recommends 1,000mg per day of EPA and DHA for people with heart disease, and higher amounts (2,000–4,000mg per day) if you need to lower triglycerides.

VEGETARIANS AND OMEGA-3S

Fish is hands down the best source of omega-3 fatty acids. So, if you rely on plants to get these fats, you'll be getting primarily ALA omega-3s. (The only plant soure of DHA is algae.) To be beneficial, ALA must be converted in our bodies to EPA and DHA. Unfortunately, we're not all that efficient with this process, so very little (10% or less) gets converted. But vegetarians needn't despair: It is possible to get enough omega-3s in your diet.

Here's how:

- **Eat more salads.** Make salads with dark, leafy greens and top with a vinaigrette made with omega-3–rich canola or soybean oil. Toss in some edamame and pumpkinseeds.
- **Find fun ways to add in ground flaxseed.** A 2-tablespoon serving has more than 3 grams of ALA omega-3s. Add it to your morning oatmeal, stir it into yogurt, or mix it into bread dough or muffin batter for a nutritional boost.
- **Buy high-omega-3 eggs.** Hint: Chickens fed a high-flaxseed diet produce eggs that are higher in omega-3 levels.
- **Consider a supplement.** It's best to get omega-3s naturally from food, but realistically it's tough to get what you need if you're really forgoing fish. Talk to your doctor about an algae-based supplement that provides DHA omega-3.

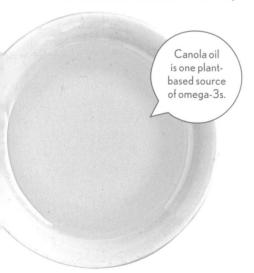

Canola oil is one plant-based source of omega-3s.

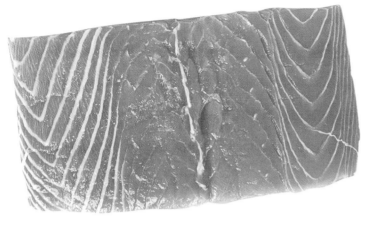

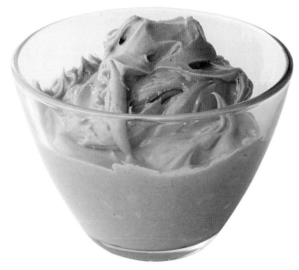

SALMON VS. PEANUT BUTTER
You'd have to consume 1,520 calories of peanut butter (1 cup) to get the same amount of omega-3s found in one 200-calorie, 4-ounce serving of salmon.

BUYER BEWARE: FORTIFIED FOODS

Omega-3s are popping up in all sorts of food, including peanut butter, yogurt, bread, and cereal. But check the label: You're probably getting less than you think. When you see omega-3 touted on a food label (and it's not fish and doesn't contain fish oil or algal oil), it's safe to assume you're only getting ALA. That means you may only get the amount of omega-3s found in a bite of salmon, and there's little evidence that ALA offers the same benefits of EPA and DHA.

One study estimates that Americans' low seafood and omega-3 intake may be responsible for about 84,000 deaths per year, making seafood deficiency the second biggest dietary contributor to preventable deaths, just behind sodium consumption.

WHAT ABOUT MERCURY?

Larger and carnivorous fish contain higher levels of mercury, which they absorb from prey. Mercury interferes with brain development in fetuses and children. The Dietary Guidelines for Americans advise women who are or may become pregnant, nursing mothers, and children to eat two servings per week of fish and avoid shark, swordfish, tilefish, and king mackerel. If you're pregnant, you should also limit albacore tuna, which is higher in mercury, to 6 ounces a week. Focus instead on seafood lowest in mercury, which includes shipped, canned light tuna, salmon, pollock, catfish, and shrimp.

Sustainable Seafood

A LAS, SOME OF THE FISH that rate highest on ecofriendly lists are also among the lowest in heart-healthy omega-3 fatty acids. But don't give up yet. Fish is the best source of two important types of omega-3s: DHA and EPA. A 4-ounce serving of one of the fish below provides a hefty dose of your daily omega-3s while also offering a great sustainable option.

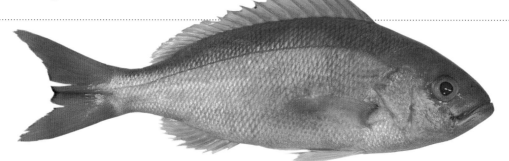

BEST FOR OMEGA-3S

- Wild-caught Alaskan salmon

- Farmed or wild-caught oysters from Canada or the Gulf of Mexico

- Wild-caught Pacific sardines

- U.S-farmed rainbow trout

- U.S.-caught fresh or frozen Pacific albacore tuna

WAYS TO SUSS OUT SUSTAINABLE SEAFOOD

- **Keep knowledge on hand.** Download free wallet-sized guides for seafood and sushi at blueocean.org and seafoodwatch.org that will give you the lowdown on the best sustainable choices for your region. You can also use your mobile phone to download the Seafood Watch app from Monterey Bay Aquarium and find out instantly if a fish you plan to buy or eat is ecofriendly.
- **Be label literate.** When you're grocery shopping and you've forgotten your Monterey Bay Guide, look for these two labels: Marine Stewardship Council and Friend of the Sea. Fish and seafood with these labels come from certified sustainable and well-managed fisheries.

- **Know your menus.** Fish2Fork.com rates restaurants by the greenness of their seafood offerings. The Seafood Watch iPhone and Android apps include Project FishMap, which lets you share the locations of restaurants where you found ocean-friendly seafood.

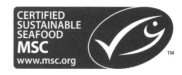

THREE REASONS YOU SHOULD GO SUSTAINABLE

1. IT'S LESS EXPENSIVE.

Sustainable products are usually very plentiful and available, so oftentimes they're the most economical option. The most sustainable seafood item in your supermarket is probably the canned fish, which is often the cheapest.

2. YOU'LL GET BETTER-QUALITY FISH.

If you walk into your local fish store and ask for the freshest fish available, chances are you'll get something sustainable. That's a much better option than insisting on salmon—which may not be in season—because the recipe you're using requires it. A lot of people don't realize that 90% of fish cookery is purchasing. There's nothing I can do as a chef to make up for poor-quality fish.

3. IT SUSTAINS THE ECOSYSTEM.

Some people wrongly assume it's better to avoid eating fish entirely, but the truth is that it does damage to our ecosystem, too. When you support and eat sustainable seafood, you encourage the restoration of ecosystems rather than just sacrificing them.

When you have the choice, substitute farmed Arctic char for farmed salmon. While they both have nice orange colors and are high in omega-3s, the char's more ecofriendly.

SUSTAINABLE LOBSTER. Opt for the species called "American lobster"—its population is well managed in Canada and the U.S. in the northeastern Atlantic states.

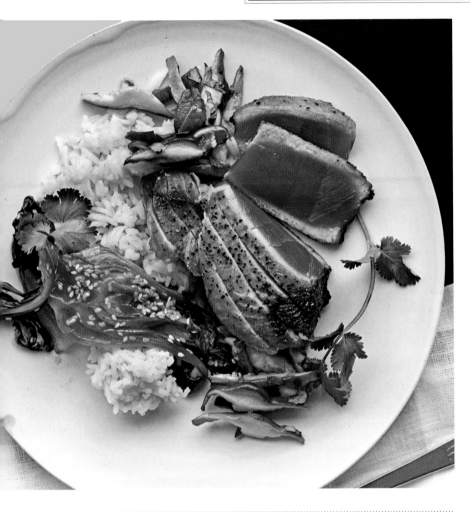

Sesame Albacore Tuna

1 tablespoon olive oil
4 cups thinly sliced shiitake mushroom caps (about 10 ounces)
$1/4$ cup organic vegetable broth
$1/4$ cup rice vinegar
2 medium baby bok choy, quartered lengthwise
1 tablespoon sesame oil
2 tablespoons lower-sodium soy sauce
2 teaspoons sesame seeds
2 tablespoons chopped fresh cilantro
1 tablespoon canola oil
4 (6-ounce) fresh or frozen albacore tuna fillets, thawed
$1/2$ teaspoon salt
$1/4$ teaspoon freshly ground black pepper
2 cups hot cooked long-grain white or brown rice

1. Heat a medium skillet over medium-high heat. Add olive oil to pan; swirl to coat. Add mushrooms, and sauté 5 minutes or until lightly browned, stirring occasionally. Add

Go for the Greenest

WHEN YOU'RE MAKING YOUR PLANS to up your weekly fish intake, start with options on the "Super Green" list created by Seafood Watch, a program run by the Monterey Bay Aquarium. To make the list, fish must have low levels of contaminants like mercury, be high in omega-3s (at least 250mg per serving), and come from a sustainable fishery.

broth and vinegar; boil 1 minute or until liquid almost evaporates. Keep warm.

2. Steam bok choy 1 minute. Heat a medium skillet over medium-high heat. Add sesame oil to pan; swirl to coat. Add bok choy, cut sides down; cook 1 minute. Add soy sauce and sesame seeds; cook 1 minute or until thoroughly heated. Add 1 tablespoon bok choy cooking liquid and cilantro to mushroom mixture; stir to combine.

3. Heat a large cast-iron skillet over high heat. Add canola oil to pan; swirl to coat. Sprinkle fish evenly with salt and pepper. Add fish to pan; sauté 1 minute on each side or until desired degree of doneness. Let stand 1 minute. Cut into ¼-inch-thick slices. To serve, place ½ cup rice on each of 4 plates; top each serving with 2 bok choy quarters. Arrange 1 tuna fillet on each plate; top each serving with ¼ cup mushroom mixture. Serves 4.

CALORIES 445; FAT 17.6g (sat 2.9g, mono 8g, poly 5.5g); PROTEIN 35.4g; CARB 36.2g; FIBER 3.2g; CHOL 47mg; IRON 2.4mg; SODIUM 760mg; CALC 145mg

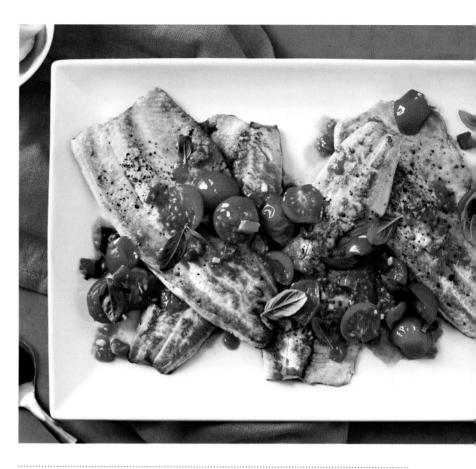

Pan-Fried Trout with Tomato-Basil Sauté

2 ounces chopped pancetta
2 cups cherry tomatoes, halved
1 teaspoon minced garlic
1 teaspoon freshly ground black pepper, divided
½ teaspoon salt, divided
¼ cup small fresh basil leaves
1 tablespoon canola oil, divided
4 (6-ounce) trout fillets, divided
4 lemon wedges

1. Heat pancetta in a medium skillet over low heat. Cook 4 minutes or just until pancetta begins to brown. Add cherry tomatoes, garlic, ½ teaspoon pepper, and ⅛ teaspoon salt; cook 3 minutes or until tomatoes begin to soften. Remove from heat, and stir in basil leaves.

2. Heat a large nonstick skillet over medium-high heat. Add 1½ teaspoons oil to pan; swirl to coat. Sprinkle fish evenly with remaining ½ teaspoon pepper and remaining ⅜ teaspoon salt. Add 2 fillets to pan; cook 2 minutes on each side or until fish flakes easily when tested with a fork. Remove fish from pan; keep warm. Repeat procedure with remaining 1½ teaspoons oil and remaining 2 fillets. Top fish with tomato mixture. Serve fish with lemon wedges. Serves 4 (serving size: 1 fillet and about ⅓ cup sauce).

Sustainable Choice: When shopping, look for U.S.-farmed rainbow trout. Avoid wild-caught lake trout.

CALORIES 388; FAT 20.5g (sat 5.9g, mono 7.9g, poly 5.5g); PROTEIN 44.3g; CARB 4.3g; FIBER 1.3g; CHOL 126mg; IRON 1.1mg; SODIUM 604mg; CALC 169mg

Arctic Char with Blistered Cherry Tomatoes

3 tablespoons extra-virgin olive oil, divided
4 (6-ounce) Arctic char fillets
¾ teaspoon coarse salt, divided
½ teaspoon black pepper, divided
4 garlic cloves, halved
3 pints multicolored cherry tomatoes
¼ cup thinly sliced fresh basil
2 shallots, thinly sliced

1. Preheat oven to 400°.
2. Heat a large ovenproof skillet over high heat. Add 1 tablespoon oil to pan; swirl to coat. Sprinkle fillets with ½ teaspoon salt and ¼ teaspoon pepper. Add fillets, flesh sides down, to pan; sauté 2 minutes. Place pan in oven; cook at 400° for 3 minutes or until desired degree of doneness.
3. Heat a large cast-iron skillet over medium heat. Add remaining 2 tablespoons oil to pan; swirl to coat. Add garlic; cook 2 minutes or until lightly browned, stirring occasionally. Increase heat to medium-high. Add tomatoes; sauté 2 minutes or until skins blister, stirring frequently. Remove pan from heat. Sprinkle tomato mixture with remaining ¼ teaspoon salt, remaining ¼ teaspoon black pepper, basil, and shallots; toss to combine. Serve with fish. Serves 4 (serving size: 1 fillet and about ¾ cup tomato mixture).

Sustainable Choice: If Arctic char is not available, substitute frozen wild Alaskan salmon.

CALORIES 380; FAT 20.4g (sat 3.8g, mono 11.7g, poly 3.6g); PROTEIN 31.4g; CARB 20g; FIBER 2.9g; CHOL 65mg; IRON 2mg; SODIUM 514mg; CALC 49mg

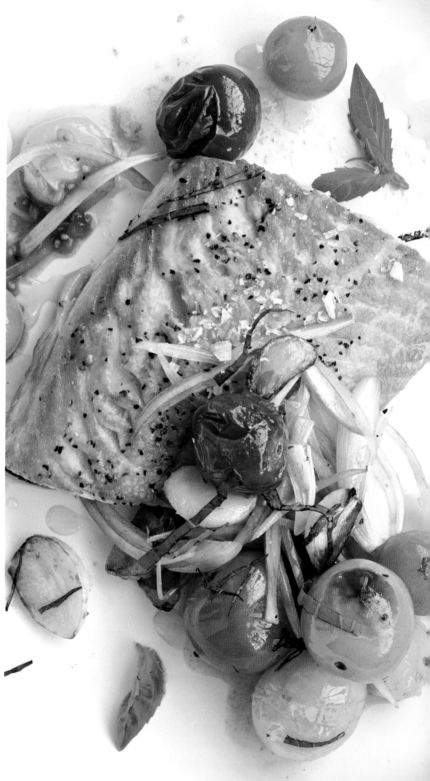

Broiled Oysters with Garlic-Buttered Breadcrumbs

1 tablespoon butter
2 teaspoons extra-virgin olive oil
2 garlic cloves, minced
1 teaspoon fresh lemon juice
1 (2-ounce) slice French bread baguette
1/8 teaspoon salt
1/8 teaspoon black pepper
24 shucked oysters
Cooking spray
1 tablespoon chopped fresh flat-leaf parsley

1. Preheat broiler.
2. Melt butter in a skillet over medium heat. Add oil and garlic; cook 1 minute, stirring occasionally. Remove from heat; stir in lemon juice.
3. Place bread in a food processor; pulse 10 times or until coarse crumbs measure 1 cup. Combine breadcrumbs, butter mixture, salt, and pepper; mix well.
4. Arrange oysters on a broiler pan coated with cooking spray; top oysters with breadcrumb mixture. Broil 5 inches from heat 3 minutes or until breadcrumbs are golden. Sprinkle with parsley. Serves 6 (serving size: 4 oysters).

Sustainable Choice: Oysters are filter feeders, so they help keep the waters they live in clean. They're a sustainable choice.

CALORIES 90; FAT 5.1g (sat 1.9g, mono 1.8g, poly 0.9g); PROTEIN 4.6g; CARB 6.4g; FIBER 0.2g; CHOL 35mg; IRON 4mg; SODIUM 232mg; CALC 39mg

Curried Coconut Mussels

Most mussels are now farm-raised, so they're easier to clean. You should still take time to rinse them under cold running water, and be sure to remove any beards. "This is amazing," said Shellycall on CookingLight.com. "If I got it in a restaurant I would go back just to eat this." Saj723 said, "My husband and I wanted to drink the broth; it was that tasty."

1 tablespoon olive oil
2 cups chopped onion
1 tablespoon finely chopped peeled fresh ginger
2 garlic cloves, minced
1 jalapeño pepper, chopped
2 teaspoons red curry paste
1 cup light coconut milk
1/2 cup dry white wine
1 teaspoon dark brown sugar
1/4 teaspoon kosher salt
2 pounds small mussels (about 60), scrubbed and debearded
3/4 cup small basil leaves, divided
3 tablespoons fresh lime juice
4 lime wedges

1. Heat a large Dutch oven over medium-high heat. Add oil to pan; swirl to coat. Add onion, ginger, garlic, and jalapeño; sauté 3 minutes, stirring frequently. Stir in curry paste; cook 30 seconds, stirring constantly. Add coconut milk, wine, sugar, and salt; bring to a boil. Cook 2 minutes. Stir in mussels; cover and cook 5 minutes or until mussels open. Discard any unopened shells. Stir in 1/2 cup basil and juice. Divide

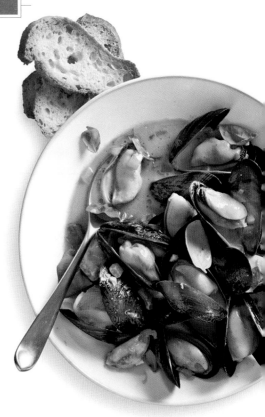

mussels mixture evenly among 4 bowls, and spoon coconut milk mixture evenly over mussels. Sprinkle each serving with remaining basil; serve with lime wedges. Serves 4 (serving size: about 15 mussels, about 1/2 cup coconut milk mixture, 1 tablespoon basil, and 1 lime wedge).

Sustainable Choice: Mussels are a good sustainable choice. Most are farmed in an environmentally responsible way, so they have healthy habitats and stocks.

CALORIES 241; FAT 9.9g (sat 4g, mono 3.2g, poly 1.3g); PROTEIN 20g; CARB 19.1g; FIBER 1.7g; CHOL 42mg; IRON 6.8mg; SODIUM 594mg; CALC 80mg

Explore Different Fish Species

MOST PEOPLE FALL INTO A HABIT of reaching for three or four familiar types of fish. Branch out and try something new. Eating a variety of fish will ensure you're eating species with varying levels of omega-3s and minimizing overexposure to environmental pollutants like mercury.

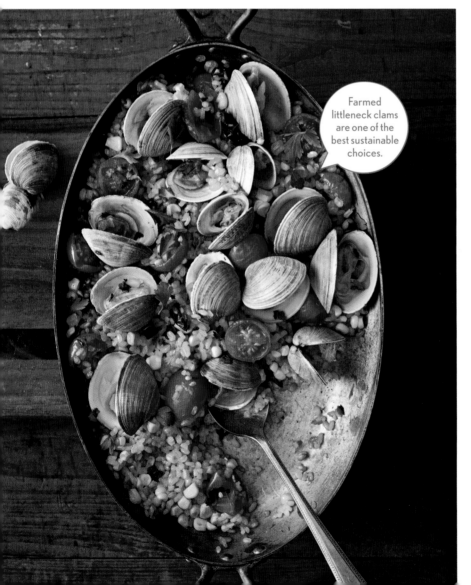

Farmed littleneck clams are one of the best sustainable choices.

Paella with Poblanos, Corn, and Clams

This classic Spanish dish uses poblanos and corn for a Mexican twist. Be sure you don't rush the last step to achieve the *socarrat*, the crisp browned rice on the bottom of the pan. The crust won't form until all of the liquid from the clams and the tomatoes has boiled off. So be patient—it's worth it.

2 tablespoons olive oil
2 cups chopped yellow onion
3 garlic cloves, minced
2 poblano chiles, seeded and chopped
1¼ teaspoons kosher salt, divided
½ teaspoon freshly ground black
  pepper, divided
¾ cup uncooked short-grain
  brown rice
¼ teaspoon saffron threads, crushed
2 cups water
⅛ teaspoon ground red pepper
1½ cups fresh corn kernels
  (about 2 ears)
1 cup halved cherry tomatoes
2 pounds littleneck clams
2 tablespoons chopped fresh
  flat-leaf parsley
8 lemon wedges

1. Preheat oven to 450°.

2. Heat a 12-inch ovenproof skillet over medium-high heat. Add oil to pan; swirl to coat. Add onion, garlic, poblanos, ½ teaspoon salt, and ¼ teaspoon black pepper; sauté 3 minutes. Add rice and saffron. Cook 2 minutes, stirring constantly. Add 2 cups water, remaining ¾ teaspoon salt, remaining ¼ teaspoon black pepper, and red pepper; bring to a boil.

3. Bake at 450° for 50 minutes or until rice is done. Stir in corn and tomatoes. Nestle clams into rice mixture. Bake at 450° for 12 minutes or until shells open, and discard unopened shells.

4. Return pan to medium-high heat, and cook without stirring 10 minutes or until liquid evaporates and rice browns. (It should smell toasty but not burned.) Top with parsley; serve with lemon wedges. Serves 4 (serving size: 1¼ cups rice mixture and about 7 clams).

Sustainable Choice: Because they help filter the water in which they live, clams and other bivalves are sustainable superstars.

CALORIES 340; FAT 9.1g (sat 1.1g, mono 5.2g, poly 1.3g); PROTEIN 14.8g; CARB 52.7g; FIBER 5.6g; CHOL 21mg; IRON 10mg; SODIUM 651mg; CALC 68mg

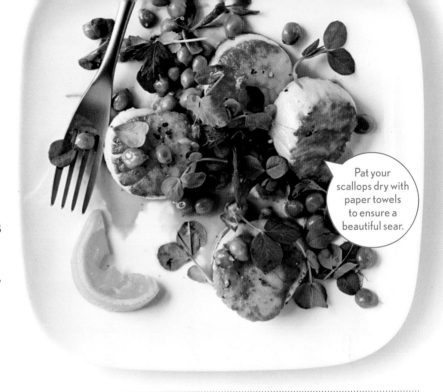

Pat your scallops dry with paper towels to ensure a beautiful sear.

Seared Scallops with Lemony Sweet Pea Relish

1 cup shelled fresh English peas
1½ teaspoons salt, divided
¼ cup extra-virgin olive oil, divided
1½ teaspoons grated lemon rind
2 tablespoons fresh lemon juice
1 tablespoon chopped fresh flat-leaf parsley
¼ cup minced shallots
½ teaspoon freshly ground black pepper, divided
2¼ pounds large sea scallops
1½ cups pea shoots
6 lemon wedges

1. Cook English peas in boiling water with 1 teaspoon salt 2 minutes. Drain and rinse with cold water; drain. Combine peas, 3 tablespoons oil, rind, juice, parsley, and shallots. Stir in ¼ teaspoon salt and ¼ teaspoon pepper; toss gently.

2. Heat a large cast-iron skillet over medium-high heat. Add 1½ teaspoons oil to pan; swirl to coat. Sprinkle remaining ¼ teaspoon salt and remaining ¼ teaspoon black pepper over scallops. Add half of scallops to pan; cook 2 minutes on each side or until browned. Repeat procedure with remaining 1½ teaspoons oil and scallops. Divide scallops evenly among 6 plates; top each serving with 2½ tablespoons pea mixture and ¼ cup pea shoots. Serve with lemon wedges. Serves 6.

Sustainable Choice: Diver-caught scallops are considered the best of the large variety (because other large scallops are dredged, harming the ocean floor).

CALORIES 260; FAT 10.4g (sat 1.4g, mono 6.6g, poly 1.4g); PROTEIN 30.2g; CARB 10.6g; FIBER 1.5g; CHOL 56mg; IRON 1.1mg; SODIUM 513mg CALC 53mg

Try Salmon Three Ways

SALMON IS ONE OF THE BEST SOURCES of heart-healthy omega-3 fats. Even better, the flavor and meaty-fatty texture make it seem luxurious and indulgent, a real treat to eat. Its high fat content keeps it moist even when slightly overcooked—so it's a perfect option for the intense heat of the grill.

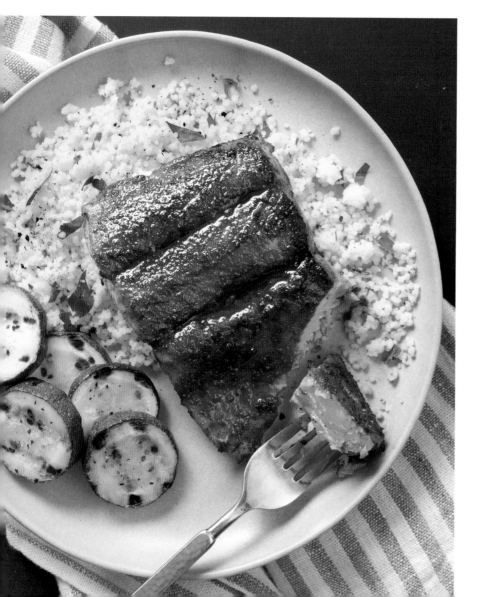

Maple-Glazed Salmon

1 teaspoon kosher salt
1 teaspoon paprika
½ teaspoon chili powder
½ teaspoon ground ancho chile powder
¼ teaspoon ground cumin
¼ teaspoon brown sugar
4 (6-ounce) wild Alaskan salmon fillets
Cooking spray
2 tablespoons maple syrup

1. Preheat broiler.
2. Combine first 6 ingredients; rub spice mixture evenly over flesh side of fillets. Place fish on a broiler pan coated with cooking spray; broil 6 minutes or until desired degree of doneness. Brush fillets evenly with syrup; broil 1 minute. Serves 4 (serving size: 1 fillet).

Sustainable Choice: Look for salmon labeled "wild Alaskan salmon." If unavailable, buy frozen Alaskan salmon. Avoid farmed Atlantic salmon. Farming salmon in ocean nets has resulted in pollution and a host of other issues, although U.S. tank-farmed coho, sake, and silver salmon are acceptable choices.

CALORIES 352; FAT 20g (sat 3.2g; mono 7g; poly 2.7g); PROTEIN 34.6g; CARB 8.6g; FIBER 0.2g; CHOL 104mg; IRON 1.6mg; SODIUM 574mg; CALC 80mg

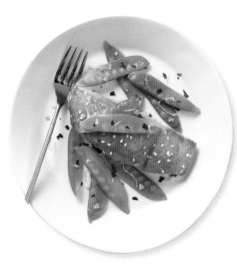

Salmon with Hoisin Glaze

2 tablespoons hoisin sauce
2 teaspoons lower-sodium soy sauce
½ teaspoon dark sesame oil
4 (6-ounce) skinless wild Alaskan
　salmon fillets
Cooking spray
1 teaspoon sesame seeds
Lemon rind strips (optional)

1. Preheat oven to 400°.
2. Combine first 3 ingredients in a shallow dish. Add fish to dish, turning to coat. Marinate at room temperature 8 minutes, turning occasionally.
3. Remove fish from marinade; discard marinade. Place fish on a baking sheet coated with cooking spray. Sprinkle fish evenly with sesame seeds. Bake at 400° for 8 minutes or until desired degree of doneness. Garnish with rind, if desired. Serves 4 (serving size: 1 fillet).

CALORIES 255; FAT 11.7g (sat 2.7g, mono 4.8g, poly 2.8g); PROTEIN 31.5g; CARB 3.9g; FIBER 0.3g; CHOL 81mg; IRON 0.7mg; SODIUM 285mg; CALC 26mg

Quick Side
Garlicky-Spicy Snow Peas

Heat a large nonstick skillet over medium-high heat. Add 1 teaspoon canola oil to pan; swirl to coat. Add 1 pound snow peas and ¼ teaspoon salt; sauté 2 minutes. Stir in 2 teaspoons bottled minced garlic and ¼ teaspoon crushed red pepper; sauté 1 minute. Stir in ¼ teaspoon sugar; sauté 1 minute. Remove from heat; drizzle with ½ teaspoon dark sesame oil. Serves 4.

CALORIES 72; FAT 2.2g (sat 0.2g, mono 1g, poly 0.7g); PROTEIN 3.2g; CARB 9.4g; FIBER 3g; CHOL 0mg; IRON 2.4mg; SODIUM 150mg; CALC 49mg

Grilled King Salmon
with Tomato-Peach Salsa

1 cup chopped peeled peach
¾ cup quartered cherry tomatoes
¼ cup thinly vertically sliced red onion
3 tablespoons small fresh mint leaves
3 tablespoons small fresh basil leaves
2 tablespoons fresh lemon juice
1 tablespoon extra-virgin olive oil
1 tablespoon honey
1 jalapeño pepper, thinly sliced (optional)
1 teaspoon kosher salt, divided
4 (6-ounce) wild Alaskan king
　salmon fillets
¼ teaspoon freshly ground black pepper
Cooking spray

1. Preheat grill to high heat.
2. Combine first 8 ingredients in a bowl; add jalapeño, if desired. Sprinkle mixture with ¼ teaspoon salt; toss gently, and set aside.
3. Sprinkle fillets evenly with remaining ¾ teaspoon salt and black pepper. Place fillets on grill rack coated with cooking spray, and grill 10 minutes or until desired degree of doneness, turning after 5 minutes. Serve with salsa. Serves 4 (serving size: 1 fillet and about ½ cup salsa).

CALORIES 325; FAT 21.9g (sat 3.3g, mono 10.2g, poly 2.8g); PROTEIN 26.7g; CARB 6.4g; FIBER 1.2g; CHOL 78mg; IRON 1.4mg; SODIUM 544mg; CALC 68mg

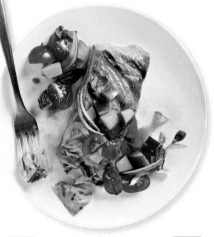

FISHING FOR FLAVORS

Versatile salmon pairs with bold and subtle tastes:

Salty: lower-sodium soy sauce, capers, miso, olives
Sweet: honey, brown sugar, maple syrup, orange juice or rind
Sour: fresh lemon, fresh lime, vinegar
Pungent: onion, shallots, garlic, ginger, horseradish, sesame
Creamy: cream cheese, yogurt, crème fraîche, butter
Smoky: chipotle chiles, smoked paprika, cumin
Green: fresh herbs (especially dill, chives, and mint), cucumber, asparagus

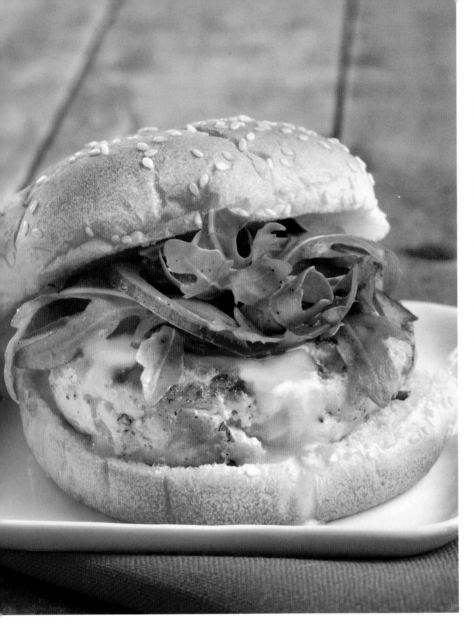

Salmon Burgers

1 pound skinless center-cut salmon
   fillets, cut into 1-inch pieces, divided
2 tablespoons Dijon mustard, divided
2 teaspoons grated lemon rind
2 tablespoons minced fresh tarragon
1 tablespoon finely chopped shallots
   (about 1 small)
$\frac{1}{2}$ teaspoon kosher salt
$\frac{1}{4}$ teaspoon freshly ground black
   pepper
1 tablespoon honey
1 cup arugula leaves
$\frac{1}{2}$ cup thinly sliced red onion
1 teaspoon fresh lemon juice
1 teaspoon extra-virgin olive oil
Cooking spray
4 (1$\frac{1}{2}$-ounce) hamburger buns, toasted

1. Place $\frac{1}{4}$ pound salmon, 1 tablespoon mustard, and rind in a food
processor; process until smooth.
Spoon puree into a large bowl. Place
remaining $\frac{3}{4}$ pound salmon in food
processor; pulse 6 times or until
coarsely chopped. Fold chopped
salmon, tarragon, shallots, salt, and
pepper into puree. Divide mixture
into 4 equal portions, gently shap-
ing each into a $\frac{1}{2}$-inch-thick patty.
Cover and chill until ready to grill.
2. Preheat grill to medium heat.
3. Combine remaining 1 tablespoon
mustard and honey in a small bowl,
and set aside.
4. Combine arugula, onion, juice,
and oil in a medium bowl. Set aside.
5. Lightly coat both sides of burgers
with cooking spray. Place patties
on grill rack; grill 2 minutes.
Carefully turn patties, and grill 1
minute or until desired degree of
doneness. Place 1 patty on bottom

Fish Up Favorite Foods

NTRODUCE FISH IN THE DISHES you and your
family already enjoy, from pizza and sandwiches
to burgers, tacos, and tostadas. Use familiar flavorings
and favorite ingredients to enhance the appeal.

half of each bun; top each serving with 1½ teaspoons honey mixture, ¼ cup arugula mixture, and top half of bun. Serves 4 (serving size: 1 burger).

CALORIES 372; FAT 16g (sat 3.2g, mono 5.9g, poly 5.8g); PROTEIN 27.3g; CARB 28.2g; FIBER 1.5g; CHOL 67mg; IRON 2.1mg; SODIUM 569mg; CALC 92mg

Broiled Tilapia Gyros

Fish:
1½ pounds tilapia fillets
1½ tablespoons olive oil
½ teaspoon freshly ground black pepper
¼ teaspoon salt
Cooking spray

Tzatziki:
¾ cup plain 2% reduced-fat Greek yogurt
2 teaspoons chopped fresh dill
1½ teaspoons fresh lemon juice
½ teaspoon freshly ground black pepper
¼ teaspoon salt
2 garlic cloves, minced

Remaining ingredients:
4 (2.75-ounce) Mediterranean-style wheat flatbreads
½ cup vertically sliced red onion (about ½ small onion)
1 ripe avocado, peeled and cut into 12 thin slices
1 medium tomato, thinly sliced
½ small English cucumber, thinly sliced (about ½ cup)

1. Preheat broiler.
2. To prepare fish, brush fish with oil; sprinkle with ½ teaspoon pepper

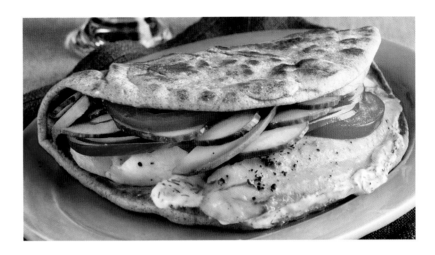

and ¼ teaspoon salt. Place fish on a broiler pan coated with cooking spray. Broil 6 minutes or until fish flakes easily when tested with a fork.
3. To prepare tzatziki, place yogurt and next 5 ingredients in a food processor or blender; pulse until smooth.
4. Spread 2 tablespoons tzatziki in center of each flatbread. Divide fish evenly among flatbreads. Top each with 2 tablespoons onion, 3 avocado slices, 2 tomato slices, and about 6 cucumber slices; fold in half. Serves 4 (serving size: 1 filled gyro).

Sustainable Choice: Avoid fillets from China or Taiwan, which are typically sold frozen. Although not abundant, U.S.-farmed tilapia is the best sustainable option. Central and South American fish are the next best alternative.

CALORIES 479; FAT 16.8g (sat 3.7g, mono 9.4g, poly 2.2g); PROTEIN 46.1g; CARB 39.7g; FIBER 9.4g; CHOL 88mg; IRON 3.5mg; SODIUM 538mg; CALC 120mg

Because tilapia is a mild-flavored fish, it's a good choice for kids and the seafood-averse.

EXPERT TIP:
Appearance Is Important

"Kids are swayed by the appearance of food, so serve your fish with style. Boost the eye appeal and get creative with your presentation: fish skewered on sticks, sautéed on a bed of pasta, grilled, baked in a boat, or crisped in the oven. Kids also like the make-your-own approach."

Jill Castle, MS, RD, blogger
Just the Right Byte

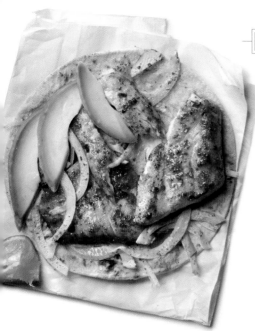

Blackened Tilapia Baja Tacos

"These were the best fish tacos I've ever had!" said BrendaLRGale on CookingLight.com. "The spices on the fish would go well with shrimp, too. All the flavors went so well together."

¼ cup reduced-fat sour cream
2 tablespoons chopped fresh cilantro
2 tablespoons fresh lime juice
1 jalapeño pepper, seeded and chopped
1 cup thinly sliced white onion
1½ teaspoons paprika
1½ teaspoons brown sugar
1 teaspoon dried oregano
¾ teaspoon garlic powder
½ teaspoon salt
½ teaspoon ground cumin
¼ teaspoon ground red pepper
4 (6-ounce) tilapia fillets
1 tablespoon canola oil
8 (6-inch) corn tortillas
½ ripe peeled avocado, thinly sliced
4 lime wedges

1. Place first 4 ingredients in a food processor; process until smooth. Combine jalapeño sauce and onion in a small bowl.
2. Combine paprika and next 6 ingredients; sprinkle evenly over fish. Heat a large cast-iron skillet over medium-high heat. Add oil to pan; swirl to coat. Add fish to pan; cook 3 minutes on each side or until fish flakes easily when tested with a fork.
3. Warm tortillas according to package directions. Divide fish, onion mixture, and avocado evenly among tortillas. Serve with lime wedges. Serves 4 (serving size: 2 tacos).

CALORIES 362; FAT 13.6g (sat 3.1g, mono 6.4g, poly 2.8g); PROTEIN 37g; CARB 27.1g; FIBER 4.9g; CHOL 79mg; IRON 1.5mg; SODIUM 388mg; CALC 74mg

Chimichurri Halibut Tacos

Top with pineapple salsa or fresh salsa.

2 cups fresh flat-leaf parsley leaves
2 tablespoons fresh oregano
¾ teaspoon ground cumin
¼ teaspoon ground red pepper
5 garlic cloves, crushed
⅓ cup extra-virgin olive oil
5 (6-ounce) halibut fillets
1 teaspoon kosher salt
½ teaspoon black pepper
Cooking spray
12 (6-inch) corn tortillas

1. Place first 5 ingredients in a food processor; process until finely chopped. Slowly pour oil through food chute; process until smooth. Place fish in a shallow dish; rub mixture over fish. Cover and chill 2 hours.
2. Preheat grill to high heat.
3. Sprinkle fish with salt and black pepper. Place fish on grill rack coated with cooking spray, and grill 4 minutes on each side or until fish flakes easily when tested with a fork. Remove from grill. Break fish into chunks. Heat tortillas according to package directions. Divide fish evenly among tortillas. Serves 6 (serving size: 2 tacos).

Sustainable Choice: Wild-caught Alaskan halibut is the best option. If not available, opt for other U.S. or Canadian wild-caught Pacific halibut.

CALORIES 266; FAT 10.4g (sat 1.3g, mono 5.8g, poly 2g); PROTEIN 24.6g; CARB 19.8g; FIBER 2.6g; CHOL 34mg; IRON 1.6mg; SODIUM 394mg; CALC 93mg

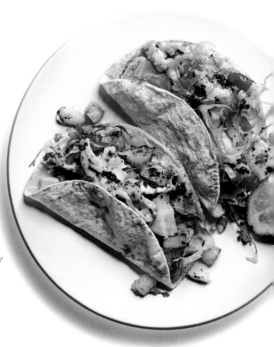

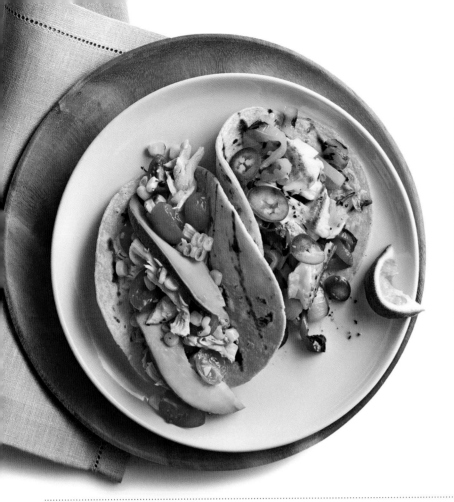

Sautéed Tilapia Tacos with Grilled Peppers and Onions

2 (½-inch-thick) slices white onion
1 (8-ounce) package mini sweet bell peppers
Cooking spray
¾ teaspoon salt, divided
½ teaspoon freshly ground black pepper, divided
4 (5-ounce) tilapia fillets
8 (6-inch) corn tortillas
1 small jalapeño pepper, thinly sliced
8 lime wedges (optional)

1. Preheat grill to high heat.
2. Arrange onion slices and bell peppers on grill rack coated with cooking spray. Grill onions 12 minutes, turning after 6 minutes. Grill bell peppers 12 minutes, turning occasionally. Remove onions and bell peppers from grill, and let stand 5 minutes. Slice onion rings in half. Thinly slice bell peppers; discard stems and seeds. Combine onion, bell peppers, ¼ teaspoon salt, and ⅛ teaspoon black pepper in a small bowl.
3. Sprinkle fish evenly with remaining ½ teaspoon salt and remaining ⅜ teaspoon black pepper. Heat a large skillet over medium-high heat. Coat pan with cooking spray. Add fish to pan, and cook 3 minutes on each side or until fish flakes easily when tested with a fork.
4. Warm tortillas according to package directions. Divide fish, onion mixture, and jalapeño slices evenly among tortillas. Serve with lime wedges, if desired. Serves 4 (serving size: 2 tacos).

CALORIES 292; FAT 4.4g (sat 1.2g, mono 1.2g, poly 1.3g); PROTEIN 32.6g; CARB 32g; FIBER 4.8g; CHOL 71mg; IRON 1.9mg; SODIUM 526mg; CALC 120mg

Give Pasta a Seafood Boost

S EAFOOD AND PASTA ARE A PERFECT MATCH, and the combination—once you add loads of vegetables—is a light and easy one-dish meal. Try cold pasta salads with seafood, or heartier, Mediterranean-inspired pasta meals with penne, linguine, or fettuccine.

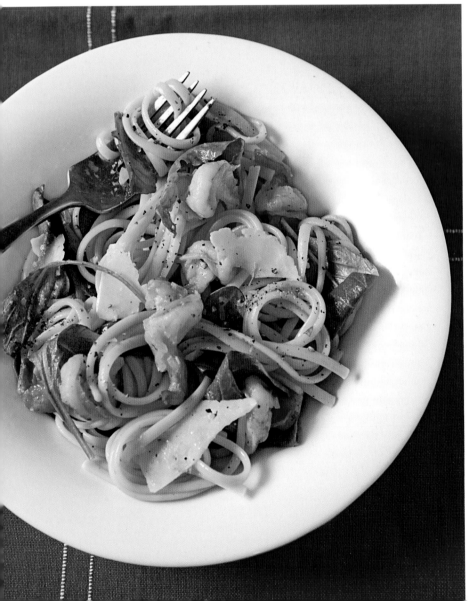

Peppery Pasta with Arugula and Shrimp

1 tablespoon minced fresh garlic, divided
1¼ teaspoons black pepper, divided
½ teaspoon salt, divided
1 (5-ounce) package fresh baby arugula
4 quarts water
8 ounces uncooked linguine
1 tablespoon olive oil
½ pound peeled and deveined medium shrimp, cut in half horizontally
2 tablespoons minced shallots
¾ cup fat-free, lower-sodium chicken broth
2 tablespoons fresh lemon juice
1 tablespoon butter
½ cup (2 ounces) shaved fresh Romano cheese

1. Combine 2 teaspoons garlic, 1 teaspoon pepper, ¼ teaspoon salt, and arugula in a large bowl; toss well.
2. Bring 4 quarts water to a boil in a large Dutch oven. Add pasta, and cook 10 minutes or until al dente; drain. Add hot pasta to arugula mixture, and toss well until arugula wilts.
3. Heat a large skillet over medium-high heat. Add oil to pan; swirl to coat. Add shrimp, remaining

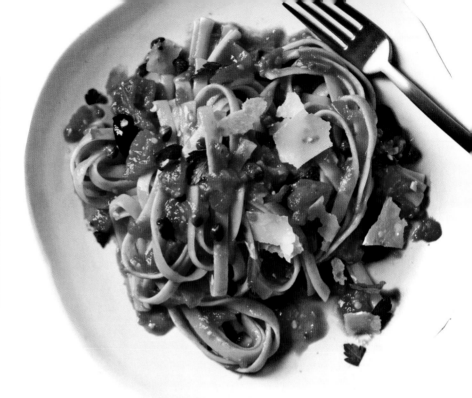

¼ teaspoon salt, and remaining ¼ teaspoon pepper, and sauté 1 minute. Add remaining 1 teaspoon garlic and shallots, and sauté 1 minute or until shrimp are done. Remove shrimp from pan. Add broth and juice to pan, scraping pan to loosen browned bits; cook 5 minutes or until liquid is reduced by half. Return shrimp to pan. Remove from heat, and stir in butter.
4. Arrange 1½ cups pasta mixture on each of 4 plates. Spoon ⅓ cup shrimp mixture over each serving. Top each serving with 2 tablespoons cheese. Serves 4.

Sustainable Choice: Look for the Marine Stewardship Council stamp to ensure you're making an eco-friendly choice. U.S.-farmed shrimp or wild northern shrimp from Canada are the best options. Avoid other imported wild and farmed species.

CALORIES 409; FAT 12.5g (sat 5g, mono 4.5g, poly 1.1g); PROTEIN 26.1g; CARB 46g; FIBER 2.1g; CHOL 107mg; IRON 3.3mg; SODIUM 671mg; CALC 231mg

Pasta Puttanesca

3 tablespoons olive oil, divided
2 garlic cloves, minced
3 anchovy fillets
1½ cups canned crushed tomatoes
¾ cup pitted kalamata olives, coarsely chopped
1 tablespoon minced fresh parsley
1 tablespoon drained capers
¼ teaspoon crushed red pepper
6 quarts water
8 ounces uncooked fettuccine
¼ cup (1 ounce) shaved fresh Parmesan cheese

1. Heat a large nonstick skillet over medium heat. Add 2 tablespoons oil to pan; swirl to coat. Add garlic; cook 30 seconds, stirring constantly. Add anchovies; mash in pan to form a paste. Stir in tomatoes and next 4 ingredients; cook 5 minutes, stirring occasionally.

2. Bring 6 quarts water to a boil. Add pasta, and cook 8 minutes or until almost al dente. Drain in a colander over a bowl, reserving ½ cup pasta water. Add pasta and reserved pasta water to tomato mixture; increase heat to medium-high. Cook 5 minutes or until pasta is al dente, tossing to combine. Spoon 1½ cups pasta mixture into each of 4 bowls. Drizzle each serving with ¾ teaspoon oil, and sprinkle with cheese. Serves 4.

CALORIES 404; FAT 17.5g (sat 3.5g, mono 11.1g, poly 2.2g); PROTEIN 13.1g; CARB 51.5g; FIBER 3.9g; CHOL 7mg; IRON 3.5mg; SODIUM 648mg; CALC 144mg

Simmer a Fish Stew

ENJOY FISH AND SEAFOOD in a flavor-packed stew or soup, a technique that's employed around the globe from New England clam chowder and New Orleans gumbo to French bouillabaisse and Asian-style fish stews.

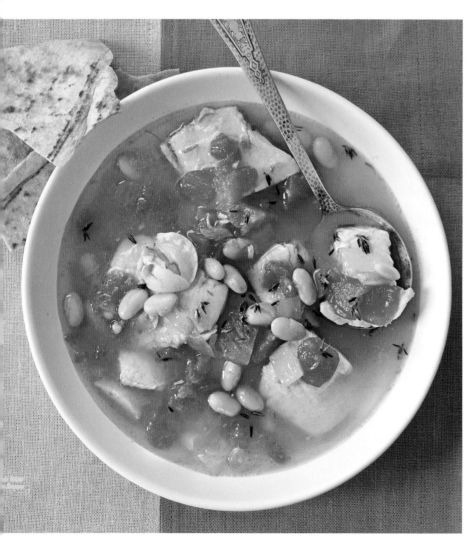

Saffron Fish Stew with White Beans

1 tablespoon extra-virgin olive oil
1 cup prechopped onion
1 teaspoon ground fennel
$\frac{1}{2}$ teaspoon ground coriander
2 garlic cloves, crushed
1 thyme sprig
$\frac{1}{2}$ teaspoon grated fresh orange rind
$\frac{1}{4}$ teaspoon saffron threads, crushed
$1\frac{1}{2}$ cups water
$1\frac{1}{2}$ cups clam juice
1 (14.5-ounce) can diced tomatoes, undrained
$\frac{1}{8}$ teaspoon salt
1 pound flounder fillet, cut into (2-inch) pieces
1 (14-ounce) can great Northern beans, rinsed and drained
Thyme leaves

1. Heat a large Dutch oven over medium-high heat. Add oil to pan; swirl to coat. Add onion, fennel, coriander, garlic, and thyme sprig; sauté 5 minutes. Stir in rind and saffron; add 1½ cups water, clam juice, and tomatoes. Bring to a boil; reduce heat, and simmer 5 minutes. Stir in salt, fish, and beans; cook 5 minutes. Top with thyme leaves. Serves 4 (serving size: 2 cups).

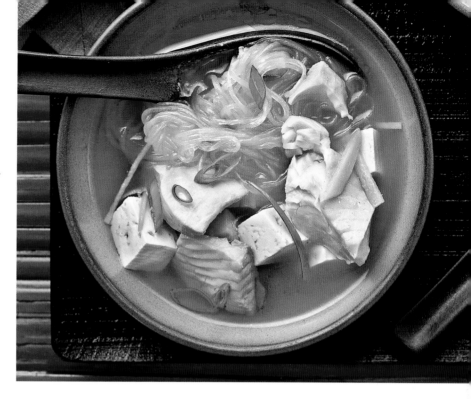

Sustainable Choice: U.S. Pacific-caught flounder is a sustainable option. Common names for these mild flatfish are sole, sanddab, and hirame.

CALORIES 249; FAT 5.1g (sat 0.9g, mono 2.8g, poly 0.9g); PROTEIN 279g; CARB 23g; FIBER 5.7g; CHOL 57mg; IRON 2.2mg; SODIUM 495mg; CALC 101mg

Shanghai-Inspired Fish Stew

Traditionally, this comfort-food stew is made with flash-fried and then long-simmered fish heads. Tilapia fillets make an excellent, quick-cooking substitute. Look for U.S.-farmed tilapia for the best sustainable option.

3 ounces uncooked bean threads (cellophane noodles)
2 cups boiling water
1 ounce dried wood ear mushrooms
4 cups fat-free, lower-sodium chicken broth
2 tablespoons julienne-cut peeled fresh ginger
1 tablespoon rice vinegar
1 tablespoon lower-sodium soy sauce
1 tablespoon Chinese black vinegar or Worcestershire sauce
1/2 teaspoon ground white pepper
1/2 teaspoon dark sesame oil
1/4 teaspoon salt
1 pound tilapia fillets, cut into bite-sized pieces
8 ounces silken firm tofu, drained and cubed
1/4 cup thinly sliced green onions

1. Prepare noodles according to package directions. Drain and rinse with cold water. Drain. Snip noodles several times with kitchen shears.
2. Combine 2 cups boiling water and mushrooms in a medium bowl, and let stand 20 minutes. Drain mushrooms in a sieve over a bowl; discard mushrooms. Combine mushroom soaking liquid, broth, and next 7 ingredients in a Dutch oven. Bring to a boil. Cover, reduce heat, and simmer 20 minutes. Add tilapia; cover and simmer 10 minutes. Stir in noodles and tofu; simmer, uncovered, 5 minutes. Ladle 1 cup soup into each of 8 bowls; sprinkle each serving with 1½ teaspoons green onions. Serves 8.

CALORIES 121; FAT 2g (sat 0.5g, mono 0.6g, poly 0.8g); PROTEIN 14g; CARB 11.1g; FIBER 0.5g; CHOL 28mg; IRON 0.8mg; SODIUM 407mg; CALC 19mg

> **EXPERT TIP:**
> *Consider the Catch of the Day*
>
> "Instead of deciding on a fish recipe and making a shopping list, be open to the catch of the day when you head to the seafood counter. Adopt the same approach you use at the farmers' market: See what's in season and what's freshest."
> —*Kate Geagan, MS, RD, blogger and author of* Go Green Get Lean

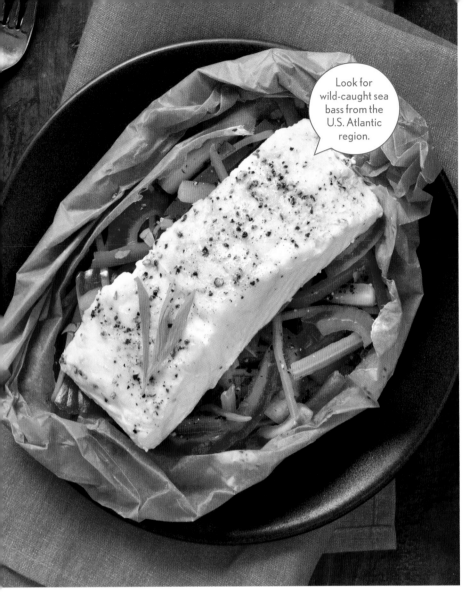

Look for wild-caught sea bass from the U.S. Atlantic region.

Gulf Fish en Papillote

1 cup matchstick-cut carrots
1 cup vertically sliced red onion
¾ cup (2-inch) julienne-cut celery
½ cup red bell pepper strips
1 teaspoon chopped fresh chervil
1 teaspoon chopped fresh tarragon
¼ teaspoon salt, divided
¼ teaspoon freshly ground black pepper, divided
2 (6-ounce) white sea bass fillets
2 teaspoons butter
¼ cup dry white wine
Tarragon sprigs (optional)

1. Preheat oven to 350°.
2. Combine first 6 ingredients, ⅛ teaspoon salt, and ⅛ teaspoon pepper in a medium bowl.
3. Sprinkle fish evenly with remaining ⅛ teaspoon salt and ⅛ teaspoon black pepper. Cut 2 (15-inch) squares of parchment paper. Fold each square in half, and open each. Place half of vegetable mixture near each fold. Top each serving with 1 fillet, 1 teaspoon butter, and 2 tablespoons wine. Fold paper; seal edges with narrow folds. Place packets on a jelly-roll pan. Bake at 350° for 18 minutes or until parchment is puffy. Place on plates, and cut open. Garnish with tarragon, if desired. Serve immediately. Serves 2 (serving size: 1 fillet and about 1½ cups vegetable mixture).

CALORIES 264; FAT 7.6g (sat 3.3g, mono 1.7g, poly 1.6g); PROTEIN 33.2g; CARB 15.4g; FIBER 3.8g; CHOL 80mg; IRON 1.2mg; SODIUM 518mg

Wrap It Up

A FRENCH COOKING METHOD known as "en papillote," steaming fish in sealed packets in the oven, results in flavorful, moist, and tender fish. It's also a great and easy way to add vegetables to your meal, cooking them right in the packet with the fish.

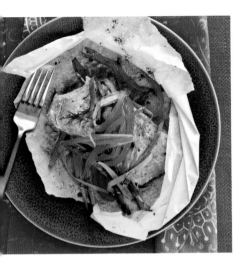

Arctic Char and Vegetables in Parchment Hearts

1½ tablespoons unsalted butter, softened
1 teaspoon grated lemon rind
1 tablespoon fresh lemon juice
1 teaspoon chopped fresh dill
2 (6-ounce) Arctic char fillets (about 1 inch thick)
¼ teaspoon kosher salt
⅛ teaspoon black pepper
¼ cup julienne-cut leeks
¼ cup julienne-cut red bell pepper
¼ cup julienne-cut carrot
¼ cup julienne-cut snow peas

1. Preheat oven to 450°.
2. Combine first 4 ingredients in a small bowl; stir until blended.
3. Cut 2 (15 x 24–inch) pieces of parchment paper. Fold in half cross-wise. Draw a large heart half on each piece, with the fold of the paper along the center of the heart. Cut out the heart, and open. Sprinkle both sides of fillets with salt and pepper. Place 1 fillet near fold of each parchment heart. Top each fillet with half of vegetables and half of butter mixture. Start at the top of heart and fold edges of parchment, sealing edges with narrow folds. Twist end tip to secure tightly. Place packets on a baking sheet.
4. Bake at 450° for 15 minutes. Place on plates; cut open. Serve immediately. Serves 2 (serving size: 1 fillet, ½ cup vegetables, and about 1 tablespoon sauce).

CALORIES 301; FAT 14.6g (sat 6.4g, mono 3.8g, poly 2.7g); PROTEIN 34.8g; CARB 6g; FIBER 1.4g; CHOL 111mg; IRON 1.8mg; SODIUM 369mg; CALC 45mg

HOW TO COOK FISH IN A PACKET

Cooking fish *en papillote* yields moist, tender results with little fuss. The key is a folded seal on the paper packet. You can use parchment or foil for your fish packet, although it's best not to use foil with acidic ingredients, as it can react with the acid and create off flavors or colors.

1. Fold parchment paper in half.
2. Draw half of a heart shape.
3. Cut out shape as shown.
4. Arrange fish and veggies on one side of paper.
5. Make small, tight, overlapping folds down the outside edge to close packet.
6. Twist tail end to seal.

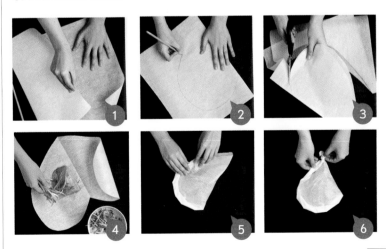

Make a Seafood Salad

MAIN ENTRÉE SALADS ARE A SUPERB WAY to work in more seafood. Try topping spinach, arugula, and other dark leafy greens with shrimp, tuna, salmon, or other fish.

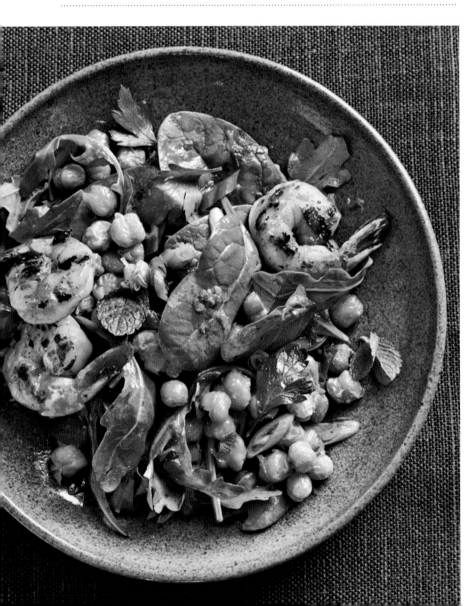

Crispy Chickpea Salad with Grilled Prawns

¼ cup extra-virgin olive oil, divided
4 teaspoons grated lemon rind, divided
¼ cup fresh lemon juice, divided
1 tablespoon chopped fresh flat-leaf parsley
2½ teaspoons crushed red pepper, divided
¾ teaspoon salt, divided
½ teaspoon freshly ground black pepper
1 garlic clove, minced
18 large shrimp, peeled and deveined (about ¾ pound)
6 cups canola oil
3 cups rinsed and drained canned chickpeas (garbanzo beans)
Cooking spray
4 cups fresh baby arugula
2 cups fresh baby spinach
½ cup fresh mint, torn
⅓ cup fresh flat-leaf parsley leaves
⅓ cup (¼-inch) diagonally cut green onions

1. Combine 1 tablespoon olive oil, 1½ teaspoons lemon rind, 1 tablespoon juice, parsley, 1 teaspoon red pepper, ½ teaspoon salt, black pepper, and garlic in a medium bowl. Add shrimp, and toss well. Marinate in refrigerator 1 hour, stirring occasionally.
2. Clip a candy thermometer onto side of a Dutch oven. Add canola oil to pan; heat oil to 385°.
3. Dry chickpeas thoroughly in a single layer on paper towels. Place 1½ cups chickpeas in hot oil;

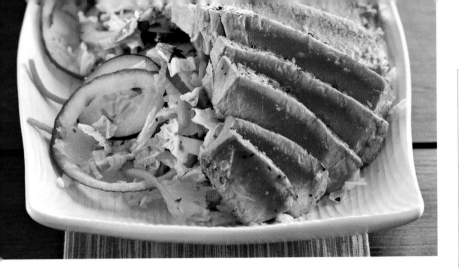

fry 4 minutes or until crisp, stirring occasionally. Make sure oil temperature remains at 375°. Remove peas from pan using a slotted spoon; drain on paper towels. Keep warm. Return oil to 385°. Repeat procedure with remaining chickpeas.

4. Remove shrimp from marinade; discard marinade. Thread 3 shrimp onto each of 6 (5-inch) skewers.

5. Preheat grill to medium-high heat.

6. Place shrimp on grill rack coated with cooking spray. Grill shrimp 2½ minutes on each side or until done.

7. Combine remaining 3 tablespoons olive oil, remaining 2½ teaspoons rind, remaining 3 tablespoons juice, remaining 1½ teaspoons red pepper, and remaining ¼ teaspoon salt in a large bowl; stir with a whisk. Add chickpeas, arugula, spinach, and remaining ingredients; toss gently to combine. Place 1¼ cups chickpea mixture in each of 6 bowls. Top each serving with 3 grilled shrimp. Serves 6.

CALORIES 262; FAT 15.8g (sat 1.7g, mono 9.6g, poly 2.5g); PROTEIN 10.2g; CARB 21.6g; FIBER 5.7g; CHOL 32mg; IRON 2.6mg; SODIUM 628mg; CALC 80mg

Pan-Grilled Thai Tuna Salad

Cooking spray
2 (6-ounce) yellowfin tuna steaks (about 1 inch thick)
¼ teaspoon salt
⅛ teaspoon black pepper
4 cups thinly sliced napa (Chinese) cabbage
1 cup thinly sliced cucumber
½ cup matchstick-cut carrots
⅓ cup presliced red onion
1 navel orange, sectioned and chopped
1 tablespoon sugar
2 tablespoons chopped fresh cilantro
2 tablespoons fresh lime juice
2 tablespoons rice vinegar
½ teaspoon dark sesame oil
¼ teaspoon sambal oelek (ground fresh chile paste) or Sriracha (hot chile sauce)

1. Heat a grill pan over medium-high heat. Coat pan with cooking spray. Sprinkle fish evenly with salt and pepper. Add fish to pan; cook 2 minutes on each side or until desired degree of doneness. Transfer to a cutting board.

2. Combine cabbage and next 4 ingredients in a large bowl. Combine sugar and remaining ingredients in a small bowl, stirring well with a whisk. Reserve 1 tablespoon dressing. Drizzle remaining dressing over salad; toss gently to coat. Divide salad mixture evenly between 2 plates. Cut each tuna steak across the grain into ¼-inch slices; arrange over salad mixture. Drizzle 1½ teaspoons reserved dressing over each serving. Serves 2.

CALORIES 307; FAT 3g (sat 0.6g, mono 0.8g, poly 1g); PROTEIN 41.8g; CARB 28.4g; FIBER 5.2g; CHOL 74mg; IRON 1.6mg; SODIUM 398mg; CALC 201mg

Expert Chatter: Talking Fish

@TanyaZuckerbrot: Fish = healthy. Fried fish, smothered in cream sauce, topped with cheese, and wedged between a bun? Not so much.

@GreenEating: Did u know risk of NOT eating fish is much greater than risk of eating it, even for kids and moms-to-be?

@RMNutrition: I like canned/ pouch salmon and tuna. Inexpensive, quick, ready to eat. Love them on top of salads.

@NourRD: I keep a bag of frozen fish fillets in my freezer at all times. Season and bake. Great when I can't go to the store.

@MarisaMoore: Quick, healthy, and inexpensive: Canned tuna or salmon w/white beans, tomatoes, arugula, or spinach, and an olive oil vinaigrette.

Use Fish Off the Shelf

STOCKING YOUR PANTRY WITH CANNED FISH can make it easier for you to make twice-a-week seafood meals. What you'll see on supermarket shelves is not your mama's canned fish. Now you can find premium tuna, salmon, crab, clams, and other fish packed in all sorts of shelf-stable containers, including cans, tins, glass jars, and pouches.

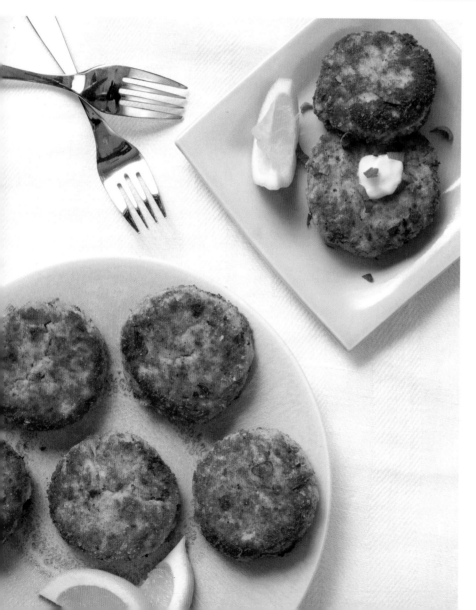

Cajun Salmon Cakes with Lemon-Garlic Aioli

"This has become one of our favorite *Cooking Light* recipes," said DaphneT on CookingLight.com. "I make the recipe exactly as written and it comes out fabulous every time, never mushy or hard to keep in cake form. The aioli is delicious as well!"

Aioli:
2 tablespoons canola mayonnaise
2 teaspoons fresh lemon juice
¼ teaspoon bottled minced garlic

Cakes:
3 (6-ounce) cans skinless, boneless pink salmon in water, drained
¼ cup sliced green onions
¼ cup canola mayonnaise
2 tablespoons dry breadcrumbs
1 teaspoon salt-free Cajun seasoning blend
2 teaspoons Dijon mustard
½ cup dry breadcrumbs
1 tablespoon canola oil
Chopped fresh parsley (optional)
Lemon wedges (optional)

1. To prepare aioli, combine first 3 ingredients in a bowl; set aside.

2. To prepare cakes, combine salmon and next 5 ingredients in a medium bowl. Divide salmon mixture into 8 equal portions, shaping each portion into a (½-inch-thick) patty. Dredge patties in ½ cup breadcrumbs.

3. Heat a large nonstick skillet over medium-high heat. Add oil to pan; swirl to coat. Place patties in pan; cook 3 minutes on each side or until lightly browned and heated through. Serve aioli over salmon. Garnish with parsley and lemon wedges, if desired. Serves 4 (serving size: 2 patties and about 1½ teaspoons aioli).

CALORIES 346; FAT 23.8g (sat 1.9g, mono 13g, poly 7g); PROTEIN 23.8g; CARB 10.2g; FIBER 0.8g; CHOL 71mg; IRON 1.3mg; SODIUM 650mg; CALC 28mg

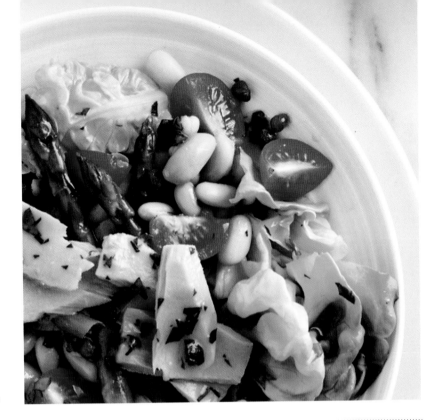

Tuna and White Bean Salad

20 asparagus spears
1 tablespoon capers, drained
1 tablespoon chopped fresh flat-leaf parsley
2 tablespoons white wine vinegar
2 tablespoons fresh lemon juice
2 tablespoons extra-virgin olive oil
1 tablespoon butter, melted
¼ teaspoon salt
¼ teaspoon black pepper
1 cup cherry tomatoes, quartered
1 (15-ounce) can organic white beans, rinsed and drained
4 cups torn butter lettuce (about 1 head)
2 (5-ounce) cans solid white tuna packed in olive oil, drained and broken into chunks

1. Snap off tough ends of asparagus spears. Steam asparagus, covered, 3 minutes. Drain and rinse with cold water; drain.

2. Combine capers and next 7 ingredients in a small bowl, stirring well with a whisk.

3. Place ¼ cup juice mixture, cherry tomatoes, and beans in a small bowl; toss gently to combine.

4. Place 1 cup lettuce on each of 4 plates, and top each serving with 5 asparagus spears. Spoon about ½ cup white bean mixture over each serving, and divide tuna evenly among servings. Drizzle each salad with about 1 tablespoon remaining juice mixture. Serves 4.

CALORIES 270; FAT 14.6g (sat 3.5g, mono 7.4g, poly 2.5g); PROTEIN 20.2g; CARB 16g; FIBER 5.6g; CHOL 24mg; IRON 2.4mg; SODIUM 467mg; CALC 65mg

It can be tricky when reading labels of canned or jarred tuna and salmon. A sustainable fish may be inside, or it may be an endangered species from overfished waters. Look for species type, and where, when, and how it was fished or raised. If that information is not there, look for a more ecofriendly option that is clearly labeled.

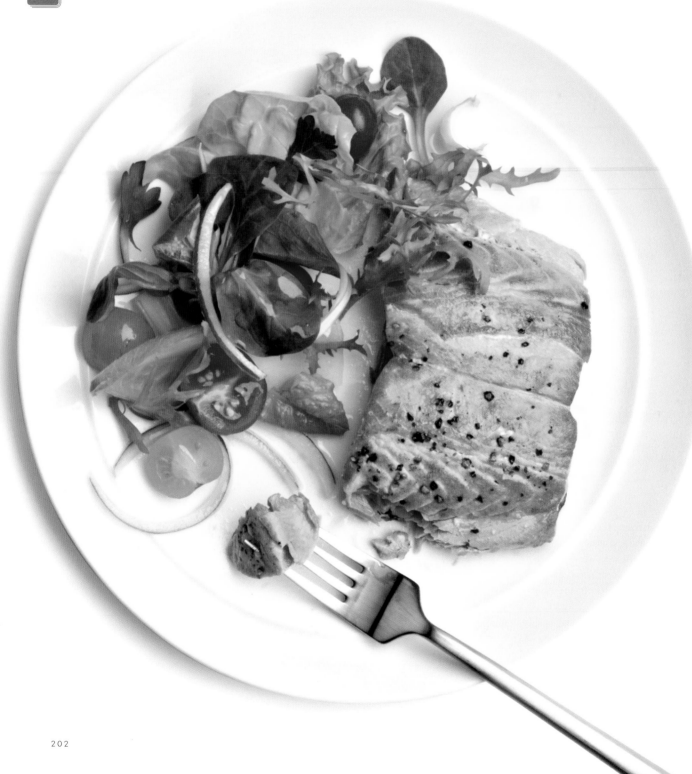

EAT MORE HEALTHY FATS

DON'T SKIP. SWAP!

I'T'S HARD TO DENY: Butter is delicious, bacon makes dishes better, and a splash of cream rarely hurts anything. Fats make food taste good. The problem is, Americans don't stop at a little, and we're eating way too much saturated fat. Then there are those people on the other end of the spectrum—leftovers from the low-fat era—who rely on fat-free or reduced-fat products that leave them unsatisfied and low on healthy fats.

Here's a primer on fats: Our bodies need fat to function properly. But saturated fats—those found in foods such as meats, butter, and other high-fat dairy products—tend, when eaten too often, to raise LDL ("bad") cholesterol levels and promote plaque buildup in your arteries. This is also true of trans fats, which are the result of the process that turns liquid fats solid for use in shortening, margarine, and processed foods. Saturated fat intake should be kept to less than 7% of total daily calories; trans fats should be avoided.

As for butter, we've got some good news: You don't have to give it up. You just need creative ways to substitute heart-healthy fats for the saturated kind more often.

The fats that we do need are the monounsaturated and polyunsaturated ones that help our bodies absorb vitamins and minerals from foods, lower LDL and total cholesterol, and keep us feeling full and satisfied. Replace unhealthy fats with good ones; those you'll find in vegetable oils, fish, nuts and nut butters, seeds, and avocados.

You'll find lots of ideas about swapping the bad for the good in this chapter, along with a plan to help you enjoy healthy fats more often.

YOUR GOAL

Increase healthy fats and decrease unhealthy fats every day.

The 12 Healthy Habits

| · 01 · GET COOKING | · 02 · BREAKFAST DAILY | · 03 · WHOLE GRAINS | · 04 · GET MOVING | · 05 · VEGGIE UP | · 06 · MORE SEAFOOD | · 07 · HEALTHY FATS | · 08 · GO MEATLESS | · 09 · GET STRONGER | · 10 · LESS SALT | · 11 · BE PORTION- AWARE | · 12 · EAT MINDFULLY |

The Facts on Fat

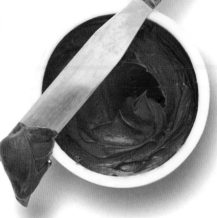

The Key Players

MONOUNSATURATED FAT

Found in: Canola, olive, and peanut oils, as well as peanuts, pecans, and avocados

What you need to know: These plant-based fats lower cholesterol when used in place of saturated fat in your diet. Research also suggests that they may have other health benefits: One study, for example, found that this type of fat helps trim weight around the waist, which is important because fat stored deep around the belly increases risk for heart disease, diabetes, breast cancer, and high blood pressure.

Smart cooking strategies: While olive oil attracts the most attention, canola and peanut oils are both good sources of monounsaturated fat and have high smoke points (the temperature where oil begins to burn); canola oil has a mild flavor, which is great for baking or sautéing, while peanut oil delivers nutty flavor to stir-fries or Asian-inspired vinaigrettes.

POLYUNSATURATED FAT

Found in: Vegetable oils like soybean, corn, and sunflower; oily fish like tuna and mackerel; and most nuts and seeds

What you need to know: These plant- and fish-derived fats lower cholesterol when they replace saturated fat in your diet. Fatty fish like salmon and tuna contain omega-3 fatty acids (a type of polysaturated fat), while certain nuts and oils offer another type.

Smart cooking strategies: Use small amounts of nuts and oils in cooking. Toast nuts and seeds to intensify flavor, and sprinkle them on top of a salad or dish to get the most textural and flavorful impact. And eat more fish—aim for at least two servings per week. See page 169 for more information.

The Not-So-Key Players

SATURATED FAT

Found in: Beef, lamb, pork, bacon, cheese, whole-milk yogurt, butter, whole milk, coconut, coconut oil, palm oil, and palm kernel oil

What you need to know: These solid fats raise LDL cholesterol and increase heart disease risk. The American Heart Association advises limiting saturated fat to less than 7% of total calories, about 15 grams for the average person on a 2,000-calorie-a-day diet. (If you're counting, a teaspoon of butter contains nearly 3 grams of saturated fat, and a 3-ounce filet mignon has about 10 grams.)

TRANS FAT

Found in: Any products with partially hydrogenated oils in the ingredient list

What you need to know: Produced when liquid oils are processed into solid shortenings and margarines, trans fats raise LDL or "bad" cholesterol, and lower HDL or "good" cholesterol. These artificial fats are also more likely to raise insulin resistance, which is a precursor to diabetes.

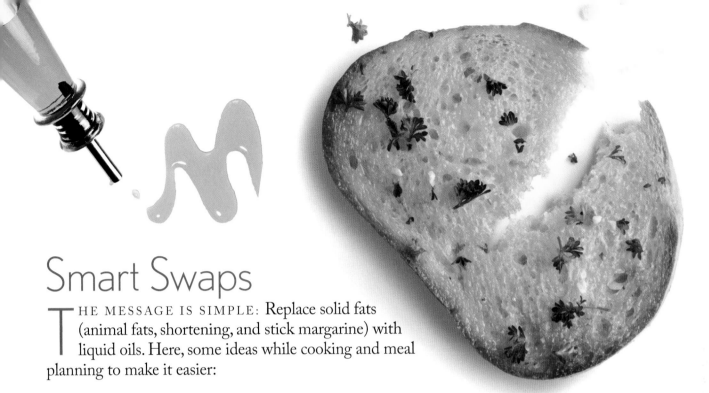

Smart Swaps

THE MESSAGE IS SIMPLE: Replace solid fats (animal fats, shortening, and stick margarine) with liquid oils. Here, some ideas while cooking and meal planning to make it easier:

Instead of butter:
Sub in olive or canola oil when you sauté or stir-fry. If you can't live without the taste of butter, cut the saturated fat in half by using equal parts olive oil and melted butter.

Instead of regular mayo:
Sub in canola or olive oil mayonnaise for dips, casseroles, and salad dressings.

Instead of creamy bottled salad dressings:
Sub in homemade vinaigrettes with extra-virgin olive oil (see pages 222–223 for tips on making your own).

Instead of dips with a sour cream base:
Sub in hummus, guacamole, or nut-based dips (like Muhammara on page 217) to serve with fresh veggies.

Just because a food is labeled "trans-fat free" doesn't mean it's a healthy choice. It might still be high in saturated fat or have lots of sugar and empty calories. So take a closer look before it lands in your shopping cart.

EXPERT TIP: *Get to Know The Nuances of Olive Oil*

"As with wines, there are many different expressions of aroma and flavor. Some olive oils have a greener, more peppery taste, while others are golden and smooth. Explore the way some mellow out the bite of dark green lettuces in a tossed salad while others add a bright note to baked chicken."

—*Carolyn O'Neil, MS, RD, blogger, Dish on Dieting*

Munchie Makeover

W ITH BUSY LIVES AND HECTIC SCHEDULES, it's no surprise your pantry may need a facelift. The problem is, crackers, cookies, and other snacky foods often harbor unhealthy trans fats, a particular type of fatty acid created during processing when hydrogen is added to liquid vegetable oil to make it solid. A labeling loophole allows food makers to list 0g trans fats if a single serving of the food has less than half a gram. Eat two servings, though, and you might have consumed nearly half the daily limit of 2 grams. Here, smart choices that will up your intake of healthy fats without sacrificing taste:

DARK CHOCOLATE AND NUTS

You'll get healthier mono- and polyun-saturated fats from the nuts; you can even add in some dried fruit to displace some of the chocolate.

OLIVES

They gratify a salty craving and help you feel satiated, yet unlike traditional salty snacks like pretzels and potato chips, they supply a decent amount of heart-healthy fats.

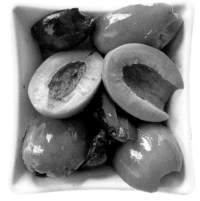

ROASTED ALMONDS

They may look high in fat, but it's really the healthy kind. In fact, studies show that consuming small amounts of nuts regularly has been linked to reduced risk of heart disease. Try roasting them with flavorful ingredients such as cinnamon, coriander, or fresh rosemary (like the recipes starting on page 212). Just prac-tice portion control: One ounce (about 20 almonds) has about 170 calories.

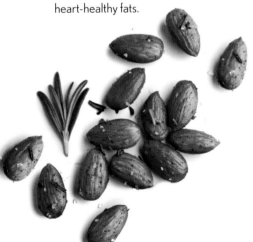

WHAT'S A SERVING?

While this chapter is all about embracing the good-for-you fats, it's important to keep an eye on your daily intake. For a 2,000-calorie diet, the daily recommendation is 2 tablespoons of oil a day. Below, the amount of healthy fat equal to 1 tablespoon of oil:

- 2 tablespoons Italian dressing
- 1 tablespoon canola mayonnaise
- 4 large olives
- ½ medium avocado
- 2 tablespoons peanut butter
- 1 ounce almonds
- 1 ounce seeds

FRUIT AND NUT BUTTER

Fresh fruit is a no-brainer when it comes to healthful snacks. But you can make it more palatable to your crew by topping it with your favorite peanut or other nut butter—a tablespoon will provide you about one-fourth of your daily healthy fat intake. (Just read the label to make sure it doesn't have any artery-clogging trans fats added in there.)

BAKED CHIPS WITH HOMEMADE GUACAMOLE

Avocados are powerhouses of healthy fats. While they're high in calories, it's worth it for their rich buttery taste. It's also supersimple to make your own guacamole.

Quick Snack
Guacamole with Fish Sauce

This recipe is for when you have perfectly ripe avocados—there's no need to add tomato or other complications. Place 2 ripe peeled and seeded avocados in a medium bowl; mash roughly with a fork. Add 1 tablespoon fresh lime juice, 1 teaspoon Thai fish sauce, and ¼ teaspoon kosher salt; mash to desired consistency. Stir in 2 tablespoons chopped fresh cilantro. Garnish with additional cilantro, if desired. Serves 4 (serving size: about ¼ cup).

CALORIES 163; FAT 14.7g (sat 2.1g, mono 9.9g, poly 1.8g); PROTEIN 2.1g; CARB 9.3g; FIBER 6.8g; CHOL 0mg; IRON 0.6mg; SODIUM 243mg; CALC 14mg

> ### READER TIP:
> *Make Your Own Nut Butter*
>
> "I love peanut butter...with chocolate, on pretzels and crackers, on bananas, on carrot sticks, or on sandwiches. I'm not limited to peanut butter, though. Any nut will do. There is nothing quite like spreading warm, fresh cashew butter onto a piece of toasted bread. In fact, once you make (and taste) your own, anything store-bought seems to pale in comparison."
>
> —*Caroline Ford*

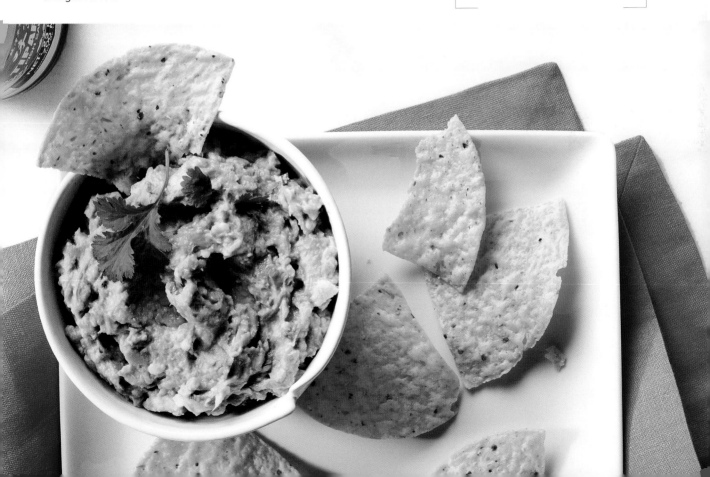

Keep It Balanced

ADDING HEALTHY UNSATURATED FATS to your meals doesn't mean completely nixing the saturated ones. "The richness fat provides, especially in butter and cream, is part of what makes comfort foods so comfy," says Tiffany Vickers Davis, assistant test kitchen director at *Cooking Light*. "You don't have to cut beloved dairy fats out of your life entirely. You just need creative ways to substitute heart-healthy fats for unhealthy saturated fats more frequently. Here, she shares what she's learned:

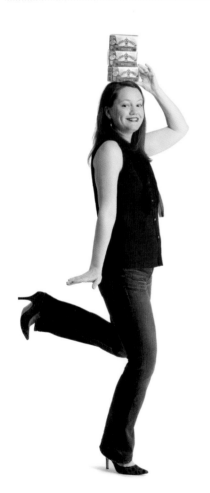

The Raised-on-Butter Cook

"I've learned how to balance my love of butter with healthier fats."

TIFFANY VICKERS DAVIS
Cooking Light *Assistant Test Kitchen Director*

➤ **HEALTHY FAT CHALLENGE:** Being a senior member of the *Cooking Light* Test Kitchen has made Tiffany Vickers Davis an expert on healthy cooking but not immune to the lure of a little extra butter. Tiffany's family emigrated from Germany when she was young. Despite the move, the kitchen remained strictly northern European. "My mother made lots of cream soups and boiled potatoes with butter." Like anyone else working in a kitchen, Tiffany is surrounded by food, including butter and cream. Here's what she's learned to keep her diet in check while not missing out on the flavors she loves:

HER ADVICE

■ **Think of a meal as a balancing act.** Indulge in one rich food, then balance it with healthier choices. If you're having ribeye (high in saturated fat), make leaner sides. Instead of baked potatoes topped with sour cream, boil or roast spuds and toss with tasty olive oil and fresh herbs. Replace creamy salad dressings with a heart-healthy vinaigrette.

■ **Use butter to finish dishes.** Cooking with butter throughout your meal ups your saturated fat intake. For maximum flavor impact, add it toward the end instead. Sauté veggies in olive or canola oil, then use a bit of butter to finish, tossing to melt and coat. Sprinkle buttered breadcrumbs on top of pasta dishes as a last touch. This way, the flavor will be up front on your palate when you bite in.

The Snack–Happy Family

"Our family loves sweets, cookies, and chips of every kind."

MONICA INGLES
Cake Shop Owner

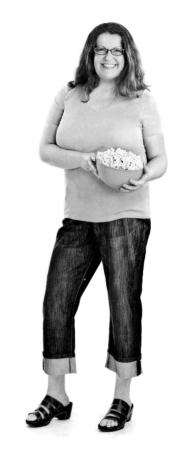

➤ **HEALTHY FAT CHALLENGE:** With Monica's hectic schedule and her family's picky palates, her pantry is filled with processed foods. "When he was small," Monica says, "my oldest son would eat a variety of healthy foods, and then it was like somebody flipped a switch: Suddenly, all he wanted was snack foods. I want what they're eating to nourish their bodies, but I don't want the constant argument that it doesn't taste good." The key to turning this situation around is finding healthy snacks that deliver on convenience, taste, and nutrition.

OUR ADVICE

■ **Don't ditch your favorite snacks; revamp them.** Try whole-grain crackers and lightly toasted almonds mixed with seasonings instead of chips and cheese curls. If your kids love stuffed pretzels, try low-sodium pretzels dipped in peanut butter. Sliced apples spread with peanut butter are a delicious alternative to sugary caramel-covered apple wedges.

■ **Pop your own popcorn.** Many microwave popcorns harbor hefty amounts of saturated and trans fats. Reduce those solid fats by popping your own: Heat kernels (¼ cup of kernels makes about 8 cups) with toasted sesame oil or peanut oil in a Dutch oven until they pop; sprinkle lightly with kosher salt. Or, if you have a sweet tooth, sprinkle on some cinnamon sugar. Bonus: Popcorn is a whole grain!

■ **Get creative with candy.** Customize your own chocolate bark using melted dark chocolate combined with chopped nuts and dried fruit. Or make a chocolate trail mix with antioxidant-rich dark chocolate chips, nuts, and whole-grain cereal. Then portion the mix into single-serve bags for easy grabbing.

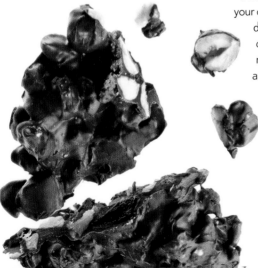

Reduce fat and sodium by baking your own pita, tortilla, and veggie chips. Make your own onion, ranch, or avocado dip using fat-free Greek yogurt and olive oil.

Nuts: An A-Z Guide

D ESPITE WHAT FAT-PHOBES MAY THINK, nuts are not a dietary no-no. These healthy-fat power players offer a satisfying crunch and a variety of health perks. Here's a rundown of some of the best (and tastiest!) options:

ALMONDS
Studies show that a handful a day—about 23 almonds—can help lower LDL cholesterol levels and fight inflammation.

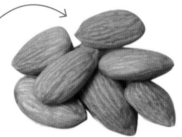

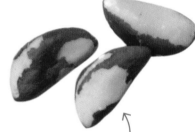

CHESTNUTS
Chestnuts contain a high amount of starch and little oil—1 ounce contains just 0.5g total fat. They also offer a healthy dose of potassium.

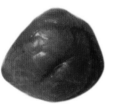

BRAZIL NUTS
They pack a punch of selenium, a mineral and antioxidant that may help prevent certain types of cancer.

CASHEWS
High in oleic acid, a monounsaturated fat also found in olive oil, cashews may help reduce blood pressure.

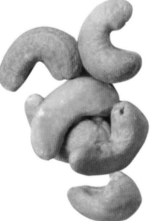

HAZELNUTS
They're an excellent source of vitamin E, dietary fiber, magnesium, and a heart-healthy compound called proanthocyanidin.

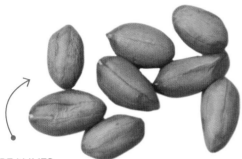

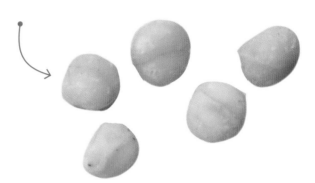

MACADAMIA NUTS

They are one of the few plant sources of palmitoleic acid, which helps lower cholestorol and reduce risk of heart disease.

PEANUTS

Studies show that eating peanuts and peanut butter can lower cholesterol levels and triglycerides, decreasing your risk of heart disease.

PECANS

They're rich in vitamin E, flavonoids, and plant sterols, natural compounds that help lower cholesterol.

PINE NUTS

Each tiny kernel packs a surprising amount of vitamin E, manganese, copper, and magnesium.

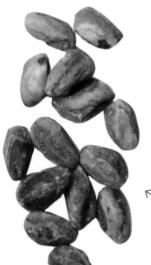

PISTACHIOS

They're rich in carotenoids, including beta-carotene and lutein.

WALNUTS

Studies show that walnuts can increase good cholesterol and decrease the bad kind.

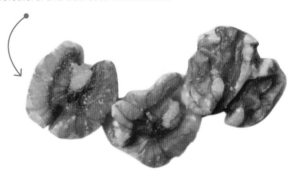

Go a Little Nuts

THERE ARE PLENTY OF REASONS TO NOSH ON NUTS: They're packed with healthy fats, plant protein, dietary fiber, and nutrients like vitamin E and folic acid. Studies show frequent nut-eaters have a lower risk of heart disease and diabetes and tend to be thinner than people who never or rarely eat nuts. Dietary guidelines recommend 4 ounces per week. Here are five easy ways to add them to your diet:

1. START YOUR DAY WITH NUTS.

Top your oatmeal or yogurt parfait with walnuts, slivered almonds, or nut butters. The extra hit of protein helps boost the staying power of your breakfast.

2. MAKE YOUR OWN TRAIL MIX.

Combine dry-roasted, lightly salted nuts (peanuts, cashews, pistachios, almonds, and macadamia nuts) with dried fruits, such as raisins, dried cranberries, chopped dried apricots, or figs.

3. ADD CRUNCH TO SALADS.

In place of croutons or bacon bits, sprinkle salads with pistachios, walnuts, pecans, or other nuts.

4. TRY NUTTY SAUCES.

Ground nuts make a flavorful base for a Mediterranean-style sauce, like Cilantro-Walnut Pesto on page 216, or a dip for veggies or to spread on pita and bruschetta.

5. BAKE THEM IN.

Add them to breads, muffins, cookies, and cakes: Sprinkling nuts on top of the batter before it bakes, rather than mixing them in, helps ensure a bit of nutty flavor.

This walnut-based sauce provides a dose of healthy fats. See recipe on page 216.

Sweet Spiced Almonds

These nuts are a wonderful addition to a salad or served as a snack.

1 cup sliced almonds
1/3 cup packed brown sugar
1 teaspoon ground cinnamon
1/2 teaspoon ground coriander
1/2 teaspoon ground cumin
1 large egg white, lightly beaten
Cooking spray

1. Preheat oven to 325°.
2. Combine almonds and next 4 ingredients in a small bowl. Stir in egg white. Spread mixture evenly onto a foil-lined baking sheet coated with cooking spray. Bake at 325° for 10 minutes. Stir mixture; bake an additional 15 minutes or until crisp. Transfer foil to a wire rack; cool almond mixture. Break almond mixture into small pieces. Serves 16 (serving size: 2 tablespoons).
Note: Store at room temperature in an airtight container for up to one week.

CALORIES 54; FAT 3g (sat 0.2g, mono 2g, poly 0.8g); PROTEIN 1.6g; CARB 5.8g; FIBER 0.8g; CHOL 0mg; IRON 0.4mg; SODIUM 6mg; CALC 22mg

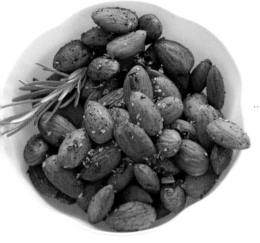

Rosemary Roasted Almonds

Fresh rosemary lends a wonderful fragrance, and chili powder provides just the right amount of spiciness. "These are my absolute favorite snack!" said KRFoodie on Cooking-Light.com. "I use dried rosemary instead of fresh."

1 tablespoon finely chopped
   fresh rosemary
1 tablespoon extra-virgin olive oil
1 teaspoon chili powder
3/4 teaspoon kosher salt
Dash of ground red pepper
1 (10-ounce) bag whole almonds
   (about 2 cups)

1. Preheat oven to 325°.
2. Combine all ingredients in a medium bowl; toss to coat. Arrange nut mixture in a single layer on a baking sheet lined with foil. Bake at 325° for 20 minutes or until lightly toasted. Cool to room temperature. Serves 16 (serving size: 2 tablespoons).

CALORIES 111; FAT 9.9g (sat 0.8g, mono 6.3g, poly 2.3g); PROTEIN 3.8g; CARB 3.6g; FIBER 2.1g; CHOL 0mg; IRON 0.8mg; SODIUM 94mg; CALC 45mg

---

Seven nuts qualify for the FDA health claim related to heart disease prevention: almonds, hazelnuts, peanuts, pecans, pine nuts, pistachios, and walnuts. Brazil nuts, cashews, and macadamias, while still healthy, do not meet the criteria because of their higher saturated fat levels.

Orange Chipotle Spiced Pecan Mix

Prepare a batch of this smoky-sweet mix to have on hand or pack into decorative jars to give as gifts. "The best!" said Carson5000 on CookingLight.com. "I think it's worth it to get the chipotle pepper; it really adds a unique flavor to the nut mix. We had these on our hors d'oeuvres table, and I swear people ate more of these nuts than anything else. The cranberries give it a nice tang and balance the spice out perfectly."

1 tablespoon grated orange rind
1 tablespoon fresh orange juice
1 large egg white
2 cups pecan halves
1 tablespoon dark brown sugar
1 teaspoon kosher salt
1/2 teaspoon ground chipotle
   chile pepper
Cooking spray
1/2 cup sweetened dried cranberries

1. Preheat oven to 225°.
2. Combine first 3 ingredients in a medium bowl; stir with a whisk. Stir in pecans. Combine sugar, salt, and pepper. Add to pecan mixture; toss well. Arrange mixture in a single layer on a jelly-roll pan coated with cooking spray. Bake at 225° for 1 hour, stirring occasionally. Remove from oven; cool completely. Stir in cranberries. Serves 20 (serving size: 2 tablespoons).
Note: Store in an airtight container for up to one week.

CALORIES 91; FAT 7.7g (sat 0.7g, mono 4.6g, poly 2.4g); PROTEIN 1.2g; CARB 4.8g; FIBER 0.8g; CHOL 0mg; IRON 0.3mg; SODIUM 98mg; CALC 1mg

---

EXPERT TIP: *Fats Have Staying Power*

"People have a tendency to fill up on foods that do not have much fat, but then they feel hungry soon after eating. Including some healthy fats will make your meal or snack more satisfying. For instance, a trail mix with almonds and dried fruit will have a lot more staying power compared to the dried fruit alone."

—*Bonnie Taub-Dix, MA, RD, blogger, Better Than Dieting*

Oops! The Biggest Fat Mistakes

YOU MIGHT THINK YOU'RE BEING HEALTHY, but these four common mistakes may be upping your intake of saturated fat and lowering your intake of good-for-you fats.

1. OOPS! You automatically swap turkey bacon for the pork kind.
Result: Bacon is a prime example of why label-reading is important. Some versions of turkey bacon contain as much saturated fat as pork bacon.
What to do: Look for lean, lower-sodium turkey bacon or opt for a lean pork kind such as center-cut.

2. OOPS! You trade ground turkey for ground beef in recipes to save saturated fat.
Result: A quarter pound of regular ground turkey contains 3 grams saturated fat, compared to only 2.5 grams in the same amount of sirloin.
What to do: Buy ground turkey breast, which has just half a gram of saturated fat.

3. OOPS! You spoon on whole flaxseeds.
Result: While flaxseeds are an excellent way to add omega-3 fatty acids to baked goods, oatmeal, and cereal, the whole seeds tend to, um, pass right through.
What to do: Grind the seeds; unlock the goodness.

4. OOPS! You buy 80/20 ground beef thinking only 20% of the calories come from fat.
Result: The 80/20 percentage refers to the proportion of fat and protein in the grind, not the proportion of calories. As a result, you're getting way more fat in your burger or meat loaf than you thought.
What to do: Buy a much leaner grind, such as 90/10, or ask for a lean whole cut like sirloin to be custom ground for you, which will be fresher anyway.

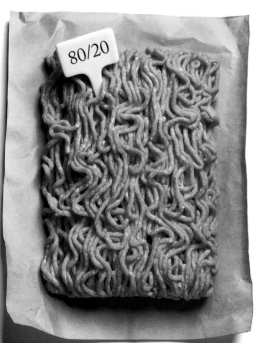

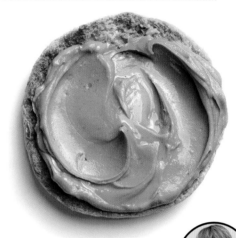

READER TIP:
Switch Up Stir-Fries

"Experimenting with stir-fries is one of the most effective ways I incorporate healthy oils. I use olive oil a lot—my husband is Greek, so you've got to use the olive oil—and I've been using sesame oil as a finishing touch for flavor in our stir-fries or in a marinade for chicken or steak."

—*Julianne Saratsis*,
Cooking Light
Healthy Habits Graduate

The Woman Who Fears Fat

"I don't understand the difference between good and bad fat."

YAEL DRINKLE
YMCA Program Director

➤ **HEALTHY FAT CHALLENGE:** In her quest to lose weight, Yael has become an obsessive label reader and tends to buy only "fat-free" or "low-fat" fare, including reduced-fat peanut butter. But her fat monitoring may actually be hampering her health, since she's probably not getting enough good-for-you fats into her overall diet.

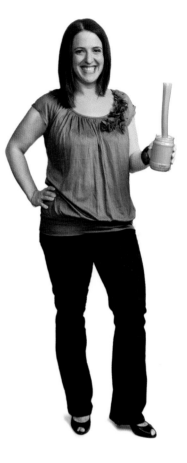

OUR ADVICE

■ **Shift your focus away from total fat.** Don't just look at the total fat on the label: It includes bad fats *and* good fats, so it's misleading. Instead, look at the specific types of fat listed under total fat. Aim for more mono- and poly-unsaturated fats, and no trans.

■ **Know a good fat when you see it.** If a fat is liquid at room temperature, such as olive and canola oils, it's likely a good fat. If the fat is solid at room temperature (butter, lard, or shortening), it's higher in saturated fat and may contain trans fats. Every rule has exceptions, though. In this case, it's dairy, which can be high in saturated fat whether solid (cheese) or liquid (cream).

■ **Low-fat isn't always better.** Don't automatically default to the low-fat version. In the case of reduced-fat peanut butter, you might be saving some calories and fat grams, but you're missing out on the healthy oils that have been stripped away. Instead, you're getting fillers like sweeteners, thickeners, and hydrogenated oils. It's not a good trade-off.

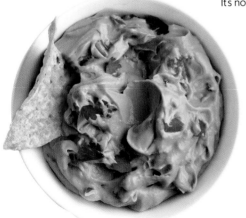

It's been touted that coconut oil fights heart disease and promotes weight loss, but there's limited evidence to back up those claims. It's true that coconut oil may not raise blood cholesterol as much as other saturated fats, but stick with vegetable oils that have reams of research supporting their benefits.

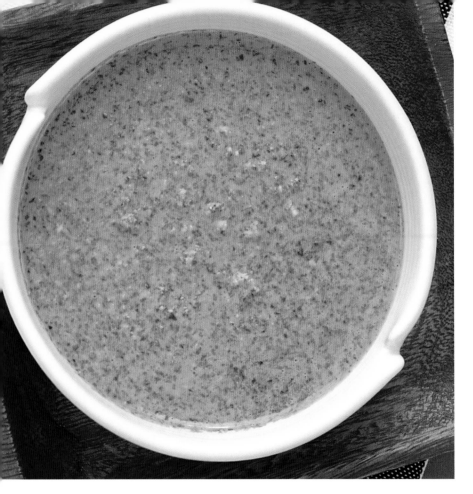

Cilantro-Walnut Pesto

3 garlic cloves
3 cups packed cilantro leaves and
   tender stems (about 3 ounces)
¼ cup chopped walnuts, toasted
2 tablespoons white wine vinegar
½ teaspoon salt
¼ cup organic vegetable broth
3 tablespoons extra-virgin olive oil

1. Place garlic in a food processor;
pulse 10 times or until minced. Add
cilantro and next 3 ingredients to
processor; process 15 seconds. Combine broth and oil in a small bowl.
With processor on, slowly pour broth
mixture through food chute; process
until well blended. Serves 16 (serving
size: 1 tablespoon).

CALORIES 37; FAT 3.9g (sat 0.5g, mono 2.1g, poly 1.2g);
PROTEIN 0.4g; CARB 0.7g; FIBER 0.3g; CHOL 0mg;
IRON 0.2mg; SODIUM 85mg; CALCIUM 6mg

Discover Nut Sauces and Dips

ONE DELICIOUS WAY TO WORK more nuts into your diet is to grind them into rich, savory sauces and dips. It's a technique used throughout the Mediterranean. Try a variety of Italian pestos with nuts and herbs or the Middle Eastern dip muhammara.

To prevent pesto
from browning
while it's stored
in the refrigerator,
place a piece of plastic
wrap directly on the
surface. Serve pesto
with fresh vegetables,
use it as a pizza topping,
or spread on crostini.

Muhammara with Crudités

Muhammara is a sweet-spicy Middle Eastern dip made with roasted bell pepper, walnuts, and, traditionally, Aleppo pepper and pomegranate molasses. To make it easy, this version is made with readily available crushed red pepper and honey.

3 red bell peppers
¼ cup walnut halves, toasted and divided
¼ cup plain dry breadcrumbs
3 tablespoons extra-virgin olive oil
2 tablespoons tomato paste
1 teaspoon ground cumin
1 teaspoon honey
½ teaspoon salt
¼ teaspoon crushed red pepper
⅛ teaspoon ground cinnamon
1 garlic clove
2 tablespoons fresh lime juice
18 radishes, halved
18 baby carrots with tops, trimmed
18 baby lettuce leaves (such as baby romaine)

1. Preheat broiler.
2. Cut bell peppers in half lengthwise; discard seeds and membranes. Place pepper halves, skin sides up, on a foil-lined baking sheet; flatten with hand. Broil 20 minutes or until blackened. Place in a zip-top plastic bag; seal. Let stand 20 minutes. Peel peppers, and discard skins.
3. Place 4 bell pepper halves, 3 tablespoons walnuts, breadcrumbs, and next 8 ingredients in a food processor, and process until smooth. Add remaining 2 bell pepper halves; pulse until coarsely chopped. Spoon dip into a bowl; stir in juice. Top with remaining 1 tablespoon walnuts. Serve with radishes, carrots, and lettuce. Serves 6 (serving size: about ½ cup dip, 6 radish halves, 3 carrots, and 3 lettuce leaves).

CALORIES 155; FAT 10.1g (sat 1.3g, mono 5.4g, poly 3g); PROTEIN 2.7g; CARB 14.5g; FIBER 3.6g; CHOL 0mg; IRON 1.5mg; SODIUM 317mg; CALCIUM 42mg

SEEK OUT SEEDS

Similar to nuts, seeds are compact packages of good-for-you fats. Get to know pumpkinseeds (pepitas), sunflower seeds, sesame seeds, and flaxseeds. Most are plentiful in protein, too. Flaxseeds have the added benefit of ALA omega-3, the plant source of this heart-healthy fatty acid.

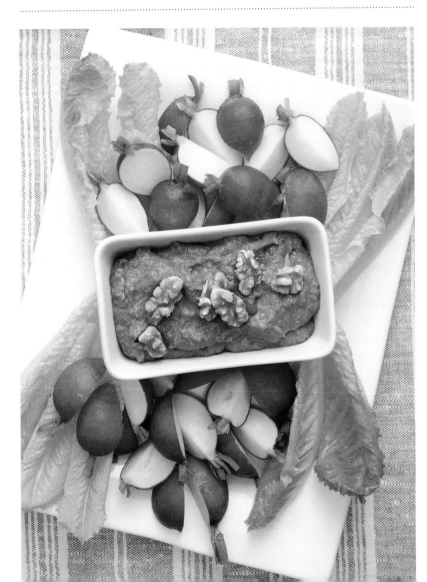

Go Beyond Guacamole

DON'T THINK OF AVOCADOS as simply a key ingredient in the classic Mexican dip. This creamy green fruit deserves a regular spot on your menu rotation. Rich, filling, and packed with healthy monounsaturated fats, avocados are the perfect addition to salads, sandwiches, soups, and entrées.

Roasted Corn and Radish Salad with Avocado-Herb Dressing

The cool creaminess of avocado helps temper the spicy bite from the radishes and adds extra flavor and texture.

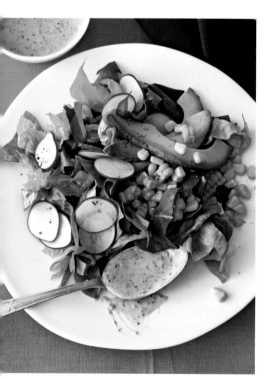

½ ripe peeled avocado, sliced
1 teaspoon fresh lime juice
2 ears yellow corn with husks
2 heads Boston or Bibb lettuce
½ cup thinly sliced radishes
½ cup Avocado-Herb Dressing
  (recipe at right)

1. Preheat oven to 450°.
2. Combine sliced avocado and juice in a small bowl; cover and refrigerate. Trim both ends of corn cobs, leaving husks from corn intact. Place corn on a baking sheet. Bake at 450° for 20 minutes or until tender. Cool. Remove husks from corn; scrub silks from corn. Cut kernels from ears of corn; discard cobs.
3. Chop lettuce to measure 4 cups. Combine chopped lettuce, avocado mixture, corn, and radishes. Serve with Avocado-Herb Dressing. Serves 4 (serving size: 1 cup salad and 2 tablespoons dressing).

CALORIES 200; FAT 15.5g (sat 2.2g, mono 8.4g, poly 3.4g); PROTEIN 3.8g; CARB 14.7g; FIBER 4.8g; CHOL 9mg; IRON 1.6mg; SODIUM 165mg; CALC 51mg

Avocado-Herb Dressing

½ cup canola mayonnaise
¼ cup finely chopped green onions
¼ cup reduced-fat sour cream
1 tablespoon chopped fresh
  flat-leaf parsley
1 tablespoon chopped fresh chives
1 teaspoon chopped fresh tarragon
1 teaspoon anchovy paste
⅛ teaspoon salt
1 garlic clove, minced
½ ripe peeled avocado
2 tablespoons water
1 tablespoon white wine vinegar
3 drops hot sauce

1. Place first 10 ingredients in a food processor; process until smooth. With processor on, pour 2 tablespoons water, vinegar, and hot sauce through food chute, processing until blended. Store dressing in an airtight container in refrigerator. Serves 20 (serving size: 1 tablespoon).

CALORIES 54; FAT 5.6g (sat 0.8g, mono 2.9g, poly 1.3g); PROTEIN 0.3g; CARB 0.8g; FIBER 0.4g; CHOL 4mg; IRON 0.1mg; SODIUM 73mg; CALC 7mg

Avocado Corn Chowder with Grilled Chicken

"I made this without the chicken and added more veggies, and it was oustanding," said TravelChickie on CookingLight.com. Jeanne1 thought it was amazing: "I did not stir in any of the toppings but instead served them in small dishes so each soup serving was a 'make it like you like it' sort of thing. It was perfect and so easy."

2 ripe avocados, divided
1½ cups water
½ cup fresh orange juice
1 teaspoon honey
1 teaspoon kosher salt, divided
½ teaspoon freshly ground
   black pepper, divided
¼ teaspoon ground red
   pepper (optional)
12 ounces skinless, boneless
   chicken breast
1 teaspoon olive oil
1 small garlic clove, cut in half
1½ cups fresh corn kernels
   (about 3 ears)
1 cup chopped red bell pepper
⅓ cup chopped green onions
¼ cup chopped fresh cilantro
4 lime wedges

1. Peel and coarsely chop 1 avocado; place in a blender. Add 1½ cups water, orange juice, honey, ¾ teaspoon salt, ¼ teaspoon black pepper, and, if desired, red pepper; blend until smooth. Place in freezer to chill while chicken cooks.

2. Heat a grill pan over medium-high heat. Brush chicken with oil; sprinkle with remaining ¼ teaspoon salt and remaining ¼ teaspoon black pepper. Add chicken to pan; cook 4 minutes on each side or until done. Remove chicken from pan; rub chicken with cut sides of garlic halves. Let chicken stand 10 minutes; cut or shred into bite-sized pieces.

3. Peel and dice remaining avocado. Stir diced avocado, corn, bell pepper, and onions into chilled avocado puree. Spoon chowder into each of 4 bowls; top with chicken and cilantro. Serve with lime wedges. Serves 4 (serving size: 1¼ cups chowder, about 2 ounces chicken, 1 tablespoon cilantro, and 1 lime wedge).

CALORIES 359; FAT 17.9g (sat 2.7g, mono 11.2g, poly 2.6g); PROTEIN 24.5g; CARB 30g; FIBER 9.7g; CHOL 49mg; IRON 2mg; SODIUM 558mg; CALC 39mg

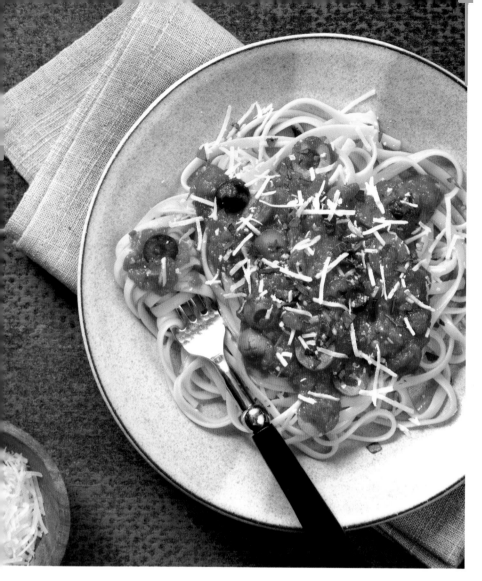

Linguine with Two-Olive Marinara

This recipe's versatile sauce can also be spooned over cheese ravioli, used as a topping for pizza, or served with breadsticks as an appetizer. Cook the linguine while the sauce simmers.

2 teaspoons olive oil
2/3 cup chopped onion
2 teaspoons fresh minced garlic
3/4 cup sliced pitted green olives (about 15)
1 (2 1/4-ounce) can sliced ripe olives, drained
1/4 teaspoon sugar
1/4 teaspoon crushed red pepper
1/4 teaspoon black pepper
1/4 teaspoon dried oregano
1/3 cup dry white wine
1 (28-ounce) can crushed tomatoes, undrained
10 ounces uncooked linguine
3/4 cup (3 ounces) grated fresh Parmesan cheese
2 tablespoons chopped fresh parsley

1. Heat a Dutch oven over medium-high heat. Add oil to pan; swirl to coat. Add onion; sauté 3 minutes or until tender. Stir in garlic; sauté 1 minute. Add olives; sauté 30 seconds. Stir in sugar, red pepper, black pepper, and oregano; cook 1 minute, stirring constantly. Add wine; cook 30 seconds. Stir in tomatoes; bring to a boil. Reduce heat; simmer 30 minutes. Remove from heat; keep warm.
2. Cook pasta according to package directions, omitting salt and fat. Drain. Arrange 2/3 cup pasta on each

Open Up to Olives

OLIVE OIL SEEMS TO GET ALL THE GLORY, but olives themselves are worthy of your attention, too. These tiny, brined fruits—one of the oldest foods known—are packed with healthy monounsaturated fat, mostly in the form of oleic acid. They're also full of vitamin E, polyphenols, and flavonoids.

of 6 plates; top each serving with ½ cup sauce, 2 tablespoons cheese, and 1 teaspoon parsley. Serves 6.

CALORIES 338; FAT 9.8g (sat 3g, mono 5g, poly 1g); PROTEIN 14.3g; CARB 48.9g; FIBER 4.3g; CHOL 10mg; IRON 3.7mg; SODIUM 808mg; CALC 246mg

Apricot, Plum, and Chicken Tagine with Olives

Moroccan stews—typically complex mixtures of spices, fruits, vegetables, and meat—provide many opportunities to balance tastes. In this dish, briny olives counter the sweetness of dried fruit and sautéed onions. Sautéeing the spices draws out their essences and makes them more potent.

1 teaspoon olive oil
1 pound skinless, boneless chicken
   thighs, halved
1 cup chopped onion (about 1 medium)
1 tablespoon grated peeled fresh ginger
3 garlic cloves, minced
1 teaspoon ground turmeric
1 teaspoon ground cumin
¼ teaspoon fennel seeds
¼ teaspoon ground cinnamon
½ cup dried apricots, halved
½ cup pitted dried plums, halved
½ teaspoon salt
20 pitted kalamata olives, halved
1 (14-ounce) can fat-free, lower-sodium
   chicken broth
3 tablespoons chopped fresh cilantro
½ teaspoon grated lemon rind
3 cups hot cooked couscous

1. Heat a large Dutch oven over medium-high heat. Add oil to pan; swirl to coat. Add chicken to pan; cook 3 minutes on each side or until browned. Place chicken on a plate, and keep warm.
2. Add onion to pan; sauté 4 minutes or until golden. Add ginger and garlic; sauté 30 seconds. Stir in turmeric, cumin, fennel seeds, and cinnamon; sauté 15 seconds, stirring constantly. Return chicken to pan. Add apricots and next 4 ingredients; bring to a boil. Cover, reduce heat, and simmer 30 minutes or until chicken is tender. Remove from heat; stir in cilantro and rind. Serve over couscous. Serves 6 (serving size: ⅔ cup chicken mixture and ½ cup couscous).

CALORIES 334; FAT 10.1g (sat 2.2g, mono 5.3g, poly 1.8g); PROTEIN 18.8g; CARB 40.5g; FIBER 3.7g; CHOL 50mg; IRON 2.4mg; SODIUM 568mg; CALC 45mg

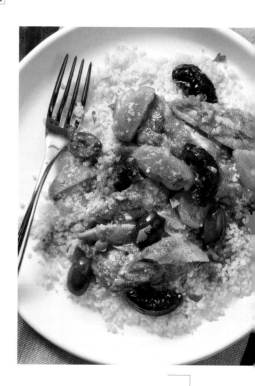

COACHING SESSION
with ALLISON FISHMAN

DON'T FEAR FATS

It's time to get over your fat phobia and embrace the notion that not all fats are bad. Here's how:

■ **Add oil at the end.** One of the easiest ways to make over a bland, low-fat diet is to add some healthy, happy fats. Start with a decorative oil dispenser, and fill it with a good-quality extra-virgin olive oil or a flavor-packed sesame oil. Then use it as a finishing oil, not a cooking oil—something to drizzle on at the end.

■ **Pair your healthy fats with veggies.** Top your salads with cubes of avocado or a sprinkling of sesame seeds, add peanut sauce to your stir-fries, and toss toasted hazelnuts over your sautéed green beans.

■ **Forgo the naked salad.** There's no need to skip dressing, or have just a tiny amount on the side. Adding a healthy oil to your greens actually helps your body absorb the nutrients, and it boosts the filling power of your salad. Instead of creamy dressings, make your own vinaigrette (check out the recipes on page 223 to get started) or try one that derives its creaminess from avocado.

DIY Vinaigrettes

SKIP THE CREAMY BOTTLED DRESSINGS and make your own. It really is easy. The ratio of oil and vinegar stays basically the same, but the variations are endless. Simply whisk ingredients in a bowl or combine in a Mason jar, close the lid tightly, and shake vigorously.

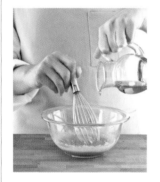

HOW TO MIX A BASIC VINAIGRETTE

The simplicity of a good vinaigrette is a thing of beauty. Grab a bowl, whisk together oil and vinegar, and add a pinch of salt to bring dull lettuces to life, give veggies a bold flavor boost, and add tang to marinated meats.

A vinaigrette may be easy to prepare, but there is a method to its magic. Success starts with good ingredients and ends with emulsification—thoroughly blending the oil's fat molecules and the watery vinegar. Adding a touch of creamy Dijon mustard eases the emulsification process. From there, flavor as you see fit. Additions can be as simple as a pinch of salt and pepper or as complex as a bit of honey, fresh herbs, or minced shallots.

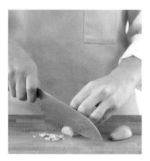

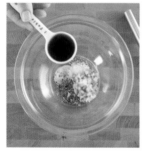

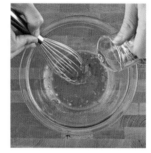

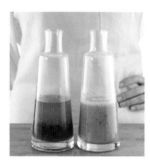

1. Build a flavor base. Finely mince 2 table-spoons shallots so pieces will incorporate easily and spread throughout your dressing. Place in a bowl with 1 teaspoon Dijon mustard.

2. Add an acid. Pour in 2 tablespoons sherry vinegar, ¼ teaspoon kosher salt, and ¼ teaspoon freshly ground black pepper; stir with a whisk to combine ingredients.

3. Whisk in oil. Slowly pour 6 tablespoons extra-virgin olive oil (almost drop by drop) into the mixture, whisking as you go to incorporate and create a creamy, emulsified finish.

4. Success! When properly emulsified, ingredients are sus-pended throughout the mix (right). A broken vinaigrette (left) will have clear separation between the oil and the vinegar.

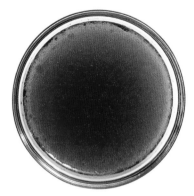

Sesame Vinaigrette

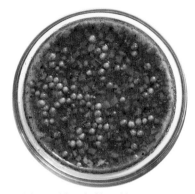

Mustard Seed–Chive Vinaigrettte

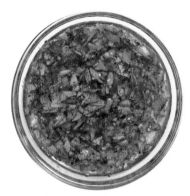

Champagne Vinaigrette

Sesame Vinaigrette

Try tossing this vinaigrette with rice noodles.

1½ tablespoons fresh lemon juice
1 tablespoon lower-sodium soy sauce
1 tablespoon honey
1½ teaspoons dark sesame oil

1. Combine all ingredients in a small bowl, stirring with a whisk. Serves 4 (serving size: 1 tablespoon).

CALORIES 35; FAT 1.7g (sat 0.2g, mono 0.7g, poly 0.7g); PROTEIN 0.3g; CARB 5.1g; FIBER 0g; CHOL 0mg; IRON 0mg; SODIUM 152mg; CALC 1mg

Mustard Seed–Chive Vinaigrette

Toss with gourmet greens or drizzle over salmon.

2 tablespoons sherry vinegar
1 tablespoon water
1 teaspoon country-style Dijon mustard
1 teaspoon honey
1 tablespoon extra-virgin olive oil
2 tablespoons chopped fresh chives
½ teaspoon kosher salt
½ teaspoon mustard seeds
½ teaspoon freshly ground black pepper

1. Combine first 4 ingredients in a small bowl; stir with a whisk. Slowly add oil, stirring constantly with a whisk until well blended. Stir in chives and remaining ingredients. Serves 5 (serving size: about 1 tablespoon).

CALORIES 32; FAT 2.8g (sat 0.4g, mono 2g, poly 0.3g); PROTEIN 0.2g; CARB 1.7g; FIBER 0.1g; CHOL 0mg; IRON 0.1mg; SODIUM 212mg; CALC 4mg

Easy Herb Vinaigrette

You can use any variety of honey that you like.

9 tablespoons white wine vinegar
1½ tablespoons wildflower honey
½ teaspoon fine sea salt
1 cup canola oil
3 tablespoons chopped fresh basil
3 tablespoons minced fresh chives

1. Combine first 3 ingredients in a medium bowl; slowly whisk in oil until combined. Stir in basil and chives. Store, covered, in refrigerator for up to 5 days. Serves 27 (serving size: 1 tablespoon).

CALORIES 160; FAT 8.6g (sat 0.6g, mono 5.1g, poly 2.6g); PROTEIN 0g; CARB 1.1g; FIBER 0g; CHOL 0mg; IRON 0mg; SODIUM 45mg; CALC 1mg

Champagne Vinaigrette

Fresh basil makes all the difference.

2 tablespoons chopped fresh basil
1 tablespoon finely chopped shallots
2 tablespoons Champagne vinegar
1 tablespoon extra-virgin olive oil
2 teaspoons sugar
½ teaspoon salt
¼ teaspoon freshly ground black pepper

1. Combine all ingredients in a small bowl, stirring with a whisk. Serves 5 (serving size: 1 tablespoon).

CALORIES 29; FAT 2.3g (sat 0.3g, mono 1.8g, poly 0.2g); PROTEIN 0.1g; CARB 2.1g; FIBER 0g; CHOL 0mg; IRON 0.1mg; SODIUM 194mg; CALC 3mg

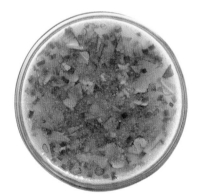

Easy Herb Vinaigrette

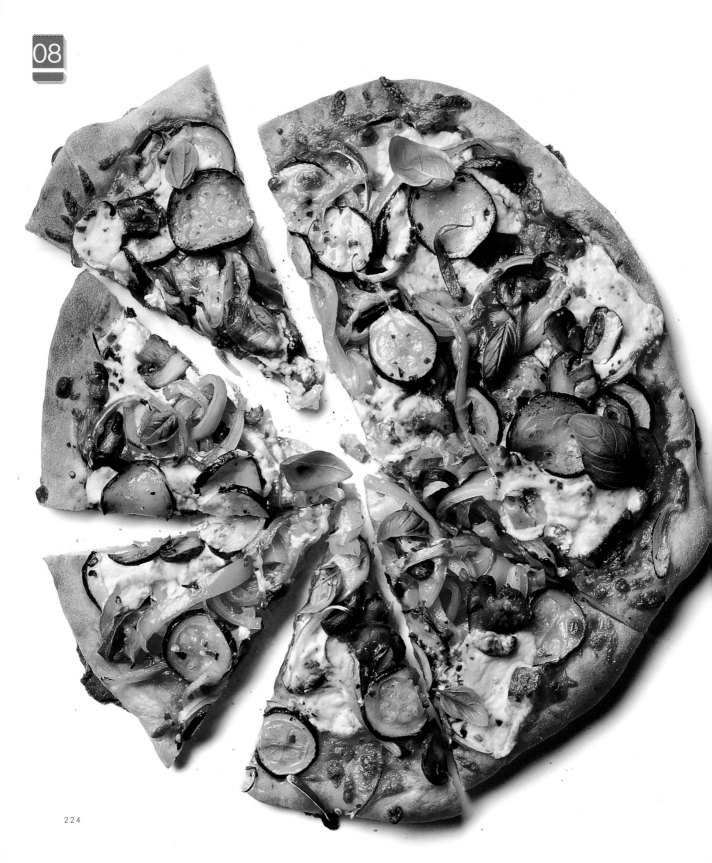

GO MEATLESS ONE DAY A WEEK

BE A PART-TIME VEGETARIAN.

T HE GROUND IS SHIFTING in America concerning vegetarian eating. Most restaurants, high and low, offer all-plant dishes. Supermarket products are changing, as well. This isn't to suggest that our beef-loving, bacon-crazy, and chicken-clucking country is thinking about giving up meat. Rather, more people are recognizing that all-plant meals can be delicious.

They're also realizing that other populations that eat more vegetables tend to be healthier, and that reducing the amount of meat in the diet doesn't mean eliminating the pleasures of eating meat: You don't have to *be* a vegetarian to eat vegetarian sometimes.

We all know that whole grains, fruits, and vegetables are among the healthiest foods you can eat—loaded with vitamins, minerals, and antioxidants, all things associated with reduced risk of cancer and heart disease. The wonderful thing about vowing to eat vegetarian at least one day a week is that it broadens your culinary horizons and encourages you to experiment with foods you might otherwise pass over.

Already eating meatless meals once a week? That's great—now aim to add in another day or two each week. And if you're a vegetarian, focus on expanding your cooking repertoire and making sure your diet is healthy and balanced with good sources of protein and fiber (and not too many saturated fats from dairy).

It's time to shift your focus and find ways to push those sides to the center of the plate. With our tips and suggestions, three more vegetarian meals a week will be a breeze, too.

YOUR GOAL

Go meatless one day a week for all three meals.

The 12 Healthy Habits

| · 01 · GET COOKING | · 02 · BREAKFAST DAILY | · 03 · WHOLE GRAINS | · 04 · GET MOVING | · 05 · VEGGIE UP | · 06 · MORE SEAFOOD | · 07 · HEALTHY FATS | 08 GO MEATLESS | · 09 · GET STRONGER | · 10 · LESS SALT | · 11 · BE PORTION-AWARE | · 12 · EAT MINDFULLY |

Make Over Family Meals

YOU MAY BE CONVINCED to jump on the meatless bandwagon...but getting your family to agree to tofu turkey may be a whole other story. Here, Chicago nutritionist Dawn Jackson Blatner, RD, author of *The Flexitarian Diet,* shares her favorite Italian, Mexican, and American family favorites that can be transformed into vegetarian meals that are no less satisfying and delicious:

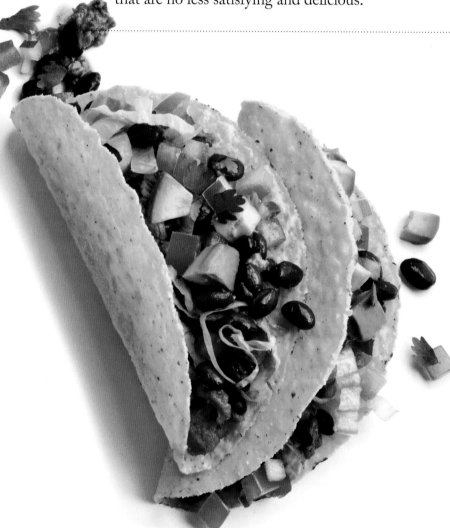

Instead of: spaghetti with meat sauce
Try: spaghetti with a white bean marinara sauce. You can still serve your favorite marinara sauce with this quick sub: For every ounce of ground beef, sub in ¼ cup beans.

Instead of: ground beef tacos
Try: tempeh tacos. Tempeh has a much meatier texture than its soy cousin tofu, so you're more likely to feel satisfied.

Instead of: chicken burritos
Try: bean burritos. Use low-fat refried beans instead of whole beans (or use a combination) for a richer flavor and texture.

Instead of: steak stir-fry
Try: edamame stir-fry. This star soybean provides 8 grams of protein per ½ cup and has a buttery, nutty flavor that will more than make up for the missing meat.

Instead of: turkey on rye
Try: a pita stuffed with protein-rich garbanzo beans or lentil salad. Pita pockets are ideal because they open up, unlike a regular sandwich that beans can roll out of.

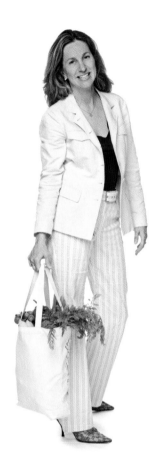

Really, No Meat?

"To me, healthy means choosing turkey chili over beef chili—not vegetarian chili."

CHERYL MARKER
Marketing Consultant

➤ **MEATLESS CHALLENGE:** Cheryl lives the busy life of a modern New York City working mom, but her thoughts on food still rest heavily in the traditional camp. "I grew up in a house where dinner was meat, potatoes, and a vegetable. I've evolved, but my family's still into the meat," she says.

OUR ADVICE

■ **Get the kids involved.** Take them to the farmers' market or grocery store, and let them choose a vegetable or fruit that interests them. When it's time to cook, let them help by stirring, pouring, and measuring ingredients.

■ **Pile veggies on pizza.** Family members won't miss the meat on a homemade pizza, and you'll find lots of veggie pies to try in this book (see pages 244–245 for some options).

■ **Swap ground beef for soy crumbles.** Mix them with rice and veggies inside a stuffed roasted pepper, rolled up in a burrito, or used to top nachos— your family may never be the wiser.

■ **Master a meatless sandwich.** Grill your favorite veggies to add a smoky (and somewhat meaty) quality, place them on a hearty bread, such as ciabatta rolls or a whole-grain loaf, and then top with cheese.

■ **Make vegetarian risotto.** Don't be intimidated by this classic rice dish. Risottos are a great way to incorporate vegetables into a meal. Any leftovers make tasty risotto cakes for tomorrow's lunch.

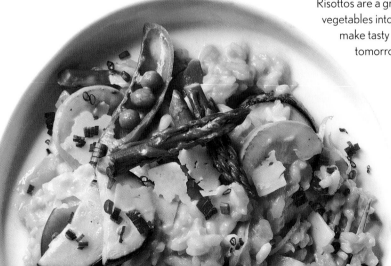

Bring Sides to the Center

I F YOU COVER YOUR PLATE with colorful veggies, beans, and whole grains, you're less likely to feel that the protein portion is missing. Here's how to do it:

AT MEALS

■ **Power up your salads.** Chickpeas, edamame, and walnuts are all healthy, filling sources of protein. Half a cup of shelled edamame will add 8g of protein to your salad. A quarter-cup of diced hard-cooked eggs boosts your salad's protein by 4g.

■ **Go for whole grains.** Brown rice, quinoa, barley, and other whole grains deliver a good helping of protein with

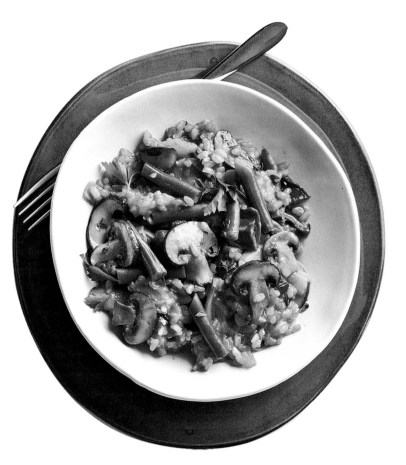

Risottos made with hearty whole grains are satisfying meat-free options. See pages 100 and 243 for recipes.

a lot less fat than meat. One cup of cooked quinoa has more than 8g of protein and less than 4g of fat; a 6-ounce rib-eye has 63g of protein but a whopping 34g of fat (more than a third is unhealthy saturated fat).

■ **Give tofu a chance.** Tofu can be a daunting ingredient to the novice vegetarian chef, but once you've tried a few recipes, you'll be thinking up your own dishes in no time. You can grill, sauté, roast, or bake tofu, just as you would any piece of meat.

■ **Experiment with beans, nuts, and soy foods.** Lentils make a great base for salads, soups, and stews, and 1 cup has nearly 18g of protein. Stir rinsed and drained canned beans into pasta dishes for a protein boost—half a cup has almost 7g of protein.

FOR SNACKS

■ **Add oomph to dips.** Enjoy fresh veggies dunked into protein-rich yogurt sauces and dips, like tzatziki or hummus. Or try bean dips, like our Artichoke, Spinach, and White Bean Dip on page 165.

■ **Partner fruits, vegetables, and whole-grain bread with protein.** Pair apples or whole-grain bread with nut butters—2 tablespoons of almond butter contain 7g of protein. Dip carrot or bell pepper strips in hummus—2 tablespoons have 3g of protein.

■ **Dish out some dairy.** A cup of low-fat cottage cheese has 28g of protein; low-fat Greek yogurt has nearly 23g in 1 cup.

Two slices of whole-wheat bread have 7.3g of protein.

Try almond, cashew, or sunflower seed butter to add variety to your snacks.

Yogurt-based dips can amp up the protein in your afternoon snack.

A NEW VIEW OF PROTEIN

Don't worry about getting enough protein—it's a hangover from earlier ideas about vegetarian diets. Protein recommendations are pretty low—46g per day for women, 56g for men—so it's difficult to be deficient. Here, three tips to make it easier:

1. Don't think of it as meals minus meat. Focus instead on swapping in plant proteins such as beans and lentils. Then add other protein sources to your plate like nuts, whole grains, and dairy foods.

2. Begin your day with a meatless meal. Whole-grain cereal and milk, Greek yogurt and fruit, or a scrambled egg and cheese sandwich on whole-wheat bread are all easy vegetarian, protein-rich meals.

3. Don't fuss over "incomplete proteins." As long as you eat a variety of protein-filled foods throughout the day, you'll get enough of the essential amino acids you need.

Maximize the Umami Factor

MOST COOKS ARE AWARE OF THE FOUR ELEMENTAL TASTES: bitter, salty, sour, and sweet. But central to Japanese cuisine is a fifth taste: umami. This Japanese word roughly translates to "delicious." The savory flavor it describes is imparted by the amino acid glutamate and ribonucleotides found naturally in vegetables and dairy (as well as fish and meats), and is what helps make certain vegetarian dishes so satisfying. Here, five meat-free foods that amp up umami flavor:

1. MUSHROOMS
Mushrooms—especially shiitake mushrooms—provide a hearty texture. Add them to pastas, risottos, casseroles, soups, salads, and sandwiches.

2. SOYBEANS
The savory taste of tofu and tempeh can be enhanced with fermented ingredients such as soy sauce, miso, and rice vinegar.

3. TOMATO PASTE AND SUN-DRIED TOMATOES
They impart depth and a rich flavor when added to sauces.

4. GREEN TEA
Think beyond the cup and try brewing green tea to use as a soup stock.

5. SWEET POTATOES
You can intensify the umami flavor of sweet potatoes by roasting, caramelizing, or stewing them. Tomatoes and carrots are also good choices.

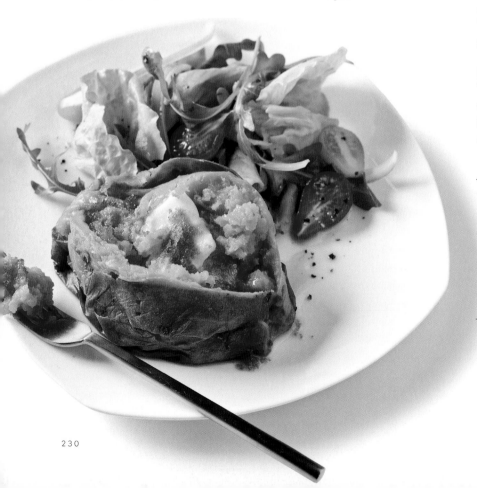

A baked sweet potato and a simple side salad make for a filling and almost-effortless meatless meal.

What Is a Serving?

MOST ADULTS NEED 5 to 6½ ounces from the protein food groups each day. It doesn't take much to reach this goal, either. Here, some amounts from various vegetarian sources that are equivalent to an ounce of meat:

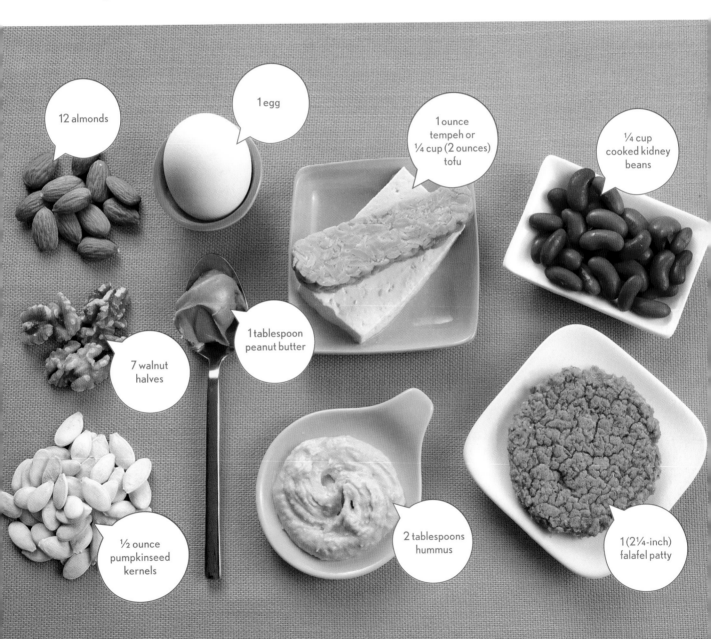

12 almonds

1 egg

1 ounce tempeh or ¼ cup (2 ounces) tofu

¼ cup cooked kidney beans

1 tablespoon peanut butter

7 walnut halves

½ ounce pumpkinseed kernels

2 tablespoons hummus

1 (2¼-inch) falafel patty

Utilize 10 All-Star Ingredients for Meatless Meals

A VEGETARIAN MEAL MAKES vegetables the center-of-the-plate star. Be sure you keep a variety of veggies on hand, including precut and frozen vegetables, which are just as nutritious as fresh. Then stock your pantry, fridge, and freezer with these essentials so that you can quickly and easily whip up a meatless meal any night of the week.

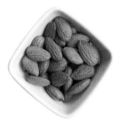

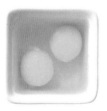

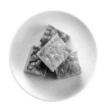

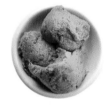

Nuts pack a hefty amount of protein and healthy fats.
Use for: a quick-energy snack or a crunchy addition to salads, grain dishes, stir-fries, and pilafs. Ground nuts add body to sauces.

Whole grains such as quinoa, farro, bulgur, and brown rice are an ideal base for meatless meals. *Use for:* whole-grain salads, risottos, curries, vegetarian stir-fries, and veggie burgers.

Large **eggs** are a high-quality protein that go far beyond breakfast.
Use for: veggie-filled quiches and frittatas, bulking up vegetarian fried rice, and hard-cooking to top entrée salads.

Made from whole soybeans, **tempeh** has a firm texture and a nutty flavor.
Use for: sandwiches, stir-fries, and kebabs.

Seitan is a high-protein meat substitute made of wheat gluten; look for it in Asian markets or refrigerated sections of specialty stores.
Use for: stir-fries, Asian-style noodle dishes, casseroles, and stews.

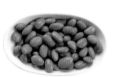

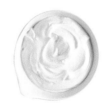

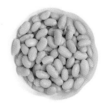

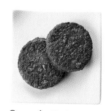

Frozen shelled **edamame** (soybeans) are a convenient way to add color, texture, and protein to most any dish. *Use for:* salads, pastas, stir-fries, and whole-grain salads.

Tofu is a meatless chameleon that takes on the flavor of whatever it's paired with; the texture varies from soft to extra-firm.
Use for: stir-fries, Asian-style noodle dishes, casseroles, and soups.

Plain **Greek yogurt** is higher in protein compared to other yogurts. *Use for:* dips, sauces, breakfast parfaits, and marinades.

Beans and lentils are a great stand-in for meat because of their high protein content. Legumes also supply fiber, folate, and iron. *Use for:* salads, pastas, pilafs, tagines, soups, stews, and dips.

Soy substitutes come in many forms: veggie crumbles, burgers, and sausages.
Use for: lasagna and other casseroles, pastas, tacos, burritos, and chili.

Show Me the Menu

"I rely on an internal database when I cook, but with vegetarian meals, I'm lost."

JANE BOUTELLE
Business Resources Manager

➤ **MEATLESS CHALLENGE:** Jane hasn't attempted a vegetarian diet in 25 years, so she feels a bit behind. "I know it's not all tofu and seitan, but if it's not that, what is it?" Jane's husband is not a fan of vegetables, but she's determined to expand the horizons of their three children.

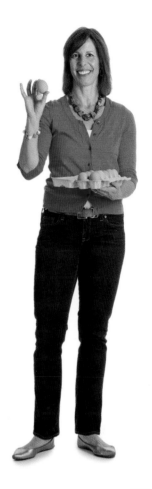

OUR ADVICE

▪ **Embrace the egg.** This low-calorie, protein-rich food is the simplest way to explore meatless meals without arousing the family's suspicions. Load up frittatas and quiches with fresh produce.

▪ **Cook family favorites, sans meat.** Start with dishes and flavor profiles that your family enjoys. Mexican food, Italian food, and many American favorites are all candidates for a meatless makeover. Instead of Beef Stroganoff, try meaty mushrooms. White or black bean enchiladas are a great alternative to traditional beef or chicken versions. Veggie nachos, loaded with fajita-style peppers, refried beans, and tomatoes, may be a big hit, too.

▪ **Then try something entirely different.** Once you've built up a bit of meatless momentum, venture outside your usual repertorie to try something like Vegetarian Moussaka (page 240), a meatless take on a classic Greek dish that uses fiber-rich bulgur wheat instead of ground meat.

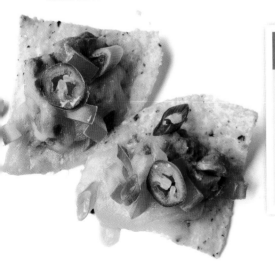

EXPERT TIP: *Forgo Faux*

"Beware of the faux-meat fixation trap. Boxes of veggie burgers, soy sausages, 'chicken' nuggets, and veggie lunchmeats are convenient and fine to include sometimes, but don't rely on them for every meatless meal. Opt instead for less-processed, lower-sodium options such as beans, nuts, and lentils to get your daily dose of plant protein."

—*Dawn Jackson Blatner, RD, blogger,* The Huffington Post, *author of* The Flexitarian Diet

Remake Family Favorites without Meat

START YOUR MEATLESS MAKEOVER with the foods and flavors that you know your family likes. You may be surprised that just a few substitutions will yield delicious meat-free entrées that everyone enjoys.

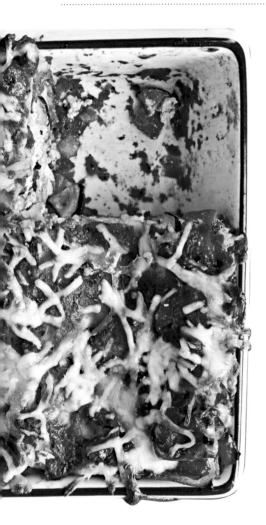

Baked Vegetable Lasagna

3 tablespoons olive oil, divided
1/2 cup chopped white onion
2 garlic cloves, minced
1 teaspoon kosher salt, divided
1 teaspoon sugar
1/4 teaspoon black pepper, divided
1/4 teaspoon crushed red pepper
1 (28-ounce) can crushed tomatoes, undrained
1/2 cup chopped fresh basil
1 tablespoon chopped fresh oregano
1 cup ricotta cheese
1/2 cup (2 ounces) grated fresh Parmigiano-Reggiano cheese
1 (14-ounce) package water-packed firm tofu, drained
1 large egg, lightly beaten
1/2 cup thinly sliced green onions
3 cups finely chopped red bell pepper (about 2 medium)
2 medium zucchini, quartered lengthwise and thinly sliced (about 3 cups)
1/3 cup finely chopped fresh parsley
Cooking spray
12 cooked lasagna noodles
3/4 cup (3 ounces) shredded part-skim mozzarella cheese

1. Preheat oven to 375°.
2. Heat a medium saucepan over medium-high heat. Add 2 tablespoons oil to pan; swirl to coat. Add white onion; sauté 5 minutes or until tender. Add garlic; sauté 1 minute or until golden. Add 1/2 teaspoon salt, sugar, 1/8 teaspoon black pepper, crushed red pepper, and tomatoes. Cover, reduce heat to low, and simmer 15 minutes or until thoroughly heated. Remove from heat; stir in basil and oregano. Cool.
3. Place ricotta, Parmigiano-Reggiano, tofu, egg, and 1/4 teaspoon salt in a food processor; process 10 seconds or until blended. Stir in green onions. Set aside.
4. Heat a large nonstick skillet over medium-high heat. Add remaining 1 tablespoon olive oil to pan; swirl to coat. Add bell pepper, zucchini, and remaining 1/4 teaspoon salt; sauté 10 minutes or until vegetables are tender and liquid evaporates. Remove from heat; stir in parsley and remaining 1/8 teaspoon black pepper.
5. Spread 1/2 cup tomato mixture in bottom of a 13 x 9–inch glass or ceramic baking dish coated with

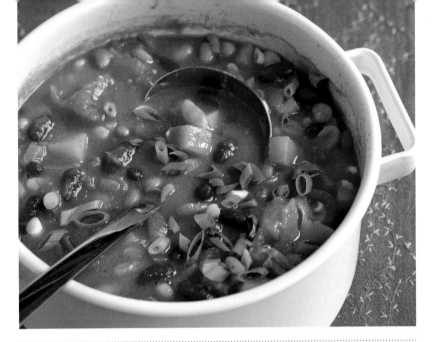

cooking spray; top with 3 noodles. Spread ¾ cup tomato mixture over noodles; top with 1 cup tofu mixture and 1 cup zucchini mixture. Repeat layers twice, ending with noodles. Spread remaining ¾ cup tomato mixture over top. Bake at 375° for 35 minutes or until bubbly; top with mozzarella cheese. Bake 5 minutes or until cheese melts. Let stand 10 minutes. Serves 8.

CALORIES 347; FAT 18g (sat 6.2g, mono 7g, poly 3.6g); PROTEIN 21.6g; CARB 28.8g; FIBER 5.3g; CHOL 53mg; IRON 8.1mg; SODIUM 543mg; CALC 595mg

---

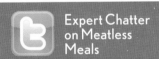 **Expert Chatter on Meatless Meals**

@EatingMadeEasy: Pick a meatless protein, then plan rest of meal around it. Beans, lentils, eggs, tofu are great meal bases.

@estachura: Use meaty veggies like portobellos and eggplant in a dish like lasagna. No one will notice the meat is missing!

@ChristysChomp: I've added lots of chopped mushrooms and soy crumbles at the end of a chili recipe. Gives it a nice "meaty" texture.

Three-Bean Vegetarian Chili

Serve a hearty salad with nuts and cheese, and corn bread on the side.

2 red bell peppers
3 tablespoons extra-virgin olive oil
1 cup chopped onion
2 teaspoons ground cumin
1 teaspoon crushed red pepper
1 teaspoon paprika
¼ teaspoon salt
4 garlic cloves, thinly sliced
2 cups organic vegetable broth
1½ cups (½-inch) cubed peeled butternut squash
1 (28-ounce) can no-salt-added diced tomatoes, undrained
1 (15-ounce) can pinto beans, rinsed and drained
1 (15-ounce) can cannellini beans, rinsed and drained
1 (15-ounce) can red kidney beans, rinsed and drained
½ cup thinly sliced green onions

1. Preheat broiler.
2. Cut bell peppers in half lengthwise. Remove and discard seeds and membranes. Place pepper halves, skin sides up, on a foil-lined baking sheet. Broil 15 minutes or until blackened. Place in a paper bag; fold to close tightly. Let stand 15 minutes. Peel and chop peppers.
3. Heat a Dutch oven over medium-low heat. Add oil to pan; swirl to coat. Add onion; cook 15 minutes, stirring occasionally. Stir in cumin and next 4 ingredients; cook 2 minutes, stirring frequently. Add bell peppers, broth, squash, and tomatoes; bring to a simmer. Cook 20 minutes, stirring occasionally. Add beans; simmer 25 minutes or until slightly thick, stirring occasionally. Sprinkle with green onions. Serves 6 (serving size: about 1½ cups).

CALORIES 264; FAT 8.3g (sat 1.2g, mono 5.2g, poly 1.3g); PROTEIN 9.5g; CARB 40.9g; FIBER 10.7g; CHOL 0mg; IRON 4.4mg; SODIUM 689mg; CALC 145mg

Make Your Own Veggie Burgers

V EGGIE BURGERS CAN BE MADE with chickpeas, black beans, white beans, potatoes, lentils, and pretty much any other vegetable that can be mashed and formed into a patty. Made right, they're delicious—but fragile. Cook them on the stovetop or under the broiler, flipping them very carefully when the time comes.

Black Bean Burgers with Mango Salsa

2 (15-ounce) cans black beans, rinsed and drained
¾ cup finely chopped fresh cilantro, divided
¾ cup (3 ounces) shredded Monterey Jack cheese
¼ cup panko (Japanese breadcrumbs)
2 teaspoons ground cumin
1 teaspoon dried oregano
½ teaspoon sea salt
½ medium jalapeño pepper, finely chopped
2 large egg whites
Cooking spray
1¼ cups chopped peeled mango (about 1 medium)
3 tablespoons chopped shallots
1½ tablespoons fresh lime juice
1 ripe avocado, peeled and chopped
1 garlic clove, minced
6 green leaf lettuce leaves
6 (2-ounce) whole-wheat hamburger buns, lightly toasted

1. Preheat oven to 350°.
2. Place black beans in a medium bowl; mash with a fork. Stir in ½ cup finely chopped cilantro and next 7 ingredients. Shape bean mixture into 6 (½-inch-thick) patties.

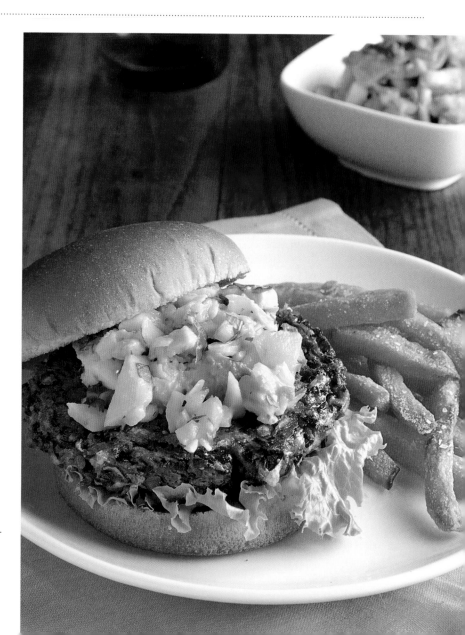

Arrange patties on a baking sheet coated with cooking spray. Bake at 350° for 20 minutes, carefully turning after 10 minutes.

3. Combine remaining ¼ cup cilantro, mango, and next 4 ingredients in a medium bowl. Place 1 lettuce leaf on bottom half of each hamburger bun; top each with 1 patty, ⅓ cup salsa, and top half of bun. Serves 6 (serving size: 1 burger).

CALORIES 320; FAT 11.9g (sat 3.9g, mono 5g, poly 1.7g); PROTEIN 13.4g; CARB 46.2g; FIBER 10.1g; CHOL 13mg; IRON 3.3mg; SODIUM 777mg; CALC 201mg

Baked Falafel Sandwiches with Yogurt-Tahini Sauce

Sauce:
1 cup plain whole-milk Greek yogurt
1 tablespoon tahini (sesame seed paste)
1 tablespoon fresh lemon juice

Falafel:
¾ cup water
¼ cup uncooked bulgur
3 cups cooked chickpeas (garbanzo beans)
½ cup chopped fresh cilantro
½ cup chopped green onions
⅓ to ½ cup water
2 tablespoons all-purpose flour
1 tablespoon ground cumin
1 teaspoon baking powder
¾ teaspoon salt
¼ to ½ teaspoon ground red pepper
3 garlic cloves
Cooking spray
Chopped fresh cilantro (optional)

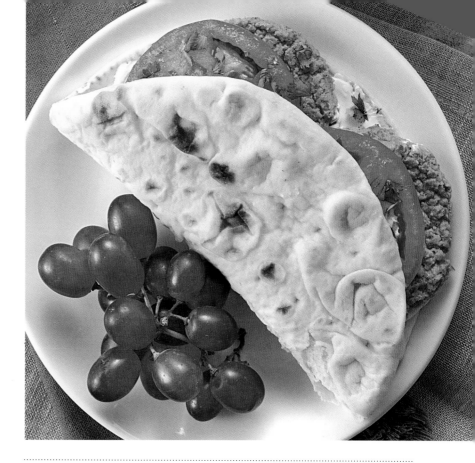

Remaining ingredients:
6 (2.8-ounce) Mediterranean-style white flatbreads
12 (¼-inch-thick) slices tomato
Chopped fresh cilantro (optional)

1. To prepare sauce, combine first 3 ingredients, stirring with a whisk until blended. Cover and chill until ready to serve.

2. To prepare falafel, bring ¾ cup water to a boil in a small saucepan; add bulgur to pan. Remove from heat; cover and let stand 30 minutes or until tender. Drain and set aside. Preheat oven to 425°.

3. Place chickpeas and next 9 ingredients in a food processor; pulse 10 times or until well blended and smooth (mixture will be wet). Spoon chickpea mixture into a large bowl; stir in bulgur.

4. Divide mixture into 12 equal portions (about ¼ cup each); shape each portion into a ¼-inch-thick patty. Place patties on a baking sheet coated with cooking spray. Bake at 425° for 10 minutes on each side or until browned. Spread about 2½ tablespoons sauce onto each flatbread. Top each flatbread with 2 falafel patties, 2 tomato slices, and, if desired, chopped cilantro. Serves 6 (serving size: 1 stuffed flatbread).

CALORIES 388; FAT 7.7g (sat 3.5g, mono 1.6g, poly 1.6g); PROTEIN 18g; CARB 64.6g; FIBER 14.7g; CHOL 7mg; IRON 5.2mg; SODIUM 535mg; CALC 181mg

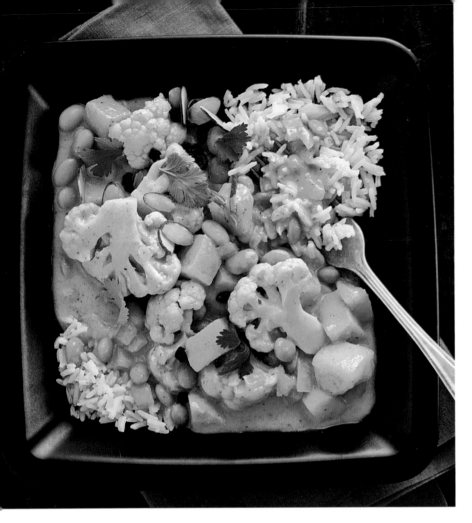

Vegetarian Country Captain

Traditionally, Country Captain is a mild chicken stew seasoned with curry powder. Myth has it that a British sea captain working in the spice trade introduced this classic, comforting dish to the Southern United States in the 19th century. Here, the chicken has been replaced with edamame and cauliflower.

1 tablespoon canola oil
1½ cups finely chopped onion
1½ cups diced peeled Granny Smith apple (about ½ pound)
1 tablespoon all-purpose flour
1 tablespoon curry powder
3 garlic cloves, minced
2 cups organic vegetable broth
2 tablespoons mango chutney
2 tablespoons whipping cream
½ teaspoon kosher salt
3 cups cauliflower florets
2 cups frozen shelled edamame (green soybeans)
3 cups hot cooked long-grain white rice
¼ cup dried currants
¼ cup sliced almonds, toasted
Chopped fresh cilantro (optional)
Sliced green onions (optional)

1. Heat a large, heavy nonstick skillet over medium heat. Add oil to pan, and swirl to coat. Add chopped onion, and cook 7 minutes or until tender, stirring frequently. Add apple, and cook 5 minutes, stirring frequently. Add flour, curry powder, and garlic; cook 1 minute, stirring

Simmer a Vegetable-Studded Stew

WHAT SAYS GOOD OLD-FASHIONED comfort food more than a pot of stew simmering on the stove? Vegetable stews typically have shorter cooking times because there's no need for long simmers to tenderize tough cuts of meat. To streamline weekday dinners even further, try cooking a pot of stew the night before for a quick reheatable meal.

constantly. Add broth, and bring to a boil. Reduce heat, and simmer 2 minutes or until slightly thick. Stir in chutney, cream, and salt. Add cauliflower and edamame; cook 8 minutes or until cauliflower is tender, stirring occasionally. Serve over rice; top with currants and almonds. Garnish with cilantro and green onions, if desired. Serves 4 (serving size: 1¼ cups cauliflower mixture, ¾ cup rice, 1 tablespoon currants, and 1 tablespoon almonds).

CALORIES 473; FAT 14.9g (sat 3.4g, mono 6g, poly 4.4g); PROTEIN 16.7g; CARB 70.6g; FIBER 5.8g; CHOL 10mg; IRON 4.4mg; SODIUM 641mg; CALC 122mg

Moroccan Chickpea Stew

2 teaspoons olive oil
1 cup diced yellow onion
  (about 1 medium)
1 cup diced carrot (about 1 large)
2 garlic cloves, minced
1 jalapeño pepper, minced
1¾ cups organic vegetable broth
1½ cups cubed peeled Yukon gold
  potato, about 1 large
2 teaspoons ground cumin
1 teaspoon chili powder
½ teaspoon ground turmeric
⅛ teaspoon salt
1 (28-ounce) can diced tomatoes,
  undrained
1 (16-ounce) can chickpeas (garbanzo
  beans), rinsed and drained
3 cups hot cooked brown rice
½ cup plain low-fat yogurt
Chopped fresh cilantro (optional)

1. Heat a large saucepan over medium-high heat. Add olive oil to pan; swirl to coat. Add onion and next 3 ingredients to pan, and sauté 6 minutes or until tender. Stir in broth and next 7 ingredients. Bring to a boil. Cover, reduce heat, and simmer 15 minutes or until potato is tender. Serve over rice. Top with yogurt, and sprinkle with cilantro, if desired. Serves 6 (serving size: 1⅓ cups stew, ½ cup rice, and about 1 tablespoon yogurt).

CALORIES 251; FAT 3.8g (sat 0.6g, mono 1.9g, poly 1g); PROTEIN 7.3g; CARB 47.5g; FIBER 6.8g; CHOL 1mg; IRON 2.2mg; SODIUM 401mg; CALC 97mg

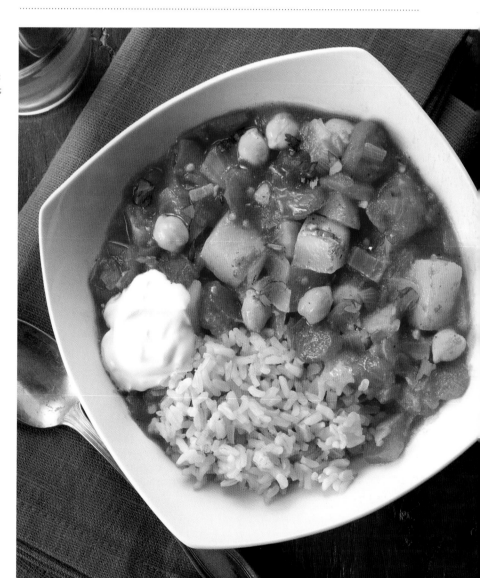

Bake a Vegetarian Casserole

WHO SAYS COMFORT FOOD can't be vegetarian? These recipes give all of the delicious flavor found in the most divine casseroles, but keep within the parameters of a vegetarian diet.

Vegetarian Moussaka

3 peeled eggplants, cut into $1/2$-inch-
   thick slices (about $2^1/2$ pounds)
2 tablespoons extra-virgin olive
   oil, divided
Cooking spray
2 cups chopped onion
4 garlic cloves, minced
$1/2$ cup uncooked bulgur
$1/4$ teaspoon ground allspice
$1/4$ teaspoon ground cinnamon
$1/8$ teaspoon ground cloves
2 cups organic vegetable broth
2 teaspoons chopped fresh oregano
1 (14.5-ounce) can no-salt-added
   diced tomatoes, undrained
1 tablespoon butter
2 tablespoons all-purpose flour
1 cup 1% low-fat milk
2 tablespoons finely grated fresh
   Romano cheese
$1/4$ teaspoon salt
1 large egg, lightly beaten

1. Preheat broiler.
2. Brush eggplant slices with
1 tablespoon oil. Place half of
eggplant on a foil-lined baking
sheet coated with cooking spray;
broil 5 minutes on each side or until
browned. Repeat procedure with
remaining eggplant. Set eggplant
aside.

3. Heat a large skillet over medium-
high heat. Add remaining 1 tablespoon oil to pan; swirl to coat. Add
chopped onion to pan; sauté 8 minutes. Add garlic; sauté 1 minute. Add
bulgur; cook 3 minutes or until bulgur
is lightly toasted, stirring frequently.
Add allspice, cinnamon, and cloves;
cook 1 minute, stirring constantly.
Stir in vegetable broth, oregano, and
tomatoes. Bring to a boil; reduce heat,
and simmer 20 minutes or until thick,
stirring occasionally.
4. Melt butter in a saucepan over
medium heat. Add flour; cook 1
minute, stirring constantly with a
whisk until well blended. Gradually
add milk, stirring constantly with
a whisk. Bring to a boil; reduce
heat to medium-low, and simmer
5 minutes or until thick, stirring
frequently. Stir in cheese and
salt. Remove from heat, and cool
slightly. Add egg, stirring well with
a whisk.
5. Preheat oven to 350°.
6. Arrange half of eggplant in an
11 x 7–inch glass or ceramic baking
dish coated with cooking spray.
Spread bulgur mixture evenly over
eggplant; arrange remaining eggplant
over bulgur mixture. Top with milk
mixture. Bake at 350° for 40 minutes,

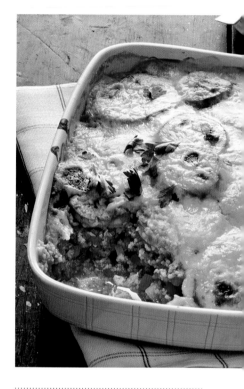

and remove from oven. Increase
oven temperature to 475°. Return
dish to oven for 4 minutes or until
top is browned. Let stand 10 minutes
before serving. Serves 4.

CALORIES 343; FAT 13.1g (sat 4.2g, mono 6.4g, poly 1.3g);
PROTEIN 11.4g; CARB 47.8g; FIBER 13.4g; CHOL 57mg;
IRON 2.3mg; SODIUM 583mg; CALC 203mg

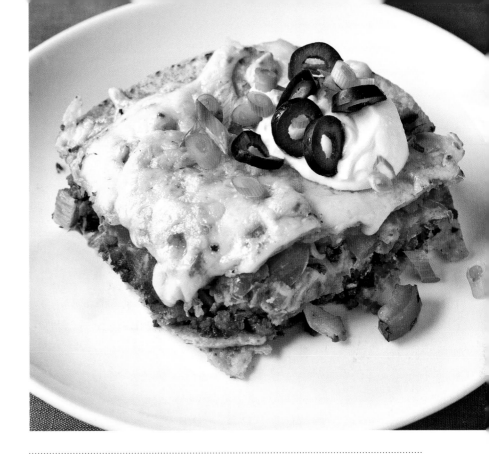

Mexican Casserole

4 teaspoons olive oil, divided
1 cup chopped onion
2 garlic cloves, minced
1 jalapeño pepper, minced
1 teaspoon chili powder
1/2 teaspoon ground cumin
1/4 teaspoon freshly ground
   black pepper
1 (12-ounce) package meatless
   fat-free crumbles
48 baked tortilla chips
Cooking spray
1 (15-ounce) can pinto beans, rinsed
   and drained
1 tablespoon fresh lime juice
2 cups chopped seeded plum tomato
2 tablespoons minced fresh cilantro
1 cup (4 ounces) shredded Monterey
   Jack cheese
2 tablespoons fat-free sour cream
2 tablespoons chopped green onions
1/4 cup sliced ripe olives

1. Preheat oven to 375°.
2. Heat a large nonstick skillet over medium heat. Add 2 teaspoons oil to pan; swirl to coat. Add onion to pan; cook 4 minutes or until tender. Add garlic and jalapeño; cook 1 minute. Stir in chili powder, cumin, black pepper, and crumbles; cook 3 minutes or until thoroughly heated. Arrange half of tortilla chips in an 11 x 7–inch glass or ceramic baking dish coated with cooking spray; top evenly with crumbles mixture.
3. Heat remaining 2 teaspoons oil in pan over medium heat. Add beans, mashing with the back of a wooden spoon until chunky and thick; cook 2 minutes or until heated, stirring constantly. Stir in lime juice.
4. Combine tomato and cilantro. Layer beans and tomato mixture over crumbles mixture in dish. Top with remaining tortilla chips, pressing to slightly crush. Sprinkle evenly with cheese. Bake at 375° for 13 minutes or until cheese is bubbly. Cut casserole into 6 equal pieces; top each serving with 1 teaspoon sour cream, 1 teaspoon green onions, and 2 teaspoons olives. Serves 6.

CALORIES 313; FAT 12.9g (sat 4.6g, mono 5.2g, poly 2.4g); PROTEIN 20.6g; CARB 30.2g; FIBER 7.4g; CHOL 18mg; IRON 3mg; SODIUM 718mg; CALC 295mg

 Are you going meatless one day a week?

"We've made a slow transition into meatless meals, less because of a conscious choice and more because we've just found awesome recipes that work for us."

—*Alyson Lewis*

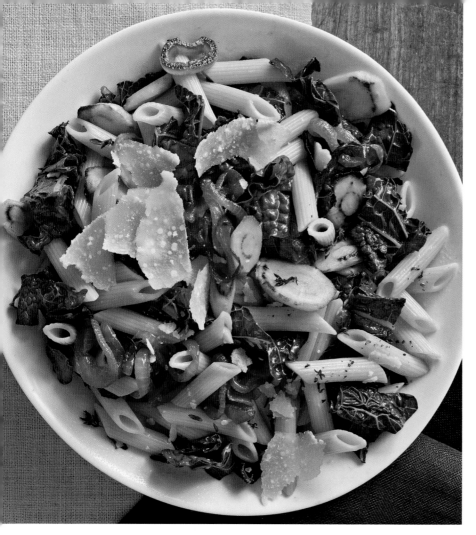

Pasta with Black Kale, Caramelized Onions, and Parsnips

If black kale is unavailable, use regular kale. "A great, hearty vegetarian dinner," said Pjdusschee on CookingLight.com. "I used regular kale; it blended well with the caramelized onions and parsnips. It takes a little while to cook, but your house will smell so good."

2 tablespoons extra-virgin olive oil, divided
3 cups ($\frac{1}{3}$-inch) diagonally cut parsnip (about 1 pound)
2$\frac{1}{2}$ cups sliced onion (about 1 large)
1 tablespoon chopped fresh thyme
4 garlic cloves, chopped
$\frac{1}{2}$ cup dry white wine
8 cups trimmed chopped black kale (about 3 bunches)
$\frac{1}{2}$ cup organic vegetable broth
8 ounces uncooked penne pasta
$\frac{1}{2}$ cup (2 ounces) shaved fresh Parmigiano-Reggiano cheese, divided
$\frac{1}{2}$ teaspoon salt
$\frac{1}{2}$ teaspoon freshly ground black pepper

1. Heat a large nonstick skillet over medium heat. Add 1 tablespoon oil to pan; swirl to coat. Add parsnip; cook 12 minutes or until tender and browned, stirring occasionally. Place in a bowl; keep warm.
2. Heat remaining 1 tablespoon oil in pan over medium-low heat. Add onion to pan; cook 20 minutes or until tender and golden brown, stirring occasionally. Stir in thyme and garlic; cook 2 minutes, stirring

Create Veggie-Rich Pastas and Risottos

PASTAS AND RISOTTOS are always crowd-pleasers: They're filling, affordable, and amazingly versatile. Opt for whole-wheat versions, which contain the nuttiness and chewiness of satisfying whole grains. Top them off with a small amount of sharply flavored, savory cheese like Parmigiano-Reggiano or pecorino Romano.

occasionally. Add wine; cook 3 minutes or until liquid almost evaporates. Stir in kale and broth; cook, covered, 5 minutes or until kale is tender. Uncover; cook 4 minutes or until kale is very tender, stirring occasionally. 3. Cook pasta according to package directions, omitting salt and fat. Drain pasta in a sieve over a bowl, reserving ¾ cup cooking liquid. Add drained pasta to kale mixture. Stir in parsnip, ½ cup reserved cooking liquid, ¼ cup cheese, salt, and pepper; cook 1 minute or until thoroughly heated. Add remaining ¼ cup reserved cooking liquid if needed to moisten. Top with remaining ¼ cup cheese. Serves 6 (serving size: 1⅔ cups).

CALORIES 324; FAT 8g (sat 2.1g, mono 4g, poly 1.1g); PROTEIN 12g; CARB 54.7g; FIBER 7.3g; CHOL 6mg; IRON 3.5mg; SODIUM 428mg; CALC 242mg

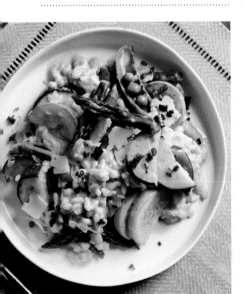

Summer Lemon-Vegetable Risotto

8 ounces asparagus, trimmed and cut into 1-inch pieces
8 ounces sugar snap peas, trimmed and cut in half
5 teaspoons extra-virgin olive oil, divided
1 (8-ounce) zucchini, halved lengthwise and cut into ½-inch-thick slices
1 (8-ounce) yellow squash, halved lengthwise and cut into ½-inch-thick slices
4¾ cups organic vegetable broth
½ cup finely chopped shallots
1 cup uncooked Arborio rice
¼ cup dry white wine
½ cup (2 ounces) grated fresh pecorino Romano cheese
¼ cup chopped fresh chives
1 teaspoon grated lemon rind
2 tablespoons fresh lemon juice
1 tablespoon unsalted butter
¼ teaspoon salt

1. Bring a large saucepan of water to a boil. Add asparagus and peas; cook 3 minutes or until crisp-tender. Drain and rinse under cold water.
2. Heat a large nonstick skillet over medium-high heat. Add 2 teaspoons oil to pan; swirl to coat. Add zucchini and squash to pan; cook 7 minutes or until lightly browned. Set aside.
3. Bring broth to a simmer in a medium saucepan (do not boil). Keep warm over low heat.
4. Heat a Dutch oven over medium heat. Add remaining 1 tablespoon oil to pan; swirl to coat. Add shallots; cook 3 minutes or until tender. Stir in rice; cook 1 minute, stirring constantly. Stir in wine; cook until liquid is absorbed (about 30 seconds), stirring constantly. Stir in 1 cup broth; cook 5 minutes or until liquid is nearly absorbed, stirring constantly. Reserve ¼ cup broth. Add remaining broth, ½ cup at a time, stirring constantly until each portion is absorbed before adding the next. Stir in vegetables; cook 1 minute or until thoroughly heated. Remove from heat; stir in reserved ¼ cup broth and remaining ingredients. Serves 4 (serving size: 1½ cups).

CALORIES 395; FAT 12.3g (sat 4.7g, mono 4.9g, poly 0.8g); PROTEIN 10.6g; CARB 56.2g; FIBER 7.1g; CHOL 18mg; IRON 3.1mg; SODIUM 512mg; CALC 191mg

EXPERT TIP:
A Perfect Meatless Pasta Formula

"Our family is eating less meat these days, and I've created a simple formula for a hearty, satisfying non-meat pasta dish that's suited for any night of the week. It's a combination of pasta + frozen or fresh veggies + a spoonful of high-quality oil or oil-based sauce + a sprinkling of hard, aged cheese + 2 tablespoons of nuts. It's easy to prepare and incredibly flexible. A favorite is whole-wheat penne, chopped spinach, pesto, sharp white cheddar, and pistachios."

—*Regan Jones, RD, blogger, The Professional Palate*

Pile Your Pizzas with Veggies

WHAT COULD BE MORE DELICIOUS—and simpler to make—than pizza sans pepperoni? A pizza crust, either homemade or ready-prepared, is the perfect canvas for a delicious vegetarian masterpiece. The options are endless.

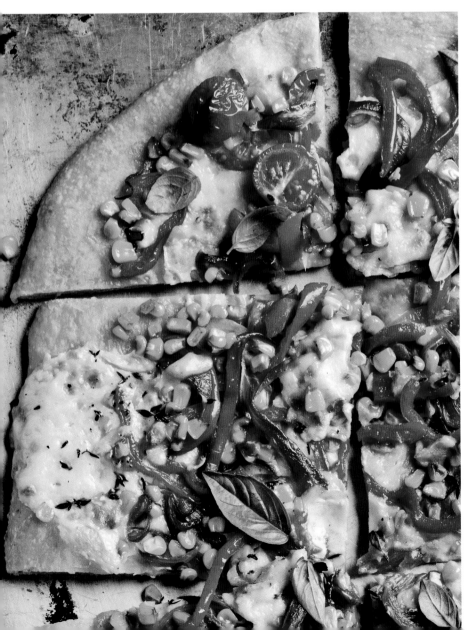

Local Farmers' Market Pizza

1 pound refrigerated fresh pizza
 dough
1 tablespoon extra-virgin olive oil
2 cups thinly sliced onion
1 teaspoon chopped fresh thyme
2 cups thinly sliced red bell pepper
5 garlic cloves, thinly sliced
1 cup fresh corn kernels (about 2 ears)
¼ teaspoon salt
¼ teaspoon black pepper
Cooking spray
5 ounces thinly sliced fresh mozzarella
 cheese
⅓ cup (1½ ounces) grated fresh
 Parmigiano-Reggiano cheese
1 cup cherry tomatoes, halved
⅓ cup fresh basil leaves

1. Remove dough from refrigerator. Let stand at room temperature, covered, 30 minutes.
2. Position an oven rack in the next to lowest setting; place a 16-inch pizza pan on rack. Preheat oven to 425°.
3. Heat a large nonstick skillet over medium-high heat. Add olive oil to pan, and swirl to coat. Add onion and thyme to pan; cook 3 minutes or until onion is tender, stirring occasionally. Add bell pepper and

garlic to pan; cook 2 minutes, stirring occasionally. Add corn, salt, and black pepper to pan; cook 1 minute or until thoroughly heated. 4. Roll dough into a 16-inch circle on a lightly floured surface. Remove pan from oven, and coat with cooking spray. Place dough on pan. Arrange mozzarella slices evenly over dough. Spread corn mixture evenly over cheese, and top with Parmigiano-Reggiano cheese. Bake at 425° for 23 minutes. Arrange tomatoes evenly over pizza; bake an additional 5 minutes or until crust is browned. Remove from oven; sprinkle with basil. Cut into 6 slices. Serves 6 (serving size: 1 slice).

CALORIES 355; FAT 11.6g (sat 4.6g, mono 1.8g, poly 1.8g); PROTEIN 14.2g; CARB 51.4g; FIBER 3.5g; CHOL 23mg; IRON 2.9mg; SODIUM 611mg; CALC 87mg

Roasted Vegetable and Ricotta Pizza

1 pound refrigerated fresh pizza dough
2 cups sliced cremini mushrooms
1 cup (¼-inch-thick) slices zucchini
¼ teaspoon black pepper
1 medium yellow bell pepper, sliced
1 medium red onion, cut into thick slices
1½ tablespoons plus 1 teaspoon olive oil, divided
1 tablespoon yellow cornmeal
⅓ cup tomato sauce
1 cup (4 ounces) shredded part-skim mozzarella cheese
½ teaspoon crushed red pepper
⅓ cup part-skim ricotta cheese
2 tablespoons small fresh basil leaves

1. Position an oven rack in the lowest setting; place a pizza stone on rack. Preheat oven to 500°.
2. Remove dough from refrigerator. Let stand, covered, 30 minutes.
3. Combine mushrooms and next 4 ingredients in a large bowl; drizzle with 1½ tablespoons oil. Toss. Arrange vegetables on a jelly-roll pan. Bake at 500° for 15 minutes.
4. Punch dough down. Sprinkle a lightly floured baking sheet with cornmeal; roll dough into a 15-inch circle on prepared baking sheet. Brush dough with remaining 1 teaspoon oil. Spread sauce over dough, leaving a ½-inch border. Sprinkle ½ cup mozzarella over sauce; top with vegetables.

Sprinkle ½ cup mozzarella and red pepper over zucchini mixture. Dollop with ricotta. Slide pizza onto preheated pizza stone. Bake at 500° for 11 minutes or until crust is golden. Sprinkle with basil. Serves 6 (serving size: 2 slices).

CALORIES 347; FAT 11.1g (sat 3.7g, mono 4.4g, poly 2g); PROTEIN 14.8g; CARB 48.5g; FIBER 2.7g; CHOL 15mg; IRON 3mg; SODIUM 655mg; CALC 193mg

BLOGGER TIP:
Step Outside Your Comfort Zone

"Going meatless were words I thought I would never say. But I have battled with weight all my life, and I wanted to reach outside my comfort zone and give something new a try. Honestly, it hasn't been as hard as I thought it was going to be. I have learned to incorporate all my CSA (community-supported agriculture) vegetables into my bean and grain dishes and pumped out a few fantastic meals. Now I've started making meatless dinners without even thinking about it. It's an amazing change that I'm really enjoying. Vegetarian eating is not just about tasteless salads. It's about eating flavorful dishes that combine grains, beans, and vegetables for the perfect balance of flavor."

—*Brandy Clabaugh, blogger, Nutmeg Nanny*

Try New Ways with Tofu

HARDWORKING SOYBEANS in the form of tofu and tempeh are often a staple in vegetarian diets, and no wonder: They have a neutral taste that can adapt to any flavor profile and work in a variety of cooking methods. They're also a powerhouse of protein and heart-healthy fats. Go ahead, have fun! Experiment with seasonings and worldly twists.

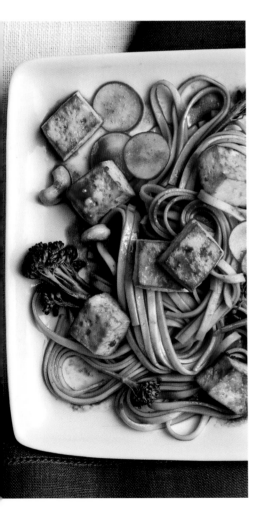

Udon Noodle Salad with Broccolini and Spicy Tofu

8 ounces water-packed
 extra-firm tofu
5 tablespoons peanut oil, divided
2 tablespoons lower-sodium tamari
 or soy sauce
1½ teaspoons Sriracha (hot chile
 sauce), divided
Cooking spray
6 ounces uncooked dried udon noodles
 (thick Japanese wheat noodles)
6 cups water
1½ teaspoons kosher salt
8 ounces Broccolini
3 tablespoons rice wine vinegar
1 tablespoon grated peeled
 fresh ginger
1 teaspoon dark sesame oil
½ cup thinly sliced radishes
 (about 3 medium)
2 tablespoons chopped dry-roasted
 cashews, toasted

1. Cut tofu into ¾-inch-thick slices. Place tofu slices in a single layer on several layers of paper towels; cover with additional paper towels. Let tofu stand 30 minutes to drain, pressing down occasionally. Remove tofu from paper towels, and cut into ¾-inch cubes.
2. Preheat oven to 350°.
3. Combine 2 tablespoons peanut oil, tamari, and 1 teaspoon Sriracha in a large bowl, stirring well with a whisk. Add tofu cubes to tamari mixture, and toss gently to coat. Let stand 15 minutes. Remove tofu from bowl with a slotted spoon; reserve tamari mixture in bowl. Arrange tofu in a single layer on a foil-lined baking sheet coated with cooking spray, and bake tofu at 350° for 10 minutes or until lightly golden.
4. Cook udon noodles according to package directions, omitting salt and fat. Drain and rinse with cold water; drain well.
5. Combine 6 cups water and salt in a large saucepan over high heat; bring to a boil. Add Broccolini to pan; cook 3 minutes or until crisp-tender. Drain and plunge Broccolini into ice water; drain well. Chop Broccolini.
6. Add remaining 3 tablespoons peanut oil, remaining ½ teaspoon Sriracha, rice wine vinegar, ginger, and sesame oil to reserved tamari mixture in bowl; stir mixture well

with a whisk. Add baked tofu, udon noodles, Broccolini, and radishes to bowl; toss gently to coat. Sprinkle salad with cashews. Serves 4 (serving size: 1¼ cups noodle mixture and 1½ teaspoons cashews).

CALORIES 438; FAT 24.7g (sat 4.1g, mono 10.1g, poly 8.2g); PROTEIN 14.3g; CARB 38.4g; FIBER 3.4g; CHOL 0mg; IRON 3mg; SODIUM 572mg; CALC 97mg

A QUICK TOFU TUTORIAL

If you've never worked with tofu, the main consideration is matching type to recipe. Tofu is made in two different ways, and each process yields different results. Once opened, you'll need to place it in an airtight container and cover it with water; change the water daily to keep it fresh. Store in the refrigerater for three to four days.

Silken Tofu

This type has a smooth texture similar to crème fraîche or yogurt. It's soy milk that's simply thickened with a coagulant.
Best for: dips, sauces, smoothies, and dessert recipes

Water-Packed Tofu

To make this variety, milk is heated and salts are added to separate the milk into curds and whey. The curds are scooped out, pressed into molds, and drained into blocks of tofu.
Best for: stir-fries and other savory applications in which you want the tofu to hold its shape after it's cooked

Tempeh and Green Bean Stir-Fry with Peanut Sauce

Tempeh is a high-protein soy product that originated in Indonesia; substitute extra-firm tofu, if desired.

Peanut sauce:
¼ cup water
1 tablespoon brown sugar
3 tablespoons natural-style, chunky peanut butter
1 teaspoon Sriracha (hot chile sauce)
1 teaspoon lower-sodium soy sauce

Stir-fry:
2 teaspoons brown sugar
5 teaspoons lower-sodium soy sauce
1 teaspoon Sriracha
4 garlic cloves, chopped
1 tablespoon plus 2 teaspoons sesame oil, divided
1 (8-ounce) package organic tempeh, cut into ⅓-inch strips
2 cups thinly sliced carrot
1 cup (2-inch) strips red bell pepper
1 pound green beans, trimmed
½ cup water
¾ cup thinly sliced green onions, divided
6 ounces mung bean sprouts

1. To prepare peanut sauce, combine ¼ cup water, 1 tablespoon brown sugar, peanut butter, 1 teaspoon Sriracha, and 1 teaspoon soy sauce in a medium bowl, stirring well with a whisk. Set aside.
2. To prepare stir-fry, combine 2 teaspoons sugar, 5 teaspoons soy sauce, 1 teaspoon Sriracha, and garlic in a small bowl, stirring with a whisk.

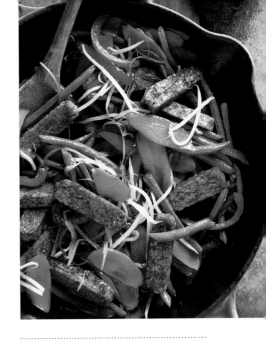

3. Heat a large heavy skillet over medium-high heat. Add 1 tablespoon sesame oil to pan; swirl to coat. Add tempeh and half of soy sauce mixture; stir-fry 5 minutes or until tempeh is golden brown. Remove tempeh mixture from pan, and keep warm. Add remaining 2 teaspoons oil to pan, swirling to coat. Add carrot, bell pepper, and green beans to pan; stir-fry 3 minutes. Add ½ cup water; reduce heat to medium. Cover and simmer 5 minutes or until beans are crisp-tender. Stir in remaining half of soy sauce mixture, tempeh mixture, half of onions, and bean sprouts; cook 2 minutes or until sprouts are tender. Serve with peanut sauce and remaining half of onions. Serves 4 (serving size: 2 cups tempeh mixture, 2 tablespoons peanut sauce, and 1½ tablespoons green onions).

CALORIES 357; FAT 18.3g (sat 2.9g, mono 7.1g, poly 6.7g); PROTEIN 18.4g; CARB 35.2g; FIBER 8.2g; CHOL 0mg; IRON 4mg; SODIUM 353mg; CALC 158mg

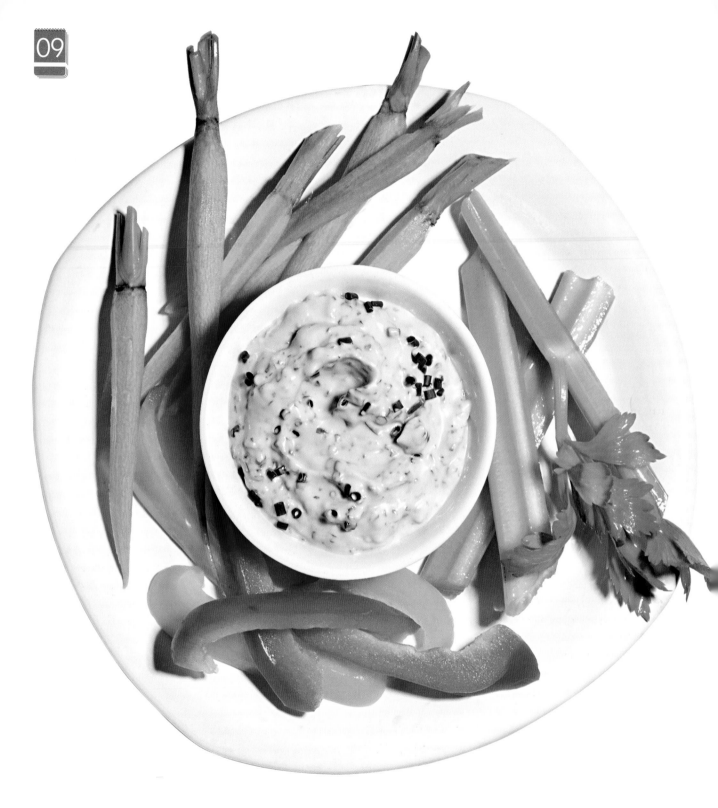

GET STRONGER

ADD STRENGTH TRAINING TWICE A WEEK.

CHANCES ARE BY NOW you've already added thirty minutes of cardio, three times a week into your schedule. But now it's time to go one step further and add strength training to your fitness regimen at least two times per week.

Put simply, strength training is defined as the use of resistance to build muscle size and strength. But the benefits of strength training go beyond that: Lean muscle burns calories more efficiently than fat, even when your body is at rest. More muscle means burning more calories, which can make it easier to reach and maintain a healthy weight. Strength training also strengthens your bones, reduces the progression and pain of arthritis, and helps control blood sugar in people with type 2 diabetes. It can help you appear younger by helping you look more toned and firm, even as your skin gradually loses elasticity.

Though you probably know how good strength training can be, 40% of you admit to not doing any form of it at all. The biggest hurdles? Believing cardio is more important, super-busy schedules, and having no clue how to get started.

Don't be intimidated. There are plenty of quick, effective workouts you can do that don't require you to step into a gym. In this chapter, we'll give you plenty of moves and motivation to make strength training a new habit. This chapter is also full of delicious recipes to help nourish your muscles and fuel your strength.

YOUR GOAL

Include strength training in your fitness regimen at least two times per week.

The 12 Healthy Habits

| · 01 · GET COOKING | · 02 · BREAKFAST DAILY | · 03 · WHOLE GRAINS | · 04 · GET MOVING | · 05 · VEGGIE UP | · 06 · MORE SEAFOOD | · 07 · HEALTHY FATS | · 08 · GO MEATLESS | · 09 · GET STRONGER | · 10 · LESS SALT | · 11 · BE PORTION-AWARE | · 12 · EAT MINDFULLY |

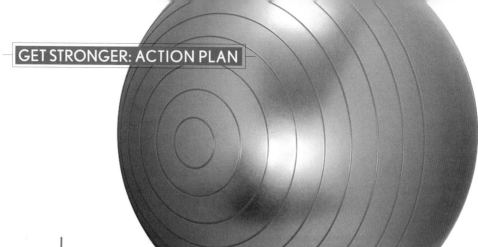

Get Equipped

YOU DON'T HAVE TO HAVE A GYM MEMBERSHIP to start strength training. Here, exercise physiologist Geralyn Coopersmith, National Director of the Equinox Fitness Training Institute, gives her top five recs for the training tools you need to get your home ready:

1. DUMBBELLS
You ideally want a variety of sizes. If you're a beginner, you may want to start at three to five pounds for arm exercises and 10 to 12 for legs. When you can easily do 12 repetitions with a particular weight, gradually increase the weight.

2. RESISTANCE BANDS
They're inexpensive, versatile, and portable so you can get a full-body workout no matter where you are. These elastic strips can be used to target your core muscles (your lower back, hips, and abdomen) as well as work your arms, shoulders, and legs.

3. STABILITY BALL
It provides a fun (or at least a more interesting) way to do sit-ups and push-ups, or you can use it as a weight bench while you lift dumbbells. It also forces you to work your core as you do basic exercises.

4. MEDICINE BALL
While you can use it like a dumbbell, you can also throw or catch this weighted leather or rubber ball to challenge your core and coordination while working both your upper and lower body.

5. VALSLIDE
This portable pair of oblong discs has a foam-like surface on one side and plastic on the other. You place your hands or feet on the foam side to create more resistance when you're doing traditional lunges or squats. (www.valslide.com)

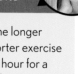

EXPERT TIP: *Schedule Shorter Sessions*

"If your workweek is hectic, schedule shorter exercises. Save the longer yoga classes and workout sessions for the weekend and do shorter exercise bursts during the week. Most people think if they don't have an hour for a workout then it's not worth it. False! Consistency matters, and the time you spend adds up."

—*Rebecca Scritchfield, MA, RD, blogger, Rebecca Thinks*

The Country Midwife

"I live far away from any gym. It's a distance problem."

JENNIFER DRAWBRIDGE
Nurse-Midwife

➤ **GET STRONGER CHALLENGE:** Jennifer lives in a rural community, and the nearest gym is a half hour away. She's able to squeeze in cardio five or six days a week with outdoor activities such as snowshoeing in the winter or hiking in the summer, but she has no idea where to start when it comes to strength training. Jen also has a family history of osteoporosis: "The women in my family have bones like Fritos—both my grandmother and mother broke their hips."

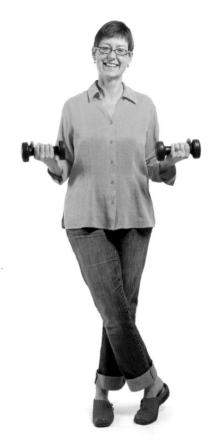

OUR ADVICE

■ **Get creative with cords.** You can do hundreds of muscle-sculpting moves using a pair of portable exercise cords. Experiment with wrapping the cords around stationary furniture, different parts of your body, or standing on them for more resistance.

■ **Do a different push-up.** The basic push-up is one of the best exercises for building upper-body strength— unfortunately, it's also one of the hardest for women to do. Try this instead: Get into a push-up position, then slowly lower yourself to the floor for a count of two. Don't push yourself up if you can't. Just get back into the up position and repeat the exercise for as many reps as you can. You'll be doing a regular push-up in no time.

■ **Don't sit when you lift.** Doing curls, presses, or triceps extensions while standing allows you to lift up to 30% more weight, which can help you develop leaner muscle faster.

■ **Try other bone-strengthening activities.** Lifting weights isn't the only way to build stronger bones. Yoga and tai chi, which work multiple muscle groups simultaneously, have been shown to improve bone growth and strengthen muscle, too. Learn a few moves or poses that you can do anywhere.

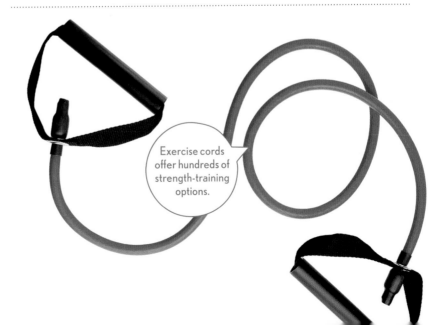

Exercise cords offer hundreds of strength-training options.

Master Your Technique

LIKE MAKING THE PERFECT ROAST or martini, strength training is all about technique. Here, exercise physiologist Geralyn Coopersmith, National Director of the Equinox Fitness Training Institute, reveals the five biggest mistakes she sees clients make:

OOPS! You skimp on your weights. If the weight isn't heavy enough, you'll see fewer results. Researchers at Grand Valley State University in Michigan found that when subjects were asked to choose weights on their own, every subject picked weights that were lighter than what they needed. A good rule of thumb: The weight should be heavy enough to tire your muscles after about 12 reps.

OOPS! You rely too much on machines.
Classic strength-training machines like leg or chest presses are great for beginners because they prevent unwanted movements, but it's also easy to "cheat" by lightening the load, changing the hand grip, or adjusting the seat. Rather than just make your way down the same old circuit, spice up your workout by adding in free weights, kettlebells, or even your own body weight (think push-ups, walking lunges, and planks).

OOPS! You always do crunches.
When you "crunch" up during your crunches you actually put strain on your back at its weakest point, the back of the spine, which can cause herniated discs. You're better off focusing on moves such as the plank, side plank, and bridges, which not only tone up your abs but also all your other core muscles such as your hips, back, and pelvis.

OOPS! You skip your warm-up.
You wouldn't jump into a sprint the minute you stepped onto the treadmill, right? The same holds true for strength training. Working cold, stiff muscles can lead to sprains and tears. Try to do at least five minutes of walking in place or simple lunges and squats to warm up muscles before starting your routine.

OOPS! You don't work opposing muscle groups.
If you don't exercise all muscles equally, you run the risk of developing strength imbalances that can leave you with back, foot, or knee pain. The solution's pretty simple: Pair every exercise that works the front of your body with one that also works your back (for example, quads with hamstrings, biceps with triceps, chest with back).

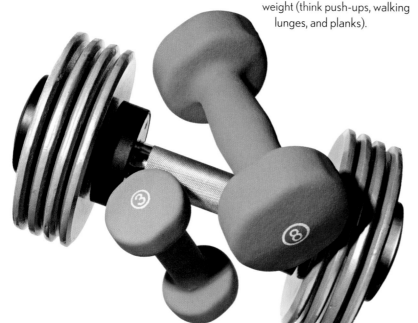

The No-Time-Whatsoever Working Mom

"I'm embarrassed to say that what I do for exercise is basically nothing."

DEBRA RICHMAN
Vice President, Communications

➤ **GET STRONGER CHALLENGE:** Debra wants to exercise, but her schedule makes it tough. During the week she's up at 4:45 and out of the house by 6:30 for an 80-minute commute into New York City. With such a killer schedule and busy weekends spent running her children to activities, sneaking strength training in takes a little creativity.

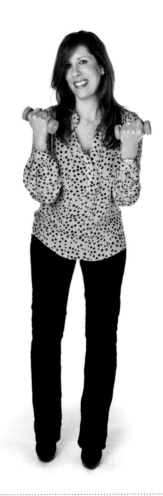

OUR ADVICE

■ **Work the whole body at once.** When time is limited, use only moves that train multiple muscle groups simultaneously, such as squats or lunges. If you must do exercises that work only one muscle group (arm curls, for example), add a lunge or squat between repetitions.

■ **Compress the sets.** Pick three exercises that work the same muscle group, and do all three back to back with no rest in between. You'll not only work your muscles 30% to 50% more thoroughly, but you'll also speed through your workout.

■ **Squeeze in some squats.** Any time you're on the phone or taking a break, kick off your heels, and stand with your feet shoulder-width apart. Slowly squat down, as if you're sitting, and stand back up. Do as many squats as you can, being sure your knees never go past your toes. Just lowering yourself a few inches strengthens all your leg muscles.

■ **Make it playtime.** Recapture your childhood, and challenge your little ones to a swing-set race. Pumping your legs works your lower body—plus the muscles in your abs, shoulders, arms, and back help keep your body stabilized. Next, work your way across the monkey bars: They target your back and biceps and strengthen your core.

Create an exercise log. Tracking each workout (weights, reps, etc.) gives you specifics about each workout for reference as you go. Plus, it can keep you motivated by revealing how far you've advanced—and you will progress, remarkably quickly.

Become A Groupie

HAVING TROUBLE GETTING MOTIVATED? Consider checking out a strength-training class at your local gym, YMCA, or community center. A recent Nielsen survey found that more than 90% of people who participate in a group fitness class like Body Pump end up going at least twice a week. An added bonus: Many classes combine cardio and strength training, so you kill two workout birds with one stone.

BOOT CAMP

These classes can vary but generally include a mix of calisthenics, such as pull-ups, push-ups, lunges, and abdominal exercises, as well as drills and sprints. Research shows that these powerful workouts can burn 9.8 calories per minute, or almost 600 calories per hour. For best results, look for one that combines equal amounts cardio and strength training.

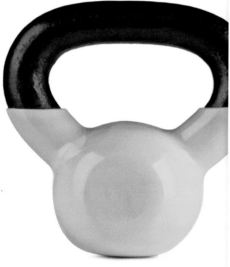

Strength training doesn't just build muscle—it may also help smokers kick the habit, according to a study funded by the National Cancer Institute. Smokers who completed a 12-week smoking cessation program that included strength training were twice as likely to quit successfully compared to those who did not regularly lift weights.

EXPERT TIP:
Women Need to Build Muscle

"Strength training is especially important for women because we naturally have less muscle than men do, and we tend to live longer. So having strong muscles and bones helps keep us healthy, vital, and independent as we grow older."

—*Miriam Nelson, PhD, Professor of Nutrition, Tufts University, and founder and director of StrongWomen*

KETTLEBELLS

Take a break from dumbbells and try a kettlebell class, which uses cannonball-shaped iron orbs as a way to build strength, balance, and endurance. You get a big bang for your buck: Research from the American Council on Exercise shows that a 20-minute kettlebell workout burns on average 273 calories. The unique shape of these weights helps you work multiple muscle groups by lifting and swinging.

BODY PUMP

This popular class is a blend of aerobics and strength training. Designed by New Zealand athlete Les Mills, Body Pump uses a barbell to work your entire body to the tune of upbeat music.

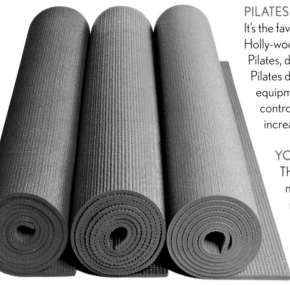

PILATES

It's the favorite fitness regimen of Holly-wood thinsters, and no wonder: Pilates, developed by gymnast Joseph Pilates during World War I, requires no equipment and forces you to rely on controlling your own body weight to increase strength and flexibility.

YOGA

The poses themselves are terrific no-impact stretches and body-resistance exercises that help you loosen up and strengthen your muscles simultaneously—using nothing more than your own sense of balance and body weight.

How do you stay motivated to do strength training?

@DietitianSherry: Schedule it on calendar as an important appt.

@Healthykids: Meeting a friend is the only way I can strength train. I hate going alone, but when I meet a friend I always get there.

@WhiskandCleaver: I put strength training above cardio so it's usually a priority for me. I do it first thing after dropping kids off at school.

@TrySeeAh: Seeing results helps me keep 2 to 3 days of strength training in my routine. #healthy-habits.

@ZenLizzie: Body Pump classes! Having someone else set the schedule makes it easier to keep the strength-training date.

STUDY THE CORRECT POSE.

Make sure you're aligning your body correctly when doing yoga or other floor exercises. It's easy to make mistakes. For instance, the Lying Bridge is a simple floor exercise that tones your body's largest muscles, but it's often done the wrong way.

➤ Don't thrust your hips.

➤ Don't lift your heels.

➤ Don't tuck your chin.

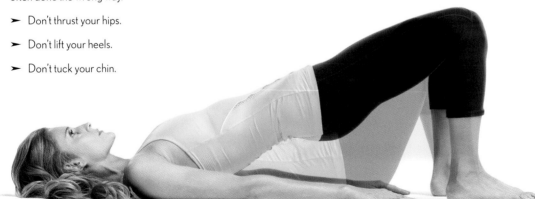

COACHING SESSION
with MYATT MURPHY, CSCS

FITNESS MADE FASTER

F OR MOST PEOPLE, it's not actually doing a strength-training regimen that's the difficult part—it's getting the time to spare to do it that's the real struggle. But you don't have to sacrifice family fun, spend fewer hours working around the house, or cut into your vacation time to accomplish your fitness goals. Feeling stronger and looking leaner by adding the right amount of weight training to your week is easy, if you take the time to simplify how you break a sweat. All you need is an exercise plan that hits all your major muscle groups from head to toe in the shortest amount of time, using as little equipment as possible. Even if you've never used weights before, this simple—yet effective—routine is all you'll need to build a body you can be proud of, without spending any more effort than you have to.

THE ROUTINE

The eight basic exercises on these pages are ideal because they utilize as many muscle fibers as possible, and target all the main muscle groups. Do one set of each exercise in the order below, performing every exercise 12 times. Rest for as long as it takes you to set up the next exercise in the circuit. Once you've completed all eight moves, rest for 60 to 90 seconds, then repeat the eight-move routine twice more. Do this 20-minute routine two to three times a week and within a month, you'll see a leaner, tighter physique in the mirror.

1. DUMBBELL SQUAT

Stand straight with your feet shoulder-width apart with a dumbbell in each hand, palms facing in. Your arms should hang down by your sides. Keeping your head and back straight, slowly squat down until your thighs are parallel to the floor. Push yourself back up into a standing position, and repeat.

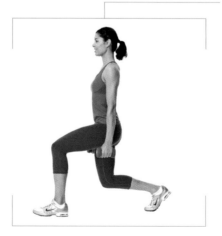

2. CHEST PRESS

Lie back on a bench with a dumbbell in each hand, the weights resting along the outside of your chest (palms facing forward). Slowly press the dumbbells straight up above your chest, elbows bent slightly. Lower the weights back down to the sides of your chest, and repeat.

3. DUMBBELL LUNGE

Stand with a dumbbell in each hand, arms hanging at your sides, feet about 6 inches apart. Keeping your back straight, step forward with your right foot and lean forward until your right thigh is almost parallel to the floor. Push yourself back up into the starting position and repeat, this time stepping out with your left foot.

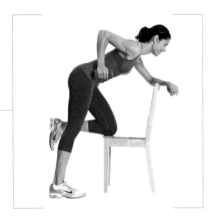

4. ONE-ARM BACK ROW

Stand with your left side to a chair, exercise bench, or the side of a high bed and a dumbbell in your right hand. Rest your left arm and knee on the chair. Bend forward at the waist until your back is almost parallel to the floor, your right arm hanging straight down toward the floor, palm facing in. Slowly draw the weight up close to the body until it reaches the outside of your chest. Lower the weight back down and repeat eight to 12 times. Afterward, switch positions to work your left arm.

5. SHOULDER PRESS

Sit on a chair, feet firmly on the floor, with a dumbbell in each hand. Bring the weights to the sides of your shoulders, palms facing out. Slowly press the weights over your head, keeping your back straight. Pause, then lower the weights back to your shoulders.

6. BICEPS CURL

Stand, holding a pair of dumbbells with an underhand grip, arms hanging down in front of you. Keeping your upper arms tucked in to your sides, slowly curl the weights up to your shoulders, then lower them back to their starting position.

7. ONE-ARM EXTENSION

Sit on the edge of a chair with a light dumbbell in your right hand. Raise the weight over your head, palm facing left, and tuck your upper arm against the side of your head. With your left hand cupping your right elbow for support, slowly lower the weight behind your head as far as you can. Raise the weight overhead until your arm is straight—repeat eight to 12 times, then switch the weight to the opposite hand to work your left arm.

8. BICYCLE CRUNCH

Lie flat, knees bent and feet together. Place your hands lightly against the sides of your head. Draw your left knee toward your chest while simultaneously extending your right leg. At the same time, curl your torso up and twist to the left, so that your right elbow and left knee touch. Lower yourself back to the floor, then repeat, this time pulling your right knee in and extending your left leg as you curl and twist your torso to the right—touching your left elbow to your right knee. Continue to alternate for the entire set of eight to 12 repetitions.

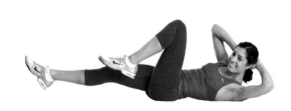

Protein: A Primer

W HEN YOU'RE TRYING TO EAT RIGHT to support your strength training, protein is crucial: This nutrient accelerates muscle growth and speeds recovery after a tough workout. Spread out protein intake throughout the day instead of eating mega doses just once or twice: Unlike carbs and fat, protein isn't stored for energy production. The best muscle-friendly sources of protein include the essential amino acid leucine: Eggs, dairy, meat, poultry, and fish top the list, but plant protein sources, such as lentils, beans, nuts, seeds, and soybeans supply some, too. Yogurt, particularly Greek yogurt, is a good source of high-quality protein. It's always a smart choice for breakfast, but there are ways you can incorporate it at any time of day, in dishes from soups and salads to snacks and desserts.

Cucumber Gazpacho with Shrimp Relish

2 teaspoons extra-virgin olive oil
¾ pound peeled and deveined medium shrimp, chopped
½ teaspoon salt, divided
½ teaspoon black pepper, divided
¼ teaspoon ground cumin
¼ teaspoon paprika
2 cups quartered grape tomatoes
⅓ cup cilantro leaves
2½ cups chopped English cucumber
1 cup fat-free, lower-sodium chicken broth
1 cup plain whole-milk Greek yogurt
¼ cup chopped onion
2 tablespoons fresh lime juice
Dash of ground red pepper
1 large garlic clove, peeled

1. Heat a skillet over medium-high heat. Add oil to pan; swirl to coat. Sprinkle shrimp with ¼ teaspoon salt, ¼ teaspoon black pepper, cumin, and paprika. Add shrimp; sauté 2 minutes or until done. Stir in tomatoes; remove from heat. Add cilantro.
2. Place remaining ¼ teaspoon salt, ¼ teaspoon black pepper, cucumber, and remaining ingredients in a blender; process until smooth. Ladle 1 cup soup into each of 4 bowls; top with ¾ cup relish. Serves 4.

CALORIES 225; FAT 9.6g (sat 5.1g, mono 1.9g, poly 0.9g); PROTEIN 22.7g; CARB 11.5g; FIBER 2.2g; CHOL 139mg; IRON 2.4mg; SODIUM 557mg; CALC 130mg

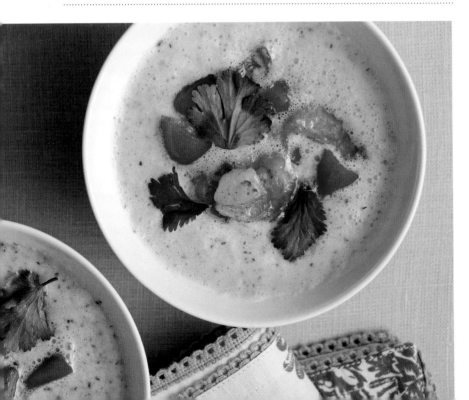

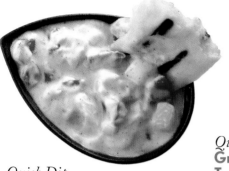

Quick Dip
Indian-Style Raita

Combine 1½ cups plain low-fat yogurt, ¾ cup chopped seeded peeled cucumber, ¾ cup chopped seeded tomato, 1 teaspoon garam masala, and ¼ teaspoon salt. Cover and chill before serving. Serves 6.

CALORIES 44; FAT 1.2g (sat 0.7g, mono 0.1g, poly 0.1g); PROTEIN 3.2g; CARB 5.5g; FIBER 0.7g; CHOL 6mg; IRON 0.8mg; SODIUM 130mg; CALC 111mg

Quick Dip
Greek-Style Tzatziki

Combine 1 cup plain 2% reduced-fat Greek yogurt, ¾ cup finely chopped seeded cucumber, 1 tablespoon chopped mint, ⅛ teaspoon salt, and ⅛ teaspoon white pepper. Cover and chill before serving. Serves 3.

CALORIES 62; FAT 1.8g (sat 1.3g, mono 0.3g, poly 0g); PROTEIN 7.8g; CARB 4.4g; FIBER 0.3g; CHOL 4mg; IRON 0.1mg; SODIUM 127mg; CALC 86mg

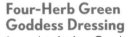

Four-Herb Green Goddess Dressing

1 cup plain fat-free Greek yogurt
½ cup reduced-fat mayonnaise
2 teaspoons Worcestershire sauce
2 teaspoons fresh lemon juice
½ teaspoon hot pepper sauce
3 canned anchovy fillets
1 garlic clove, minced
⅔ cup fresh parsley leaves
¼ cup fresh tarragon leaves
¼ cup chopped fresh chives
¼ cup fresh chervil leaves (optional)

1. Place first 7 ingredients in a blender or food processor; process until smooth. Add parsley, tarragon, chives, and, if desired, chervil; process until herbs are minced. Serves 10 (serving size: about 2½ tablespoons).

CALORIES 36; FAT 1.8g (sat 0g, mono 0.1g, poly 0.8g); PROTEIN 2.6g; CARB 3.6g; FIBER 0.1g; CHOL 1mg; IRON 0.4mg; SODIUM 171mg; CALC 30mg

THINGS TO KNOW ABOUT YOGURT

■ **Look for the seal.** The "Live & Active Cultures" symbol was established by the National Yogurt Association to confirm that a yogurt contained at least 100 million cultures per gram at the time it was manufactured. It's not policed by the FDA, though, and not all companies pay the yearly fee to use the package symbol.

■ **Love the whey.** The clear liquid that often separates and floats to the top of many yogurts contains a little protein and tart flavor. Don't pour it off—stir it in. Whey protein has the highest concentration of leucine compared to other proteins. This amino acid stimulates protein synthesis in muscles. That's why it's the source of protein in many bodybuilding powders. (But you're better off sticking with yogurt.)

■ **Be careful about the yogurt health-halo.** Look out for "yogurt" coatings on pretzels, candies, or other snack foods. It's likely oil and sugar with just a bit of yogurt powder, and any good-for-you bacteria on these snacks do not always survive the spray-drying process.

Power Up with Bean Protein

BEANS PROVIDE A HEALTHY TRIFECTA of protein, complex carbohydrates, and fiber, which makes them a superb choice for a post-workout meal. Each cup of cooked beans provides about 15 grams of protein. You'll also get a notable amount of iron, folate, magnesium, and potassium.

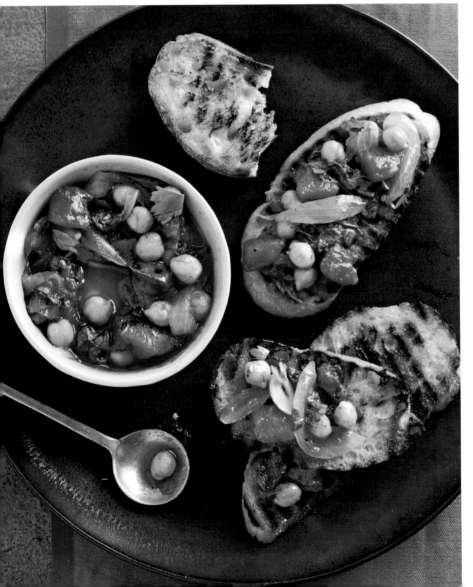

Chickpeas and Spinach with Smoky Paprika

If you don't have smoked paprika, substitute 1 teaspoon sweet paprika and ¼ teaspoon ground red pepper. Serve this mixture on grilled or toasted bread for a small-plate appetizer or side.

1 tablespoon olive oil
4 cups thinly sliced onion
5 garlic cloves, thinly sliced
1 teaspoon Spanish smoked paprika
½ cup dry white wine
¼ cup organic vegetable broth
1 (14.5-ounce) can fire-roasted diced
   tomatoes, undrained
1 (15-ounce) can chickpeas (garbanzo
   beans), rinsed and drained
1 (9-ounce) package fresh spinach
2 tablespoons chopped fresh
   flat-leaf parsley
2 teaspoons sherry vinegar

1. Heat a large Dutch oven over medium heat. Add oil to pan; swirl to coat. Add onion and garlic to pan; cover and cook 8 minutes or until tender, stirring occasionally. Stir in smoked paprika, and cook 1 minute. Add white wine, vegetable broth, and tomatoes; bring to a boil.

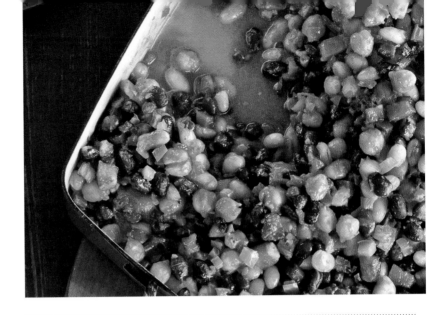

Add chickpeas; reduce heat, and simmer until sauce thickens slightly (about 15 minutes), stirring occasionally. Add spinach; cover and cook 2 minutes or until spinach wilts. Stir in parsley and vinegar. Serves 10 (serving size: about ⅔ cup).

CALORIES 86; **FAT** 1.9g (sat 0.2g, mono 1g; poly 0.2g); **PROTEIN** 3.1g; **CARB** 14.6g; **FIBER** 3.5g; **CHOL** 0mg; **IRON** 1.8mg; **SODIUM** 168mg; **CALC** 64mg

Smoky Three-Bean Bake

Three kinds of beans take the classic dish from ho-hum to fun with different shapes and pleasing textures—from the al dente bite of chickpeas to the creaminess of Great Northern beans. If you happen to use hot smoked paprika, you can omit the ground red pepper.

4 applewood-smoked bacon slices, chopped
2 cups finely chopped onion
1 cup finely chopped green bell pepper
6 garlic cloves, minced
¾ cup no-salt-added tomato sauce
⅓ cup packed brown sugar
1 tablespoon cider vinegar
1 tablespoon honey
1 tablespoon Dijon mustard
1 teaspoon smoked paprika
¾ teaspoon kosher salt
½ teaspoon freshly ground black pepper
¼ teaspoon ground red pepper
1 (15-ounce) can organic black beans, rinsed and drained
1 (15-ounce) can organic chickpeas, rinsed and drained
1 (15-ounce) can organic Great Northern beans, rinsed and drained
Cooking spray

1. Preheat oven to 325°.
2. Heat a large nonstick skillet over medium-high heat. Add bacon to pan, and sauté 5 minutes or until crisp. Remove bacon from pan with a slotted spoon, reserving 1½ tablespoons drippings in pan. Set bacon aside. Add onion, bell pepper, and garlic to drippings in pan, and sauté 6 minutes or until tender, stirring occasionally. Remove from heat, and cool slightly.
3. Combine tomato sauce and next 8 ingredients in a large bowl, stirring with a whisk. Stir in onion mixture and beans. Spoon bean mixture into an 11 x 7–inch glass or ceramic baking dish coated with cooking spray, and sprinkle with reserved bacon. Cover and bake at 325° for 30 minutes. Uncover; bake an additional 30 minutes. Serves 8 (serving size: about ¾ cup).

CALORIES 204; **FAT** 4.7g (sat 1.4g, mono 1.8g, poly 0.5g); **PROTEIN** 7.3g; **CARB** 33.2g; **FIBER** 6g; **CHOL** 6.8mg; **IRON** 1.7mg; **SODIUM** 382mg; **CALC** 71mg

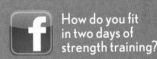

How do you fit in two days of strength training?

"I have a list of exercises taped to the back of my iPod so I don't forget the order."
—*Tricia Fitzgerald*

"Seriously, kettlebells are the BEST strength, overall body shaping, and cardio workout ever."
—*Debbie Gail Trout*

"I've had a lot of success with the Body Pump class at my gym. I go 3 times a week and love it! It's an hour of strength training mainly using a bar, and it works your whole body. I've been amazed at the difference in my body and how strong I am from going for only a few months."
—*Brittany Lee Botti*

Load Up on Lentils

LENTILS MAY BE THE RUNT of the legume family, but they have a lot going for them: They contain about a steak's worth of protein and are packed with metabolism-boosting B vitamins, magnesium for bone health, and iron for healthy red blood cells. Plus, they cook in half the time of other legumes.

Turkish Carrots and Lentils

3 tablespoons extra-virgin olive oil
1½ cups thinly sliced onion
1 garlic clove, minced
1 tablespoon tomato paste
½ teaspoon ground Aleppo pepper
1 pound carrots, halved lengthwise and thinly sliced (about 3 cups)
¾ teaspoon sea salt, divided
3 cups water
1 cup uncooked dried green lentils
¼ teaspoon freshly ground black pepper
¼ cup plain 2% reduced-fat Greek yogurt
Dill sprigs (optional)

1. Heat a large saucepan over medium heat. Add oil to pan; swirl to coat. Add onion; cook 9 minutes or until lightly browned, stirring occasionally. Add garlic; cook 1 minute. Stir in tomato paste and Aleppo pepper; cook 30 seconds. Stir in carrots and ¼ teaspoon salt; cook 1 minute. Remove from heat.

2. Combine 3 cups water and lentils in a large saucepan; bring to a boil. Cover, reduce heat, and simmer 30 minutes. Uncover, increase heat to medium-high, and stir in onion mixture; cook 2 minutes or until liquid almost evaporates. Stir in remaining ½ teaspoon salt and black pepper. Cover with a kitchen towel; cool to room temperature. Serve with yogurt. Garnish with dill, if desired. Serves 4 (serving size: about 1 cup lentil mixture and 1 tablespoon yogurt).

CALORIES 357; FAT 12.2g (sat 2.8g, mono 7.7g, poly 1.2g); PROTEIN 17.4g; CARB 48.6g; FIBER 10.6g; CHOL 3mg; IRON 5mg; SODIUM 549mg; CALC 64mg

EXPERT TIP:
Reclaim Yourself

"Exercise for me came to a screeching halt when I got pregnant and then the challenge of being a new mom and generally running on fumes. I canceled my gym membership and put fitness on the shelf. But a funny thing happened: I missed it. So I dusted off some old hand weights and set a 30-day goal—the first exercise-related goal.

On day one, I thought my ankles would snap during the warm-up jumping jacks. By the second week I was far less winded, and by day 20, I could push both kids uphill in the double stroller without feeling nauseous. By the end, I felt like a new person. I had reclaimed a piece of my pre-baby self: I was, once again, Someone Who Exercised."

—*Sally Kuzemchak, MS, RD; blogger, Real Mom Nutrition*

Sloppy Lentils in Pita

This Middle Eastern-inspired sandwich combines brown lentils and ground lamb, and is topped with cooling yogurt, cucumber, and mint.

1 tablespoon olive oil
¾ cup finely chopped onion
1 tablespoon minced garlic
¼ teaspoon salt
¼ teaspoon freshly ground
   black pepper
8 ounces lean ground lamb
¾ cup dried brown lentils
1 teaspoon ground cumin
1 teaspoon dried thyme
1 cup water, divided
2 cups diced plum tomatoes or
   boxed diced tomatoes, undrained
1 bay leaf
4 (6-inch) whole-wheat pitas,
   cut in half
½ cup plain 2% reduced-fat
   Greek yogurt
1 cup thinly sliced cucumber
Mint leaves

1. Heat a large skillet over medium-high heat. Add olive oil to pan; swirl to coat. Add onion, garlic, salt, pepper, and lamb; cook 5 minutes or until lamb is browned and vegetables are tender, stirring occasionally to crumble lamb.
2. Add lentils, cumin, and thyme; stir until seasonings become fragrant. Add ½ cup water, tomatoes, and bay leaf; bring to a boil. Cover, reduce heat to medium, and cook 15 minutes. Stir lentil mixture; add remaining ½ cup water. Cover and cook 15 minutes or until lentils are

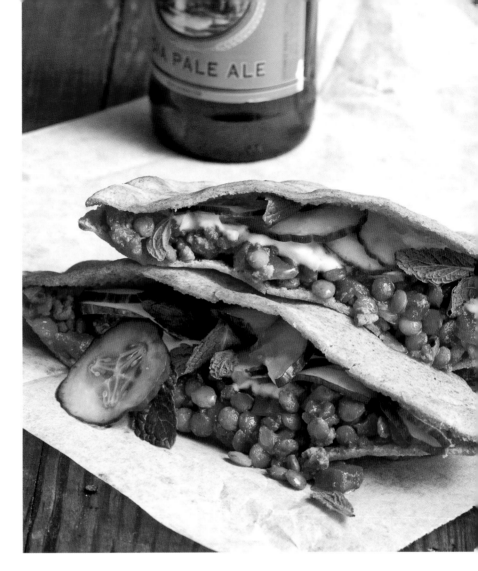

tender and mixture is thick (add additional water as needed). Discard bay leaf. Fill each pita half with ½ cup lentil mixture. Spoon 1 tablespoon yogurt into each pita half; top with 2 tablespoons cucumber. Sprinkle with mint, if desired. Serves 4 (serving size: 2 filled pita halves).

CALORIES 454; FAT 13.8g (sat 4.4g, mono 5.8g, poly 1.4g); PROTEIN 28.2g; CARB 57.4g; FIBER 11.6g; CHOL 39mg; IRON 4.9mg; SODIUM 568mg; CALC 115mg

When traveling, rely on two travel-friendly classics. Push-ups and lunges utilize your body weight to build and strengthen muscle without any exercise equipment.

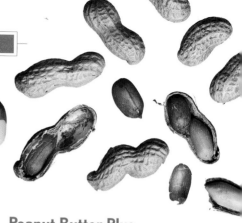

In Praise of Peanuts

ALTHOUGH "NUT" IS PART of their name, peanuts are more closely related to beans than to walnuts. Proof that peanuts are legumes comes every time you crack the shell with your hands: They're lined up just like, well, peas in a pod. Peanuts provide 7g of protein per ounce—not that far short of beef—and they're full of healthy monounsaturated fat, too.

Peanut Butter Plus Sandwiches

Half a sandwich makes a great post-exercise snack, or enjoy a whole sandwich for lunch. Mix up a batch of the spread (it will keep in the refrigerator for several days), and make sandwiches as needed or use to top whole-grain bagels or waffles. The filling doubles as a tasty dip for apple wedges, celery, or strawberries.

3 tablespoons creamy peanut butter
2 tablespoons honey
3 tablespoons golden raisins
1 tablespoon roasted salted sunflower
   seed kernels
8 (1-ounce) slices whole-wheat bread
1 large banana, sliced

1. Combine peanut butter and honey in a small microwave-safe bowl. Microwave at HIGH 20 seconds. Stir in raisins and sunflower seeds. Spread about 2 tablespoons peanut butter mixture on each of 4 bread slices. Top evenly with sliced banana and remaining bread slices. Cut each sandwich into 4 triangles. Serves 8 (serving size: 2 triangles).

CALORIES 152; FAT 4.9g (sat 1g, mono 2g, poly 1.5g); PROTEIN 4.8g; CARB 25.3g; FIBER 3g; CHOL 0mg; IRON 1.2mg; SODIUM 181mg; CALC 26mg

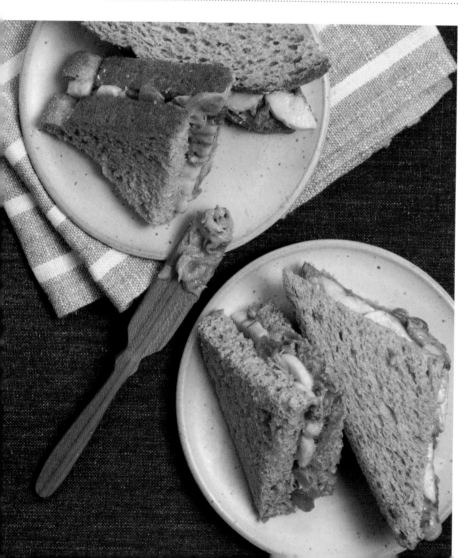

EXPLORE A NEW NUT BUTTER

Creamy, protein-packed nut butters go far beyond peanut butter, and they're not difficult to make at home. Here's the scoop: If you buy raw nuts, you'll need to roast them in a 375° oven for 15 to 20 minutes, just until they're lightly browned. Then place the nuts in a food processor, and grind until they form a paste. The higher the fat of the nut, the smoother the butter will be. You can add canola oil to the mixture as is grinds to help get a smoother consistency.

Homemade nut butters taste fresher but are more perishable than commercial varieties, so make them in small batches. Store in an airtight container in the refrigerator for up to a month.

1. Cashew
The smooth butter forms after about 2 minutes of processing. It's ideal for sandwiches, but you can also substitute it for tahini when making hummus.

2. Almond
When the almonds start to come away from the sides of the food processor, the butter is ready. Slivered, toasted almonds take about 3½ minutes to form a butter, but roasted whole almonds have additional oil and will be ready in just 2½ minutes. This mild, sweet butter is adaptable in sweet and savory dishes.

3. Hazelnut
This thick, grainy butter is fruity and naturally sweet. If nuts are whole, toast them at 375° for 5 minutes or until they start to look shiny and the skins begin to loosen. You can leave the skins on to toast them, then just rub the nuts in a dish towel to remove skins. Process in a food processor for about 2½ minutes.

4. Pecan
Pecans process into butter in about a minute. The loose paste spreads easily, but skins give it a slightly bitter aftertaste, so it's best used in recipes.

5. Peanut
Use plain roasted peanuts rather than dry-roasted peanuts, which are seasoned with paprika, garlic, and onion powder. This smooth nut butter has distinctive fresh peanut flavor, and the nuts take about 2 minutes to process. It is grainier than commercial brands.

6. Pistachio
A very dry, crumbly butter, it's best combined with something else, like softened cream cheese. Cream cheese–pistachio spread is nice on French or egg bread. It takes about 3½ to 4 minutes to grind into butter, and it tends to clump during processing.

7. Walnut
Like pecan butter, this soft, oily butter is ready in about a minute. Like pecan butter, it has a bitter aftertaste from the skins, making it good for recipes but not on sandwiches. Walnut halves are expensive, so look for pieces.

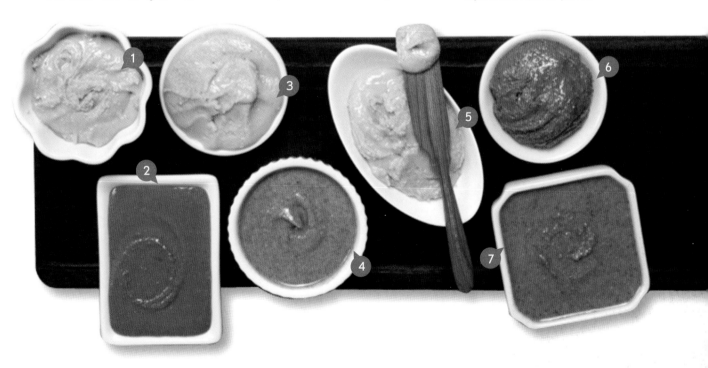

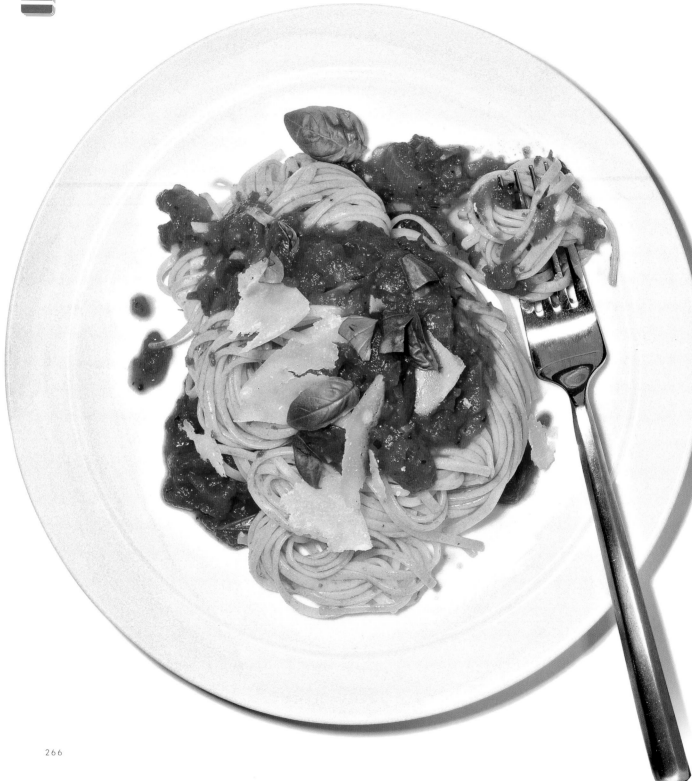

EAT LESS SALT

KEEP YOUR SHAKER, BUT BEWARE SNEAKY SOURCES.

MOVE OVER TRANS FAT. Ciao, carbs. Salt is having its day in the nutrition hot seat. But beyond the salt we add in the kitchen and at the table, most of us don't know where salt lurks, nor do we know the recommended limits, or why it even matters anyway. Even the terminology muddles things up: "Salt" and "sodium" are used almost interchangeably, but salt is only 40% sodium (the rest is chloride).

Our bodies need sodium to maintain the right balance of fluids and to help with muscle movement and contraction. The problem is, we're getting too much: The average American gets 3,400mg a day, about one and a half times more than the maximum allotted by the Dietary Guidelines for Americans. High levels of sodium can elevate blood pressure, which damages the body's circulatory system. The challenge is that not everyone has the same sensitivity to sodium, so a direct correlation between high or low sodium in the diet and cardiovascular disease risk has been difficult to prove.

Still, national guidelines recommend adults limit their daily intake to less than 2,300mg, the equivalent of just 1 teaspoon of salt. The limit for those at risk of high blood pressure—African-Americans, people with hypertension, and anyone over the age of 51—was lowered to 1,500mg.

Your goal for this chapter is to become salt-aware—to prudently monitor and reduce your intake even if you're not hypertensive, and to actively reduce it if you are. You'll find guidance about sneaky sources of sodium and how to use spices and other low-sodium ingredients for maximum flavor.

YOUR GOAL

Reduce the amount of sodium you eat every day.

The 12 Healthy Habits

| · 01 · GET COOKING | · 02 · BREAKFAST DAILY | · 03 · WHOLE GRAINS | · 04 · GET MOVING | · 05 · VEGGIE UP | · 06 · MORE SEAFOOD | · 07 · HEALTHY FATS | · 08 · GO MEATLESS | · 09 · GET STRONGER | · 10 · LESS SALT | · 11 · BE PORTION-AWARE | · 12 · EAT MINDFULLY |

Focus on Fresh

NEARLY 80% OF THE SODIUM WE CONSUME comes from restaurant meals and packaged foods. You can significantly slash that by focusing on fresh, unprocessed foods that you can make easily at home, like these six:

1. SALAD DRESSING

Just two tablespoons of some prepared dressings add 500mg of sodium to your otherwise healthy salad. Whisk up your own vinaigrette instead, like the Easy Herb Vinaigrette on page 223.

2. TOMATO SAUCE

Almost any tomato that isn't fresh (like jarred pasta sauce, salsa, and canned tomatoes) is soaked with sodium. Try making Basic Marinara sauce on page 278, which has 270mg of sodium per serving, compared to 500mg or more in jarred versions. The recipes for Pico de Gallo and Tomatillo-Lime Salsa on page 277 have half the sodium of typical store-bought salsas.

3. PICKLES

Store-bought pickles are sodium bombs. Six bread-and-butter slices can have almost 200mg sodium, whereas a quarter-cup of Easy Refrigerator Pickles (see page 279) has only 64mg.

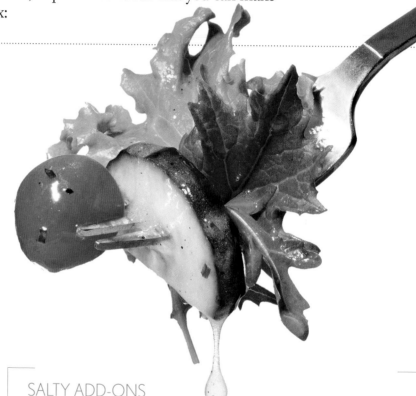

SALTY ADD-ONS

You may not realize just how easily sodium can sneak into your meal. Keep an eye out for these culprits:

1 beef bouillon cube	900mg
2 ounces deli ham	600mg
2 tablespoons barbecue sauce	450mg
1 pickle spear	320mg
1 tablespoon steak sauce	280mg
2 tablespoons sauerkraut	180mg
1 teaspoon capers	105mg

READ THE LABEL

Many foods we consider healthy contain a not-so-healthy dose of sodium. Here, three surprising offenders:

- **Whole-wheat bread**
Some have as much as 400mg per slice—which means you're getting 800mg in your sandwich without even adding in your sodium-heavy lunchmeat. Look for a brand that provides less than 170mg per slice of bread.

- **Breakfast cereal**
You probably carefully check the cereal's food label for calories, fiber, and sugar, but some brands also pack 170 to 280mg of sodium per serving. Look for lower-sodium options. Shredded wheat brands and plain oatmeal fit the bill.

- **Cottage cheese**
With an average of 400mg sodium per ½-cup serving, it can change a healthy dish into a high-sodium one. Choose no-salt-added cottage cheese for just 60mg sodium per serving.

4. NUT BUTTER

An average 2-tablespoon serving of nut butter can have as many as 125mg of sodium. Get into the habit of buying a no-salt-added nut butter or break out the food processor and make your own. See page 265 for recipes.

5. FROZEN MEALS

Dedicate an hour every week to cook one freezable meal, and you'll get huge payoffs. Baked Vegetable Lasagna on page 234, for example, has only 543mg of sodium compared to the more than 700mg found in many store-bought frozen lasagna meals. Really don't have time to cook? Cut the sodium of takeout or frozen family meals by adding equal amounts of fresh steamed vegetables.

6. CANNED SOUPS

Yes, they're convenient, but many are also loaded with added salt. Soups are ideal make-ahead meals, and you can save yourself and your family hundreds of milligrams of sodium (and money, too). See pages 280–281 for some ideas.

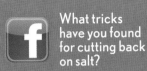

What tricks have you found for cutting back on salt?

"My motto is steering clear of the drive thru. I make a lot of Mexican food at home, and make my own seasonings, rather than buying 'taco seasoning' for example; that way, I control the sodium."

—*Aimee Jackson Fortney*

"Instead of buying premade seasoning mixes (which contain mostly salt) I started making my own: taco seasoning, Italian seasoning, chili seasoning, etc. Now I can have all the flavor with virtually no salt!"

—*Chris O'Malley*

FORGO STORE-BOUGHT SAUCES to pair with your meals in favor of easy-to-make at-home versions that slash sodium. See pages 276–277 for ideas.

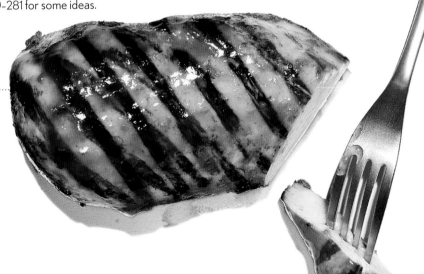

Pump Up the Produce

FRUITS AND VEGGIES are naturally low in sodium and high in potassium, a mighty mineral that helps counter sodium's effect on blood pressure. Here, six ways to help you get more of this super substance:

REACH FOR THE STARS.

Oranges, bananas, potatoes, tomatoes, dried apricots, melon, and kidney beans all have the highest levels of potassium, so aim to include at least a couple of them in meals and snacks every day.

MAKE YOUR OWN CONDIMENTS.

Try replacing ketchup, which has 190mg of sodium per tablespoon, with a fresh homemade salsa. Chop roasted bell peppers, drizzle with olive oil, and sprinkle with black pepper, and use as a flavorful relish for burgers, chicken, or fish.

KEEP THE CONVENIENCE.

It's not necessary to give up all convenience products to keep sodium levels in check. Most plain frozen vegetables are salt-free. Ditto for dried beans, chickpeas, and vegetables canned without salt. You can also cut sodium by 40% by simply rinsing canned beans. (See page 281 for more information.)

EAT SEASONALLY.

Rely on the season's freshest produce for more flavor satisfaction. Because the produce is fresh, the flavor will be at its best.

SPICE IT RIGHT.

Instead of frozen French fries doused with salt, try baked potato wedges finished with fresh sage or thyme or a toasted nut oil.

SPLASH IT UP.

Roasting carrots, eggplant, tomatoes, or any vegetable with a splash of olive oil and a grind of fresh pepper can result in rich-flavored side dishes that don't need salt.

THE POWER OF POTASSIUM

This mineral helps lower risk of high blood pressure and possibly even stroke. So don't just focus on ways to cut sodium; look for ways you can increase potassium in your diet. Few of us get the recommended 4,700mg every day.

10 Big-Time Potassium Players

1 small baked potato, flesh and skin	738mg
½ cup white beans, canned	595mg
8 ounces plain fat-free yogurt	579mg
1 medium sweet potato, baked in skin	542mg
1 cup fresh orange juice	496mg
3 ounces halibut, cooked	490mg
1 medium banana	422mg
1 cup fat-free milk	382mg
3 ounces pork loin, roasted	371mg
½ cup cooked lentils	365mg

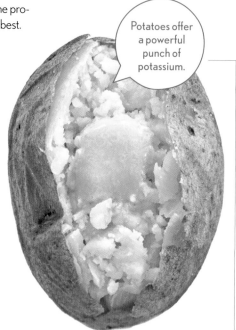

Potatoes offer a powerful punch of potassium.

LESS SALT DOESN'T MEAN LESS FLAVOR

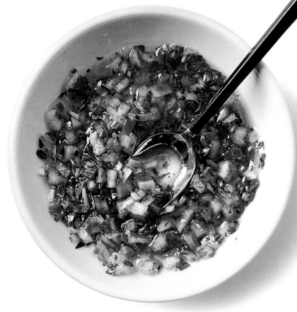

It's a scientific fact that salt is an acquired taste—the more you eat, the more you get used to it. But you can turn the tables by gradually cutting back: Every two weeks, measure out all the salt called for in a recipe, put 25% of it back, and cook with the remaining 75%. Your palate will adjust.

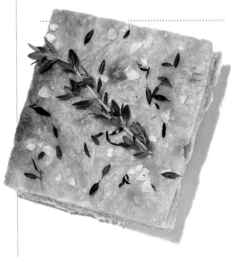

There are loads of ways to reduce your reliance on salt without sacrificing flavor.

■ **Make your own spice blends instead of buying premade seasoning mixes, which are often laced with salt.** When you amp up the flavor with robust spices (such as cumin, cayenne, and curry powder), you'll find that you need less salt.

■ **Put a bowl of cut lemons and limes on the table.** Instead of salting your vegetables, salads, and fish, add a perky hit of something acidic.

■ **Let fresh herbs lend a helping hand.** Basil pesto, chimichurri, and other herb sauces can brighten up a dish without a lot of salt. You'll find that a little goes far, whether you're tossing your pasta in pesto or using chimichurri sauce with your seared skirt steak. Plus, herb sauces are a great way to use up those big bunches of herbs, and they'll keep for a week in your fridge.

■ **Adjust your salt attitude.** Instead of making salt a source of guilt, turn it into a pleasure. Skip the salting during cooking and save it for the table where you can salt with style. Buy a decorative salt cellar for kosher or sea salt and gracefully spoon or pinch it onto your plate. You'll likely use less and enjoy it more.

How to Read Salt Labels

W HEN FOOD COMPANIES make sodium claims, they
have to follow labeling rules. That's where it gets tricky.
Here's our guide:

"NO SALT ADDED" OR "UNSALTED"

No salt is added during processing. This does
not always mean sodium-free; some foods
contain sodium naturally.

For example:
Land O' Lakes Unsalted Butter
(0mg)
vs.
Land O' Lakes Salted Butter
(95mg)

Sodium savings:
95mg per tablespoon

"REDUCED SODIUM" OR "LESS SODIUM"

Must contain at least 25% less than the original food, a
competitor's product, or another reference.

For example:
Kikkoman Less Sodium Soy Sauce
(575mg)
vs.
Kikkoman Soy Sauce
(920mg)

Sodium savings:
345mg per tablespoon

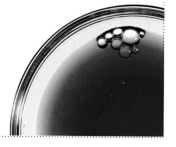

"LOW SODIUM"

This is the most stringent reduced-sodium
label. Each food can have only 140mg or
less sodium (natural or added) per serving.

For example:
Nabisco Wheat Thins Hint of
Salt (60mg)
vs.
Nabisco Original Wheat Thins
(230mg)

Sodium savings:
170mg per 16 crackers

"LIGHT IN SODIUM" OR "LIGHTLY SALTED"

Must contain 50% less than the original food, a competitor's product, or another reference.

For example:
Lay's Lightly Salted Potato Chips
(85mg)
vs.
Lay's Classic Potato Chips
(180mg)

Sodium savings:
95mg per ounce

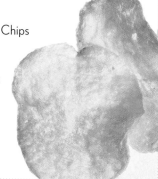

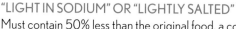

BOTTOM LINE: Always check the nutrition label for sodium per serving.

Show Me the Flavor

"I have a healthy diet, but my blood pressure is still higher than I would like."

MARY IHLA
Web Designer

➤ **SALT CHALLENGE:** Mary misses salt—a hankering that dates back to childhood. "I crave it. When other kids were buying candy bars, I was buying sunflower seeds," she says. However, Mary fears that recently losing 50 pounds has only compounded the sodium problem. "I have noticed that when products are low in fat, they're high in sodium. They put sodium in to add flavor."

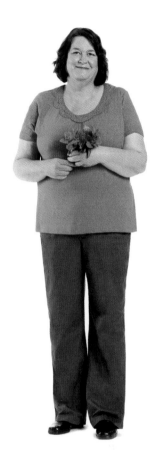

OUR ADVICE

■ **Low fat can mean more salt.**
Mary caught on to a trick of some low- and no-fat foods: swapping salt (or sugar) for missing fat. Reduced-fat and fat-free sour cream have twice the sodium of regular, but with half the calories and fat. Be a label reader!

■ **Watch for salty soups.** Canned soup is often very salty, so start making your own (freeze extra for busy nights). But know that store-bought broths can be high in sodium. Use reduced-sodium versions— it's an easy switch. Our Turkey and Bean Chili on page 280, which uses lower-sodium chicken broth, has only 474mg sodium per serving—half the amount of some canned soups.

■ **Identify one salty component.** When using a high-sodium food (like a store-bought marinade), make the other parts of the meal low-sodium, like opting to dip your bread in olive oil instead of a salty garlic-butter spread.

Use lower-sodium broths and stocks in soups and stews, like Turkey and Bean Chili (page 280).

■ **Focus on other flavors.** Glaze chicken breasts with sweet apricot preserves, top grilled meats with car-melized onions, serve Beef Tenderloin with Horseradish Chive Sauce (page 320), or Roast Pork Tenderloin with Plum Barbecue Sauce (page 321).

Monitor Kids' Sodium

PARENTS NEED TO WATCH THE AMOUNT of sodium their kids are taking in—kids have lower calorie needs, which means they also need less sodium. The daily sodium intake limit for children 1 to 3 is 1,000mg; 1,200mg for kids 4 to 8; and 1,500mg to 2,300mg per day for adolescents and adults up to age 51.

Kids need lunches for school on average 180 times a year. These lunch ideas are a few options built around some core preferences.

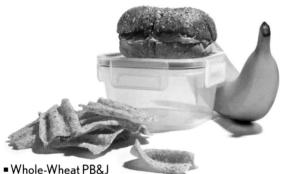

▪ Whole-Wheat PB&J

1 tablespoon peanut butter, 2 teaspoons jam on 1 mini whole-wheat bagel + 1 oz. whole-grain chips (about 16) + 1 small banana
413 mg sodium

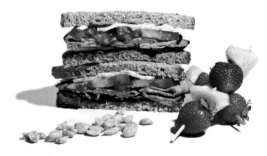

▪ Beefy Sandwich

2 oz. lower-sodium roast beef, lettuce, 2 slices tomato, ½ oz. slice white cheddar, 2 teaspoons light mayo on whole-grain bread + 2 pineapple and strawberry fruit kebabs + ½ oz. unsalted peanuts
508 mg sodium

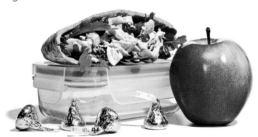

▪ Chicken Salad

½ cup Herbed Chicken Salad (page 130) with 1 tablespoon sweetened dried cranberries and ½ cup mixed greens in half a 6-inch whole-wheat pita + 1 medium apple + 4 milk chocolate kisses
381 mg sodium

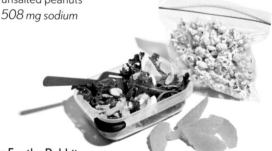

▪ For the Rabbits

Mixed greens, 2 oz. rotisserie chicken, 1 tablespoon sliced almonds, ¼ cup chopped tomatoes, 1 hard-cooked egg, 2 tablespoons oil-and-vinegar dressing + 2 cups 94%-fat-free popcorn + 1 orange, peeled
460mg sodium

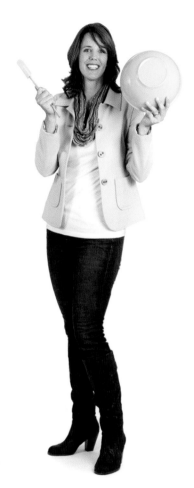

The Sodium-Clueless Mom

"When it comes to salt, I really haven't paid attention at all."

BLAKE KOHN
Preschool Director

➤ **SALT CHALLENGE:** Blake loves to cook and takes great joy in the fact that she provides a homemade dinner almost every night for her husband and two young children. She pays attention to fat and calories when she cooks, but she's not sure how salt fits into the health equation.

OUR ADVICE

■ **Pare down the packages.** Building meals and snacks around fruits and vegetables, whole grains, and lean, unprocessed meats will help keep sodium levels in check. The saltiness sneaks in with those snack bags of crackers and chips, hot dogs, cold cuts, canned foods, frozen pizzas, and packaged meats.

■ **Pick a smarter salt.** Because of its larger crystal size, a teaspoon of kosher salt contains almost 25% less sodium than a teaspoon of table salt. You can use the same amount when cooking and automatically reduce your intake by about a quarter.

■ **Rinse canned foods.** Draining and rinsing may wash away more than a quarter of the sodium. In one study, adding this step cut more than 40% of the sodium from canned beans.

■ **Add salt in stages.** Start with less, then slowly add it throughout the cooking process, tasting as you go. You may end up not needing all the salt the recipe suggests.

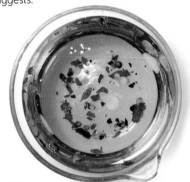

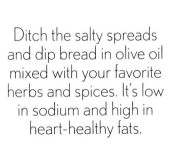

Ditch the salty spreads and dip bread in olive oil mixed with your favorite herbs and spices. It's low in sodium and high in heart-healthy fats.

Make Your Own Sauces

Y OU CAN FIND AN ASTOUNDING array of sauces and salad dressings at the grocery store these days, but these products often have a hefty dose of sodium lurking inside. The following flavor enhancers are easy to prepare with just a touch of salt and a ton of taste:

Sicilian Pesto

¼ cup pine nuts
3 garlic cloves
4 cups loosely packed basil leaves
   (about 2 ounces)
¼ cup extra-virgin olive oil
½ teaspoon kosher salt
¼ teaspoon freshly ground
   black pepper
⅛ teaspoon crushed red pepper
½ cup (2 ounces) grated fresh
   Parmigiano-Reggiano cheese
2 cups chopped seeded tomato,
   drained (about 2 large)

1. Heat a small skillet over medium heat. Add nuts to pan; cook 4 minutes or until lightly toasted, stirring constantly. Remove from pan.
2. Place nuts and garlic in a food processor; process until minced. Add basil, oil, salt, and peppers; process until blended, scraping sides occasionally. Add cheese; process until smooth. Spoon into a bowl; fold in tomato. Serves 20 (serving size: 2 tablespoons).

CALORIES 51; FAT 4.6g (sat 0.8g, mono 2.7g, poly 0.9g);
PROTEIN 1.4g; CARB 1.5g; FIBER 0.6g; CHOL 1mg;
IRON 0.4mg; SODIUM 82mg; CALC 41mg

Zingy Chimichurri

1½ cups finely chopped red onion
½ cup red wine vinegar
¼ cup chopped fresh oregano
2 tablespoons extra-virgin olive oil
1 teaspoon crushed red pepper
½ teaspoon kosher salt
2 garlic cloves, minced
3 tablespoons chopped fresh cilantro

1. Combine first 7 ingredients in a small bowl; let stand 30 minutes. Stir in cilantro. Serves 12 (serving size: about 1½ tablespoons).

CALORIES 32; FAT 2.3g
(sat 0.3g, mono 0g, poly 0g);
PROTEIN 0g; CARB 0g;
FIBER 0g; CHOL 0mg;
IRON 0mg;
SODIUM 82mg;
CALC 0mg

Aromatic herbs and seasonings like fresh oregano, garlic, and ginger add flavor to a dish without adding any additional sodium to the meal. Dried herbs work, too.

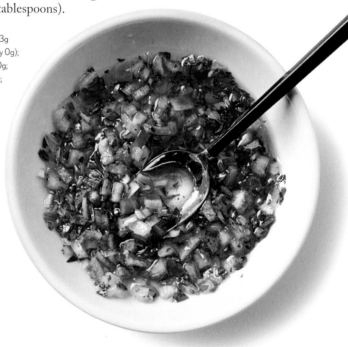

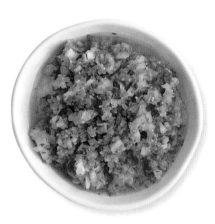

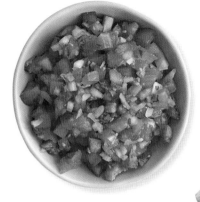

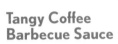

Tomatillo-Lime Salsa

1 pound tomatillos
2 to 3 tablespoons fresh lime juice
   (about 1 lime)
1 jalapeño pepper, seeded and minced
½ cup chopped onion
½ cup chopped fresh cilantro
1 teaspoon kosher salt

1. Discard husks and stems from tomatillos. Place tomatillos, lime juice, and pepper in a food processor; pulse until tomatillos are coarsely chopped. Add onion, cilantro, and salt; pulse until combined. Serves 16 (serving size: 2 tablespoons).

CALORIES 12; FAT 0.3g (sat 0g, mono 0.1g, poly 0.1g); PROTEIN 0.4g; CARB 2.5g; FIBER 0.7g; CHOL 0mg; IRON 0.2mg; SODIUM 118mg; CALC 4mg

Pico de Gallo

2½ cups chopped seeded plum
   tomato (about 6 medium)
⅔ cup finely chopped onion
2 tablespoons chopped fresh cilantro
2 tablespoons finely chopped jalapeño
   pepper (1 large)
2 tablespoons fresh lime juice
½ teaspoon salt
½ teaspoon garlic powder

1. Combine all ingredients in a serving bowl; toss well. Let stand 30 minutes before serving. Serves 14 (serving size: ¼ cup).

CALORIES 8; FAT 0.1g (sat 0g, mono 0g, poly 0g); PROTEIN 0.3g; CARB 1.8g; FIBER 0.4g; CHOL 0mg; IRON 0.1mg; SODIUM 86mg; CALC 4mg

Tangy Coffee Barbecue Sauce

1 cup no-salt-added ketchup
1 cup brewed coffee
2 tablespoons dark brown sugar
1 teaspoon onion powder
1 teaspoon garlic powder
1 teaspoon chili powder
1½ tablespoons balsamic vinegar
1½ teaspoons black pepper
1½ teaspoons lower-sodium soy sauce

1. Combine first 6 ingredients in a small saucepan; bring to a boil. Reduce heat; simmer 10 minutes or until slightly thick stirring occasionally. Remove from heat; stir in vinegar, pepper, and soy sauce. Serves 12 (serving size: about 2½ tablespoons).

CALORIES 47; FAT 0g (sat 0g, mono 0g, poly 0g); PROTEIN 0g; CARB 0g; FIBER 0g; CHOL 0mg; IRON 0mg; SODIUM 24mg; CALC 0mg

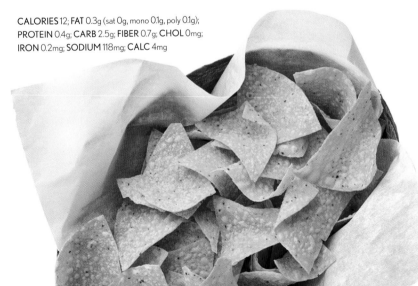

Create Your Own Convenience Foods

SOMETIMES IT'S THOSE little convenience items that can dramatically hike up the sodium in a meal. Look for lower-sodium versions of your favorite pantry staples and try your hand at making your own.

Basic Marinara

3 tablespoons olive oil
3 cups chopped yellow onion
    (about 3 medium)
1 tablespoon sugar
3 tablespoons minced garlic (about 6
    cloves)
2 teaspoons salt
2 teaspoons dried basil
1½ teaspoons dried oregano
1 teaspoon dried thyme
1 teaspoon freshly ground black pepper
½ teaspoon fennel seeds, crushed
2 tablespoons balsamic vinegar
2 cups fat-free, lower-sodium chicken
    broth
3 (28-ounce) cans no-salt-added
    crushed tomatoes, undrained

1. Heat a large Dutch oven over medium heat. Add oil to pan; swirl to coat. Add onion; cook 4 minutes, stirring frequently. Add sugar and next 7 ingredients; cook 1 minute, stirring constantly. Stir in vinegar; cook 30 seconds. Add broth and tomatoes; bring to a simmer. Cook over low heat 55 minutes or until sauce thickens, stirring occasionally. Serves 24 (serving size: about ½ cup).

CALORIES 50; FAT 1.8g (sat 0.2g, mono 1.3g, poly 0.2g); PROTEIN 1.3g; CARB 8g; FIBER 2.1g; CHOL 0mg; IRON 0.5mg; SODIUM 270mg; CALC 28mg

MARINARA BASICS

To store in the freezer: Ladle room-temperature or chilled sauce into plastic containers or zip-top plastic bags. Seal and freeze for up to four months. Consider freezing the sauce in 1-cup increments (two servings' worth). That way, you can pull out exactly as much as you want for future meals.

To thaw sauce, try one of three methods:
1. Thaw in the refrigerator overnight.
2. Place frozen blocks in a saucepan. Cover and bring to a low simmer over medium heat, stirring occasionally.
3. Place frozen blocks in a microwave-safe bowl. Cover and microwave at HIGH 1 minute at a time, stirring after each increment, until thawed.

To boost taste: Long stints in the freezer can dull the taste of tomatoes. To perk up thawed sauce, add ½ teaspoon finely grated lemon rind or 1 teaspoon balsamic vinegar while reheating.

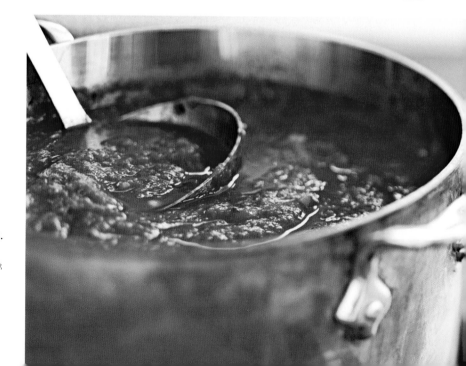

Roasted Chicken Stock

7 pounds chicken wings
Cooking spray
3 cups coarsely chopped onion
2½ cups coarsely chopped celery
2¼ cups coarsely chopped carrot
1 tablespoon olive oil
5 quarts plus 1 cup water, divided
15 parsley sprigs
15 black peppercorns
8 thyme sprigs
3 bay leaves

1. Preheat oven to 450°.
2. Arrange chicken in a single layer on a jelly-roll pan coated with cooking spray. Combine onion and next 3 ingredients in a bowl; toss well to coat vegetables. Arrange vegetable mixture in a single layer on another jelly-roll pan coated with cooking spray. Roast chicken and vegetables at 450° for 1 hour and 20 minutes or until browned, turning occasionally.
3. Place wings and vegetables in a stockpot. Pour ½ cup water into each baking sheet, scraping to loosen browned bits. Pour water mixture into pot. Add remaining 5 quarts water and remaining ingredients to pot. Place pot over medium-high heat. Bring to a boil. Reduce heat to low, and simmer 4 hours, skimming off and discarding foam as needed. Strain stock through a fine sieve into a large bowl; discard solids. Cool stock to room temperature. Cover and refrigerate 5 hours or overnight. Skim solidified fat from surface; discard fat. Serves 24 (serving size: ½ cup).

CALORIES 25; FAT 1.4g (sat 0.3g, mono 0.7g, poly 0.3g); PROTEIN 2.6g; CARB 0.3g; FIBER 0.1g; CHOL 11mg; IRON 0.2mg; SODIUM 13mg; CALC 4mg

When you buy cans or cartons of chicken broth, be sure to look for lower-sodium versions. Some regular chicken broth contains 900mg per cup.

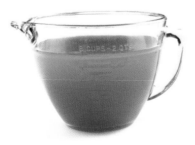

Easy Refrigerator Pickles

6 cups thinly sliced pickling cucumbers (about 2 pounds)
2 cups thinly sliced onion
1½ cups white vinegar
¾ cup sugar
¾ teaspoon salt
½ teaspoon mustard seeds
½ teaspoon celery seeds
½ teaspoon ground turmeric
½ teaspoon crushed red pepper
¼ teaspoon freshly ground black pepper
4 garlic cloves, thinly sliced

1. Place 3 cups cucumber in a medium glass bowl; top with 1 cup onion. Repeat layers with remaining 3 cups cucumber and remaining 1 cup onion.
2. Combine vinegar and remaining ingredients in a small saucepan; stir well. Bring to a boil; cook 1 minute. Pour over cucumber mixture; let cool. Cover and chill at least 4 days. Serves 28 (serving size: ¼ cup).
Note: Pickles may be stored in the refrigerator for up to one month.

CALORIES 28; FAT 0.1g (sat 0g, mono 0g, poly 0.1g); PROTEIN 0.3g; CARB 7g; FIBER 0.3g; CHOL 0mg; IRON 0.1mg; SODIUM 64mg; CALC 7mg

Slash the Sodium in Soup

OOK FOR REDUCED-SODIUM VERSIONS of canned soup, or start making your own (and freeze for busy nights). The sodium savings can be immense.

Turkey and Bean Chili

1 cup prechopped red onion

⅓ cup chopped seeded poblano
    pepper (about 1)

1 teaspoon bottled minced garlic

1¼ pounds ground turkey

1 tablespoon chili powder

2 tablespoons tomato paste

2 teaspoons dried oregano

1 teaspoon ground cumin

¼ teaspoon salt

¼ teaspoon black pepper

1 (19-ounce) can cannellini beans,
    rinsed and drained

1 (14.5-ounce) can diced tomatoes,
    undrained

1 (14-ounce) can fat-free, lower-sodium
    chicken broth

½ cup chopped fresh cilantro

6 lime wedges

1. Heat a large saucepan over medium heat. Add first 4 ingredients; cook 6 minutes or until turkey is done, stirring to crumble. Stir in chili powder and next 8 ingredients; bring to a boil. Reduce heat; simmer 10 minutes. Stir in cilantro. Serve with lime wedges. Serves 6 (serving size: about 1 cup chili and 1 lime wedge).

CALORIES 211; FAT 6.5g (sat 1.7g, mono 1.9g, poly 1.6g); PROTEIN 22.5g; CARB 16.4g; FIBER 4.7g; CHOL 54mg; IRON 3.4mg; SODIUM 474mg; CALC 52mg

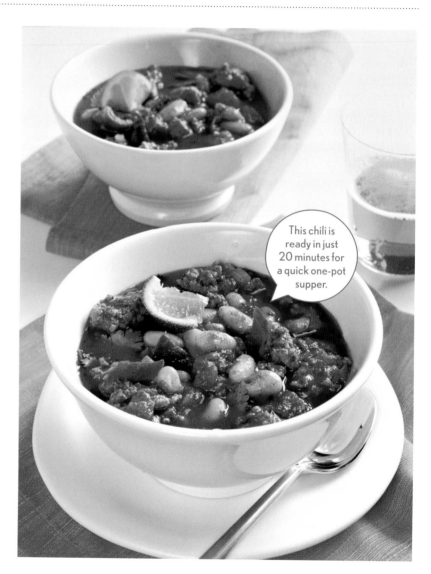

This chili is ready in just 20 minutes for a quick one-pot supper.

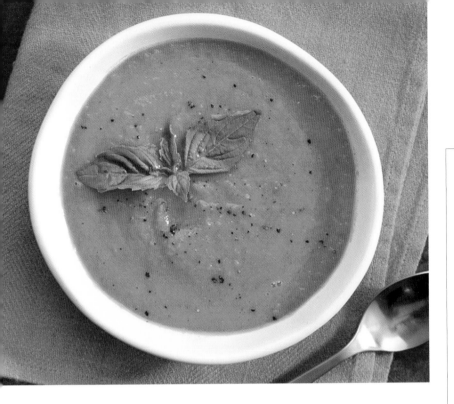

DRAIN AND RINSE CANNED FOODS

By simply draining and rinsing canned foods, you can cut a significant chunk of sodium. Consider this: A 15-ounce can of chili beans contains 1,570mg sodium. Draining the beans can reduce the sodium count by about 40%. The combination of draining and rinsing reduces sodium by another 5%. That shaves off about 644mg sodium—almost 30% of your daily allowance.

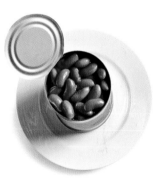

Undrained: 1,570mg sodium

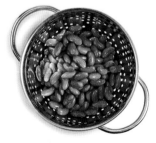

Rinsed and drained: 926mg sodium

Double Tomato Soup

1 tablespoon butter
1 cup chopped onion (1 medium)
³/₄ cup shredded carrot
1 tablespoon minced garlic
1 tablespoon minced shallots
1 teaspoon sugar
¹/₄ teaspoon freshly ground black pepper
¹/₈ teaspoon salt
10 large basil leaves, divided
3 drained sun-dried tomato halves, packed in oil with herbs
2 (14.5-ounce) cans organic diced tomatoes, undrained
1 (14-ounce) can fat-free, lower-sodium chicken broth

1. Melt butter in a large saucepan over medium heat. Add chopped onion, shredded carrot, garlic, and shallots to pan, and cook 5 minutes or until vegetables are tender, stirring frequently. Add sugar, pepper, salt, and 4 basil leaves, and cook 5 minutes. Add sun-dried tomatoes, diced tomatoes, and broth, and bring to a boil. Reduce heat, and simmer 1 hour. Remove from heat. Place half of soup in a blender. Remove center piece of blender lid (to allow steam to escape); secure blender lid on blender. Place a clean towel over opening in blender lid (to avoid splatters). Blend until smooth. Pour into a large bowl. Repeat procedure with remaining soup. Divide soup evenly among 6 bowls. Garnish each serving with 1 basil leaf. Serves 6 (serving size: ¾ cup).

CALORIES 76; FAT 2.5g (sat 1.3g, mono 0.7g, poly 0.1g); PROTEIN 2.2g; CARB 9.4g; FIBER 2g; CHOL 5mg; IRON 1.1mg; SODIUM 229mg; CALC 14mg

Shave Salt from Your Snacks

PREPACKAGED SNACKS CAN BE serious sodium offenders, especially salted nuts, microwave or prepopped popcorn, pretzels, crackers, and chips. We've got some tasty solutions that satisfy the craving with a lot less salt.

Sweet Chipotle Snack Mix

¼ cup sugar
1 teaspoon salt
1 teaspoon ground chipotle chile pepper
½ teaspoon ground cumin
½ teaspoon dried oregano
½ teaspoon chili powder
1 large egg white
1 cup slivered almonds
1 cup unsalted cashews
1 cup unsalted pumpkinseed kernels

1. Preheat oven to 325°.
2. Combine first 6 ingredients in a small bowl; stir with a whisk.
3. Place egg white in a bowl; stir with a whisk until foamy. Add almonds, cashews, and pumpkin-seeds; toss well to coat. Sprinkle with spice mixture; toss well to coat. Spread nuts in an even layer on a baking sheet lined with parchment paper. Bake at 325° for 15 minutes, stirring once. Turn oven off. Remove pan from oven; stir nut mixture. Immediately return pan to oven for 15 minutes (leave oven off). Remove pan from oven and place on a wire rack; cool completely. Serves 19 (serving size: 3 tablespoons).

CALORIES 130; FAT 9.7g (sat 1.4g, mono 5.8g, poly 2g); PROTEIN 4.5g; CARB 7.3g; FIBER 1.1g; CHOL 0mg; IRON 1.1mg; SODIUM 175mg; CALC 23mg

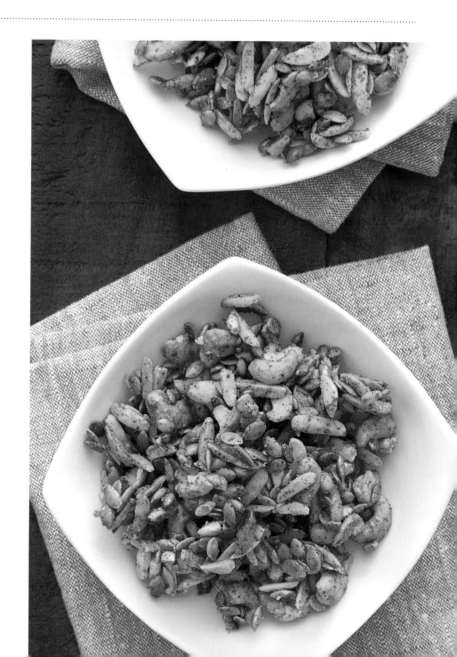

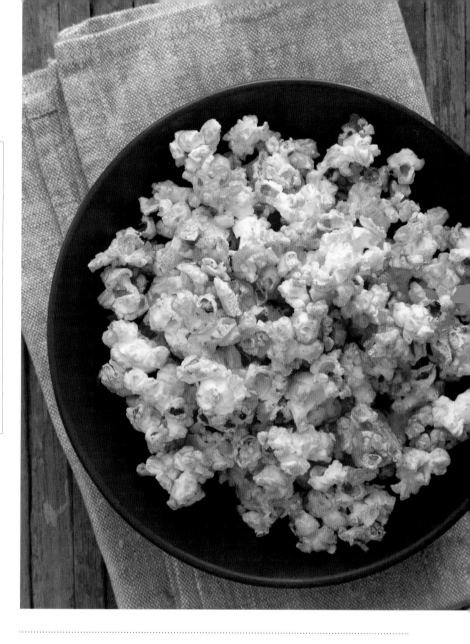

Maple-Chile Popcorn

"Very quick and easy to make, and so much better for you than store-bought caramel corn," said AngelaV on CookingLight.com.

Cooking spray
8 cups popcorn (popped without salt or fat)
½ cup maple syrup
1 tablespoon butter
½ teaspoon salt
½ teaspoon ground red pepper

1. Preheat oven to 300°.
2. Coat a 15 x 10–inch jelly-roll pan or other large rimmed baking pan with cooking spray. Place popcorn in a large metal or glass bowl lightly coated with cooking spray.
3. Combine syrup and next 3 ingredients in a saucepan over medium heat. Bring to a boil, stirring just until combined. Cook, without stirring, 2 minutes. Pour syrup mixture over popcorn in a steady stream, stirring to coat.
4. Spread popcorn mixture in an even layer into prepared pan. Bake at 300° for 15 minutes. Remove from oven, and cool completely in pan. Serves 16 (serving size: ½ cup).

CALORIES 48; FAT 0.9g (sat 0.5g, mono 0.2g, poly 0.1g); PROTEIN 0.5g; CARB 9.9g; FIBER 0.6g; CHOL 2mg; IRON 0.2mg; SODIUM 79mg; CALC 7mg

Replicate Restaurant and Packaged Favorites

I'S TOUGH TO EAT OUT without blowing your sodium budget, especially with all the deep-fried appetizers, French fries, and jumbo portions. Frozen entrées and packaged foods are also notoriously high in sodium. Try these substitutes that deliver the flavor but aren't doused with salt.

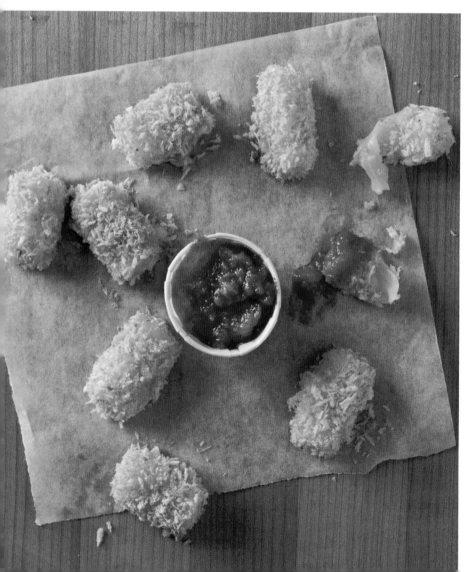

Baked Mozzarella Bites

HeatherL said on CookingLight.com, "Oh my goodness…these are divine! And easy to make." Quinn16 said, "These are so good! I will totally make them again. My kids loved them."

⅓ cup panko (Japanese breadcrumbs)
3 (1-ounce) sticks part-skim mozzarella string cheese
3 tablespoons egg substitute
Cooking spray
¼ cup lower-sodium marinara sauce

1. Preheat oven to 425°.
2. Heat a medium skillet over medium heat. Add panko to pan, and cook 2 minutes or until toasted, stirring frequently. Remove from heat, and place panko in a shallow dish.
3. Cut mozzarella sticks into 1-inch pieces. Working with 1 piece at a time, dip cheese in egg substitute; dredge in panko. Place cheese on a baking sheet coated with cooking spray. Bake at 425° for 3 minutes or until cheese is softened and thoroughly heated.

4. Pour marinara sauce into a microwave-safe bowl. Microwave at HIGH 1 minute or until thoroughly heated, stirring after 30 seconds. Serve with mozzarella pieces. Serves 4 (serving size: 3 bites and 1 tablespoon sauce).

CALORIES 91; FAT 5.1g (sat 2.8g, mono 1.3g, poly 0.3g); PROTEIN 7.2g; CARB 6.7g; FIBER 0.1g; CHOL 12mg; IRON 0.3mg; SODIUM 162mg; CALC 162mg

Truffled Roasted Potatoes

"These potatoes are outstanding!" said Lizlee on CookingLight.com. "I couldn't have been happier with the way they turned out. These would be a perfect, easy side dish for a dinner party."

2 (20-ounce) packages refrigerated
    red potato wedges
2 tablespoons olive oil
1 tablespoon minced garlic
½ teaspoon kosher salt
½ teaspoon freshly ground
    black pepper
1 tablespoon white truffle oil
2 teaspoons thyme leaves

1. Preheat oven to 450°.
2. Place potatoes on a jelly-roll pan; drizzle with olive oil, and sprinkle with garlic, salt, and pepper. Toss well to combine. Bake at 450° for 35 minutes or until potatoes are browned and tender. Remove from oven. Drizzle potatoes with truffle oil, and sprinkle with thyme. Toss gently to combine. Serves 8 (serving size: about ¾ cup).

CALORIES 134; FAT 5.1g (sat 0.7g, mono 3.7g, poly 0.5g); PROTEIN 3.6g; CARB 18g; FIBER 3.6g; CHOL 0mg; IRON 0.8mg; SODIUM 269mg; CALC 3mg

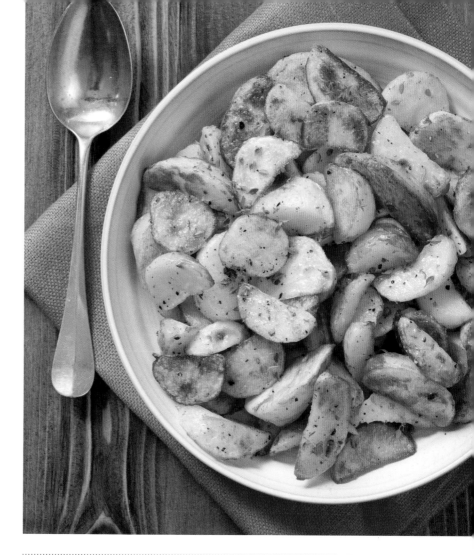

A SPUD SPECTRUM

Potatoes, like other vegetables, start out with very little sodium, but once they turn "instant" in a package or they're all dressed up on a restaurant menu, all bets are off. Here's how big the sodium difference can be:

1 medium potato —————————————→ 25mg
½ cup Hungry Jack Creamy Butter Mashed Potatoes —→ 420mg
½ cup Betty Crocker Potatoes Au Gratin ————→ 610mg
Chili's Loaded Mashed Potatoes ————————→ 1,160mg
Denny's Loaded Baked Potato Soup —————→ 1,710mg
Applebee's Potato Twisters ———————————→ 3,520mg

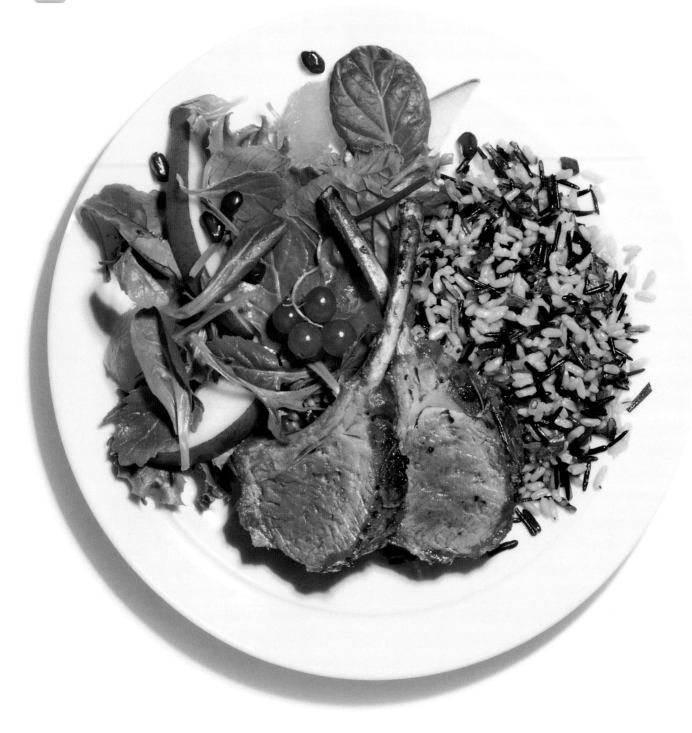

BE PORTION-AWARE

MANAGE AMOUNTS AT EVERY MEAL.

IN A WORLD of triple-stacked hamburgers, double-stuffed cookies, and super-sized sodas, it's no wonder most Americans struggle to control portions—we're not entirely sure what one should be. Plus, there are all sorts of factors that unconsciously influence the portions we choose, from the size of our plates and the bulk of a box to the messages on TV commercials.

While the terms "portion size" and "serving size" are often used interchangeably, there is a difference: A portion is the amount of food you put on your plate. A serving is the amount you need, a USDA-recommended amount defined in terms of meaurements, such as ounces, cups, and tablespoons. A rib-eye portion in a local steak-house, for example, may be 6 to 18 ounces, but the USDA—and *Cooking Light*—serving size for steak is just 3 ounces (cooked).

Our escalating portions are at the core of our country's growing girth. It's not so much what we're eating that's to blame—it's how much. Yet experts estimate that eating just 100 fewer calories a day may be all it takes to curtail weight gain. It's a small change that can be enough to cause you to lose (or gain) 10 pounds a year.

The challenge of this habit is to be portion-aware—to read labels and recipes and learn what the recommended servings are. This chapter is full of strategies to help you keep your portions in check and under control, without obsessively counting calories or relying on measuring cups and scales for the rest of your life. You'll learn what influences how much you eat and what you can do to cut back painlessly. You'll also find an array of portion-friendly recipes, ranging from bite-sized appetizers and single-serve entrées to small treats to savor.

YOUR GOAL

Find strategies to help you eat a little less without even thinking about it.

The 12 Healthy Habits

| • 01 • GET COOKING | • 02 • BREAKFAST DAILY | • 03 • WHOLE GRAINS | • 04 • GET MOVING | • 05 • VEGGIE UP | • 06 • MORE SEAFOOD | • 07 • HEALTHY FATS | • 08 • GO MEATLESS | • 09 • GET STRONGER | • 10 • LESS SALT | • 11 • BE PORTION-AWARE | • 12 • EAT MINDFULLY |

Divide and Conquer

THE BIGGER YOUR SERVING BOWL or package, the more you'll eat. Studies show people unintentionally consume more calories when faced with larger amounts of food. Here's how to avoid falling into that trap:

PORTION TEMPTING TREATS.
The bigger the package, the more food you'll pour out of it. When two groups were given half- or 1-pound bags of M&Ms to eat while watching TV, those given the 1-pound bag ate nearly twice as much.

LIMIT YOUR CHOICES.
The more options you have, the more you want to try. In one study, researchers gave two groups jelly beans to snack on while they watched a movie. One group got six colors, neatly divided into compartments; jelly beans for the other group were jumbled together. Those given a mix ate nearly two times more.

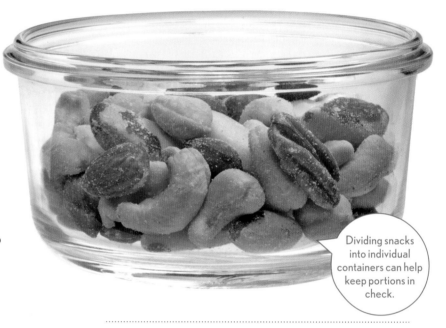

Dividing snacks into individual containers can help keep portions in check.

Homemade muffins can be a wonderful preportioned meal. You'll find recipes on page 66.

When it comes to portion control, you can count on your brain not being very well calibrated. Incremental over-eating adds up to weight gain.

SLICE MEATS.

Instead of plating two slab-sized 8-ounce chicken breasts or steaks, cook one and slice it on the bias, divide in half, then plate. Slicing meats and fanning them out helps fill up the plate.

FORGET FAMILY STYLE.

Fill plates in the kitchen. When serving dishes were kept off of the table, people ate 20% fewer calories.

EXPERT TIP: *Create a Meal Midpoint*

"Once you have the amount of food you think you'll need, physically divide it in half on your plate to remind yourself to stop halfway and check in again. This little 'speed bump' will slow you down so you can reconnect with your hunger and fullness level."

—*Michelle May, MD, author of* Eat What You Love, Love What You Eat *and founder of amihungry.com*

THE FUZZY MATH OF FOOD LABELS

Serving size
The serving size is the most important thing to read on the label in order for the rest of the numbers to make sense.

Servings per container
Be sure you check how many servings are in the package. This bag contains 4.5 servings. That means if you down the whole thing, you've devoured 540 calories.

Ingredients
You might think this food is mostly healthy popcorn... but it's not. Ingredient lists go by weight, so sugar and corn syrup take top billing.

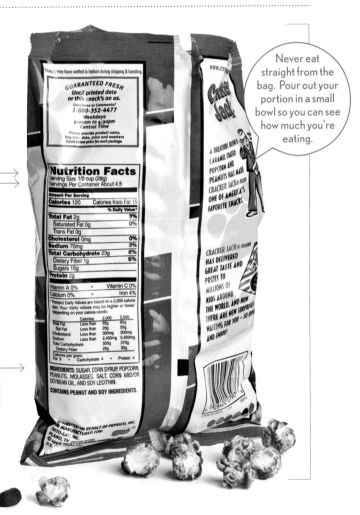

Never eat straight from the bag. Pour out your portion in a small bowl so you can see how much you're eating.

Change Your Visual Cues

RESEARCH SHOWS THAT THE SIZE of your dinner plate or the shape of your cocktail glass can influence how much you eat and drink. Even how you stock your pantry and organize your fridge can play a role.

DOWNSIZE YOUR DISHES.
If you're one of the 54% of Americans who eat until their plates are clean, make sure those plates are modestly sized. On a standard 8- to 10-inch dinner plate (instead of the typical 12-inch variety), a portion of spaghetti looks like a meal. When researchers gave study participants 34- or 17-ounce bowls and told them to help themselves to ice cream, those with the bigger bowls dished out 31% more ice cream.

AVOID A SEE-FOOD DIET.
Office workers who kept candy in clear dishes on their desks dipped in for a sample 71% more often than those who kept their candy out of sight. Or better yet, replace your candy dish with a fruit bowl instead.

THINK BEFORE YOU DRINK.
Pour your drinks into tall, narrow glasses rather than short, wide ones. One study found that people poured 19% more cranberry juice into a short glass rather than a tall one because the eye is a poor judge of volume in relation to height and width.

SERVE GOOD-FOR-YOU FOODS FAMILY-STYLE.
Place the foods you want your family to eat more of—salads and vegetable sides—within easy reach on the dining table. One study found that people who kept baby carrots in plain sight ate 25% more during a day.

...AND HIDE THE NOT-SO-GOOD ONES.
When you bake a pan of brownies, even a *Cooking Light* recipe, cut them into small pieces, and store out of view, on a higher shelf (don't worry, you'll remember they're there). Put fresh fruit in view instead—you're much more likely to take and eat something off a fridge or cupboard shelf at eye level.

What Is a Serving?

THERE'S NO NEED TO WEIGH AND MEASURE everything you eat, but a few visual aids can be handy reminders to help you calibrate your portions when dining out or dishing up meals.

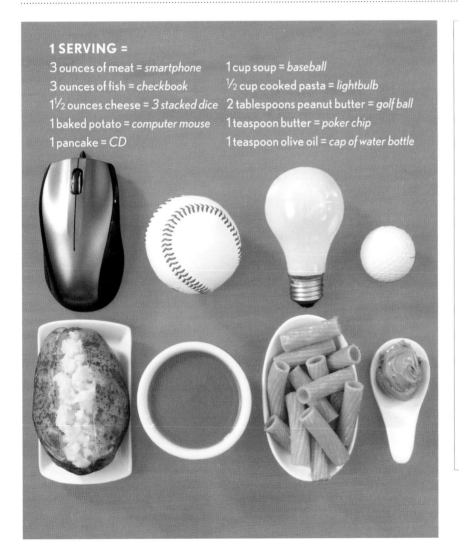

1 SERVING =

3 ounces of meat = *smartphone*

3 ounces of fish = *checkbook*

1½ ounces cheese = *3 stacked dice*

1 baked potato = *computer mouse*

1 pancake = *CD*

1 cup soup = *baseball*

½ cup cooked pasta = *lightbulb*

2 tablespoons peanut butter = *golf ball*

1 teaspoon butter = *poker chip*

1 teaspoon olive oil = *cap of water bottle*

A DAY'S WORTH

Here's how your total servings should add up for the full day (based on a 2,000-calorie diet):

Vegetables	*2½ cups*
Fruits	*2 cups*
Grains	*6 ounces*
Dairy	*3 cups*
Protein	*5½ ounces*
Oils	*6 teaspoons*

Visit choosemyplate.gov to find the number of servings for each food group needed for various calorie levels, from 1,000 to 3,500 calories. For grains, 1 ounce equals ½ cup of cooked rice, pasta, or cooked cereal; 1 ounce of dry pasta or rice; 1 slice of bread; 1 small muffin; or 1 cup of ready-to-eat cereal. For protein, 1 ounce equals 1 ounce of lean meat, poultry, or fish; 1 egg; ¼ cup of dry beans or tofu; 1 tablespoon of peanut butter; or ½ ounce of nuts or seeds.

Pump Up the Volume

I F YOU SIMPLY EAT TEENY-TINY PORTIONS, you may end up feeling hungry and deprived. The key is to focus on eating more high-volume foods that are loaded with water, such as fiber-rich fruits and veggies, says Barbara Rolls, PhD, Guthrie Chair of Nutrition at Penn State University and author of *The Ultimate Volumetrics Diet*. Here, her top five tips to help keep you full and satisfied:

1. WHIP IT UP.

Foods that are puffed up with air (like air-popped popcorn, smoothies, and puffed cereal) help prevent you from overeating. In one study, Rolls blended strawberry milkshakes for differing periods of time and found that subjects who consumed the biggest shakes ended up eating 12% less a half hour later at lunch than those who had the smallest.

2. SERVE SOUP WITH DINNER.

While soup's mostly water, our bodies perceive it as food, especially if it contains tiny pieces of food your stomach needs to break down. The result: You feel fuller than if you'd just sipped a glass of water. Rolls' research has found that people who enjoy a first course of soup eat on average 100 fewer calories during the meal than those who don't.

3. START WITH A SALAD.

Load up on a large, low-calorie salad (about three cups) before you even touch your entrée. Studies show that people who eat a salad before the main meal end up eating fewer calories than if they'd had none at all.

4. DOUBLE THE VEGGIES IN YOUR ENTRÉES.

A 200-calorie serving of pasta, for example, will be almost twice the size if you cut the serving by one-third and simply double the amount of vegetables you toss in. Research shows that adding a second or third veggie works better than increasing the portion size of one of them.

5. SAVOR SOMETHING SWEET AT THE END.

Rolls confesses to a craving for chocolate, but rather than eating it as a snack—when she's hungry and tempted to overindulge—she lets herself enjoy a small square at the end of her meal, when she's satiated.

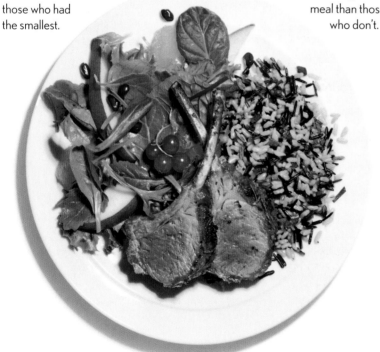
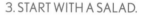

"You call that a portion?"

"Sometimes the proper portion of food just looks so small."

JENNIFER CHINN
Corporate Event and Promotions Coordinator

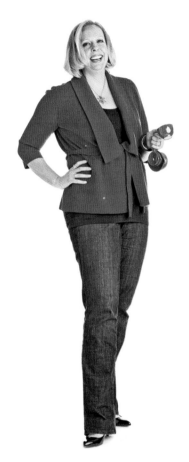

➤ **PORTION CHALLENGE:** When it comes to portions, Jen and her husband, Mark, raise a white flag. Dinner is the main struggle—recipes often make four to six servings, but it's just the two of them at the table. "When I'm giving him a big plate of food and I'm getting my girly portion, I tend to feel deprived," she says. Plus, she asks herself that all-important question: "Where does ice cream fit into this?"

OUR ADVICE

■ **Eat before you eat.** Grab a piece of fresh fruit or a handful of nuts before you sit down to a meal. Curbing your hunger just a bit will help you slow down so you won't devour everything on your plate once you get to the table.
■ **Lower your calorie density.** Building your meals around less-calorie-dense foods like vegetables and fruits will help you feel full on fewer calories. That means you can bulk up your plate with several portions of these foods.

■ **Add freebie foods.** Vegetables and fruits are less calorically dense than meat or carbohydrates, meaning you can add several portions of them to your plate and still not eat too many calories.
■ **Go ahead and take a trip down that Rocky Road.** Enjoy your ice cream; just stick to a half-cup serving (and don't eat straight from the carton unless it's one of those 4-ounce single-serve cups). Scoop your single portion of ice cream into a French demi bowl or soufflé cup, and savor every spoonful.

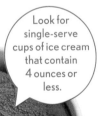

Look for single-serve cups of ice cream that contain 4 ounces or less.

EXPERT TIP: *Build in a Stopping Place*

"Think of portion sizes as a place to start. It builds in an automatic stopping place that gives you the opportunity to think if you really want more. Then pay attention to your internal hunger cues. If you decide you want more, it's fine to have a second helping. But you're making a conscious decision rather than just eating all that's on your plate."

—*Marsha Hudnall, MS, RD, blogger, A Weight Lifted*

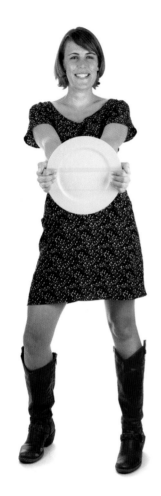

The Clean-Plate Champion

"I always end up finishing everything in front of me."

MARILYN TUSHAR
Nanny

➤ **PORTION CHALLENGE:** At the Ohio dinner table where Marilyn formed her eating habits, the food was healthy, and the rules were firm: Finish everything on your plate or you don't get dessert. "I guess I just really have taken that on," says Marilyn, who admits that she pretty much hates left-overs in any form and finds it's tough cooking for one. Marilyn is able to limit her snacks to small servings and also buys portion-controlled packs. But she's worried about the long-term effects of her eat-it-all mentality.

If you're a member of the clean-plate club, make sure you're using 8- to 10-inch plates. On modestly sized dishes, 4 ounces of fish looks like the best deal in the world.

OUR ADVICE ▪ **Learn great one-person meals.** Fish en papillote is perfect for one. Add your choice of veggies and possibly even some starch for a quick meal, or try a half recipe of Arctic Char and Vegetables in Parchment Hearts on page 197. For a single-serve pasta dish, measure out 2 ounces of dried pasta and toss with sauce, veggies, and cheese. Or go for an omelet stuffed with wilted greens or sautéed mushrooms.
▪ **Use portion-control tools.** At first, measuring portions can be tedious, but as you repeat the same measurements each day (a cup of milk with breakfast, 2 ounces of dried pasta), you'll be able to better estimate what a true serving is. That way, instead of whipping out mea-suring cups when you're at a restaurant, you'll have a clearer mental picture of a proper portion.
▪ **Cleverly reuse leftovers.** With a little planning, you can make one recipe for dinner and have enough leftovers to make a different meal for the next day

that doesn't feel like leftovers. Grilled meat or salmon, for example, can always translate into next day's lunch sandwich. And leftover rotisserie chicken is always great for easy one-person meals like tacos, sandwiches, salads, pita pizzas, and pasta tosses.

EXPERT TIP:
One Isn't Always One

"People eat in units—one bagel, one muffin, one soda, or one steak—and they don't really pay attention to how big that unit is. Just because you're eating one of something, it doesn't mean that's the appropriate amount of food you should be eating."
—*Lisa R. Young, PhD, RD, blogger, author of* The Portion Teller Plan

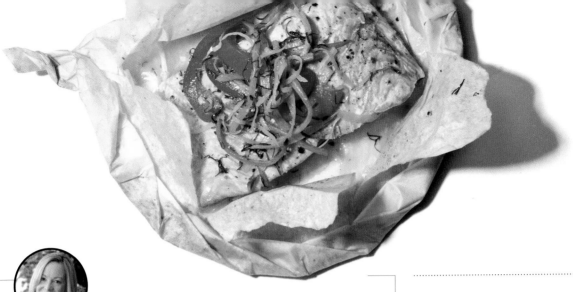

COMBATING THE MINDLESS MARGIN

When it comes to portions, making changes may be easier (and less noticeable) than you think. James O. Hill, PhD, and colleagues at the University of Colorado estimate that eating just 100 fewer calories each day could prevent weight gain in 90% of the population. Closing this "energy gap" may be all it takes to avoid the one or two pounds that many Americans gain each year.

Brian Wansink, PhD, of Cornell University's Food and Brand Lab, calls this the "mindless margin." Our body and mind fight restrictive diets that dramatically cut calories, but they don't notice a 100-calorie difference here and there.

Here are some simple ways you can shave off 100 calories:

■ Use nonstick spray in place of butter when cooking your eggs.

■ Downsize your bagel, or eat only half; some are equivalent to five slices of bread.

■ Order a slice of thin-crust pizza instead of thick-crust pizza, and remove four pieces of pepperoni from your slice.

■ Choose a 12-ounce can of soda instead of a 20-ounce bottle, or drink one fewer can of soda a day.

■ Leave three or four bites on your plate each time you eat.

We often overeat in 100- or 200-calorie increments, which over time adds up to a weight gain that seems like a mystery to the eater. But according to Brian Wansink, PhD, of Cornell University's Food and Brand Lab, most of us know what we're supposed to eat, and how much of it. We just ignore what we know. We eat, he says, "mindlessly."

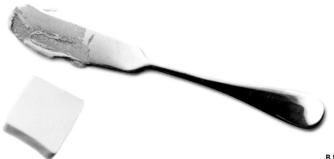

Create Single-Serve Meals

Small ramekins, soufflé cups, and individual gratin dishes can be handy portion-control tools. These single-serve dishes make for an attractive presentation, too.

Moroccan Shepherd's Pie

Sweet potatoes provide a nice foil for the full-flavored lamb, tangy olives, and earthy spices. Assemble this dish up to a day ahead, cover, refrigerate, and bake just before serving.

1 tablespoon olive oil
1 pound bone-in lamb shoulder, trimmed and cut into 1/2-inch pieces
1 teaspoon ground cumin, divided
1/4 teaspoon kosher salt, divided
1 1/2 cups chopped onion
4 garlic cloves, minced
1 tablespoon tomato paste
1 1/2 cups fat-free, lower-sodium chicken broth
1/2 cup water
1/3 cup sliced pimiento-stuffed green olives
1/3 cup raisins
2 tablespoons honey
1/2 teaspoon ground red pepper
1/4 teaspoon ground turmeric
1/2 teaspoon ground cinnamon, divided
1 cup frozen green peas
4 cups chopped peeled sweet potato
1 large egg, lightly beaten
Cooking spray

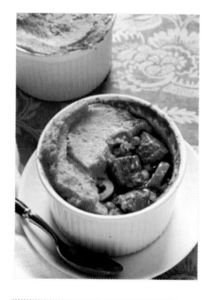

1. Heat a large skillet over medium-high heat. Add oil to pan; swirl to coat. Sprinkle lamb evenly with 1/2 teaspoon ground cumin and 1/8 teaspoon salt. Add lamb to pan; sauté 4 minutes, turning to brown on all sides. Remove lamb from pan. Add onion to pan; sauté 3 minutes, stirring occasionally. Add garlic; sauté 30 seconds, stirring constantly. Stir in tomato paste, and sauté 30 seconds, stirring frequently.

2. Add chicken broth and 1/2 cup water to pan, and bring to a boil, scraping pan to loosen browned bits. Return lamb to pan. Stir in remaining 1/2 teaspoon ground cumin, olives, raisins, honey, red pepper, and turmeric. Stir in 1/8 teaspoon cinnamon. Reduce heat, and simmer 30 minutes, stirring occasionally. Remove from heat; stir in peas.

3. Preheat oven to 350°.

4. Cook potato in a large saucepan of boiling water 10 minutes or until tender; drain. Cool 5 minutes. Place potato in a bowl. Sprinkle potato with remaining 1/8 teaspoon salt and remaining 3/8 teaspoon ground cinnamon. Beat potato with a mixer at high speed until smooth. Add egg; beat until combined. Spoon lamb mixture into 4 (10-ounce) ramekins coated with cooking spray; spread potato mixture evenly over lamb mixture. Place ramekins on a baking sheet; bake at 350° for 25 minutes or until bubbly. Serves 4 (serving size: 1 ramekin).

CALORIES 491; FAT 18.5g (sat 6.1g, mono 8.9g, poly 2.1g); PROTEIN 24.3g; CARB 58.8g; FIBER 7.7g; CHOL 110mg; IRON 3.9mg; SODIUM 728mg; CALC 101mg

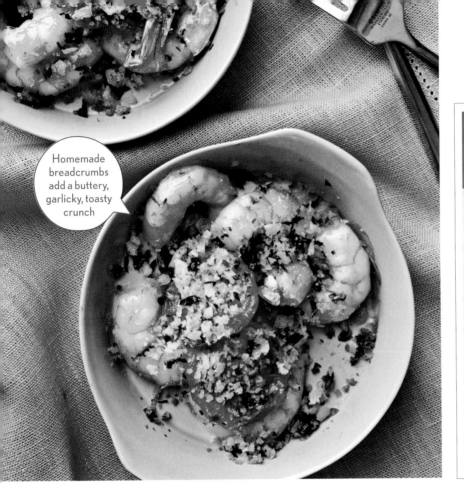

Homemade breadcrumbs add a buttery, garlicky, toasty crunch

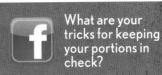

What are your tricks for keeping your portions in check?

"I've been trying out the recipes from your magazine so long and following the serving size indicated in each recipe that now I do it with any magazine recipe I find or meals I cook on my own. My tummy got in the *Cooking Light* portion habit."

—*Debbie Harry*

"When I'm at a restaurant, I decide how much of what's on the plate I'm going to eat before I start eating, and then eat slowly!"

—*Day Kibilds*

Baked Shrimp with Tomatoes

1 (2-ounce) piece French bread baguette
⅓ cup finely chopped fresh parsley
1 garlic clove, minced
4 teaspoons butter, divided
4 teaspoons olive oil, divided
1 pound large shrimp, peeled and deveined
⅛ teaspoon salt, divided
⅛ teaspoon black pepper, divided
2 small tomatoes, cut into ¼-inch-thick slices (about 11 ounces)
4 teaspoons balsamic vinegar

1. Preheat oven to 450°.
2. Place bread in a food processor; pulse until fine crumbs measure 1 cup. Combine breadcrumbs, parsley, and garlic. Heat 2 teaspoons butter and 2 teaspoons oil in a large skillet over medium-high heat. Add breadcrumb mixture, and cook 3 minutes or until golden brown and garlic is fragrant, stirring frequently.
3. Coat 4 individual gratin dishes with remaining 2 teaspoons oil. Arrange shrimp in a single layer in dishes; sprinkle with dash of salt and dash of pepper. Sprinkle with ½ cup breadcrumb mixture, and top with tomato slices. Sprinkle with remaining dash of salt and dash of pepper. Top with remaining ½ cup breadcrumb mixture; dot with remaining 2 teaspoons butter. Bake at 450° for 12 minutes or until shrimp are done. Drizzle with vinegar. Serves 4 (serving size: about 5 shrimp, ¼ cup breadcrumb mixture, and 2 tomato slices).

CALORIES 364; FAT 16.5g (sat 5.4g, mono 7.1g, poly 2.7g); PROTEIN 37.1g; CARB 16g; FIBER 1.8g; CHOL 274mg; IRON 5.5mg; SODIUM 563mg; CALC 140mg

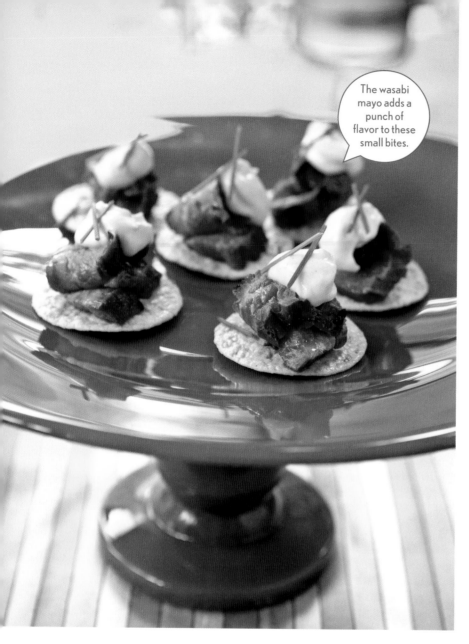

The wasabi mayo adds a punch of flavor to these small bites.

Beef Teriyaki Crisps with Wasabi Mayonnaise

Steak:
¼ cup fresh orange juice
¼ cup lower-sodium soy sauce
2 tablespoons mirin (sweet rice wine)
2 tablespoons honey
2 teaspoons grated peeled fresh ginger
½ pound flank steak, trimmed
Cooking spray

Remaining ingredients:
½ cup canola mayonnaise
2 teaspoons wasabi paste
2 teaspoons rice vinegar
24 baked rice crackers
Fresh chive pieces (optional)

1. To prepare steak, combine first 6 ingredients in a large zip-top plastic bag; seal. Marinate in refrigerator 24 hours, turning occasionally.
2. Remove steak from bag, and discard marinade. Heat a grill pan over medium-high heat. Coat pan with cooking spray. Add steak to pan; grill 6 minutes on each side or until desired degree of doneness. Remove steak from pan; let stand 10 minutes. Cut steak diagonally across grain into thin slices; cut slices into 2-inch pieces.
3. Combine mayonnaise, wasabi paste, and vinegar, stirring well. Spoon ¾ teaspoon mayonnaise mixture onto each cracker. Divide steak evenly among crackers; top each with ¼ teaspoon mayonnaise mixture. Garnish with chives, if desired. Serves 12 (serving size: 2 topped crisps).

CALORIES 125; FAT 8.6g (sat 1.1g, mono 4.4g, poly 2g); PROTEIN 4.5g; CARB 5.8g; FIBER 0g; CHOL 10mg; IRON 0.3mg; SODIUM 148mg; CALC 5mg

Savor Cocktail Hour

WHEN HOSTING A PARTY, proper portions are possible. These small bites prove you can have bold flavor without overindulging.

Smoked Salmon and Cheese Mini Twice-Baked Potatoes

6 small Yukon gold or red potatoes (about 2 pounds)
1 teaspoon olive oil
½ teaspoon salt, divided
Cooking spray
½ cup (2 ounces) finely grated white cheddar cheese
2 tablespoons fat-free milk
1 tablespoon butter
½ teaspoon black pepper
2 tablespoons finely chopped smoked salmon (1 ounce)
Chopped fresh chives (optional)

1. Preheat oven to 400°.
2. Rub potatoes with oil; sprinkle with ¼ teaspoon salt. Place potatoes on a jelly-roll pan coated with cooking spray. Bake at 400° for 35 minutes or until tender. Remove from oven; cool 10 minutes.
3. Cut potatoes in half crosswise; cut off a small portion of rounded edge so potato will stand upright. Carefully scoop out about 1 teaspoon pulp from each half, leaving shells intact. Combine potato pulp, cheese, milk, butter, pepper, and remaining ¼ teaspoon salt in a bowl. Spoon about 1 heaping teaspoon potato mixture into each potato shell. Arrange stuffed potatoes on a jelly-roll pan; top each with ½ teaspoon chopped salmon. Bake at 400° for 15 minutes or until thoroughly heated. Sprinkle with chives, if desired. Serves 12 (serving size: 1 stuffed potato half).

CALORIES 96; FAT 2.9g (sat 1.7g, mono 0.6g, poly 0.1g); PROTEIN 3.5g; CARB 13.6g; FIBER 0.9g; CHOL 8mg; IRON 0.7mg; SODIUM 159mg; CALC 37mg

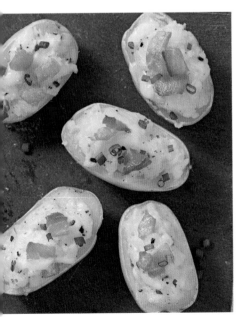

Sparkling Pear Cocktail

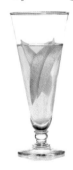

This beautiful aromatic sipper is surprisingly stout. Combine 1⅓ cups chilled brut sparkling wine and ⅔ cup chilled pear liqueur. Garnish with Seckel pear slices, if desired. Serves 4 (serving size: ½ cup).

CALORIES 142; FAT 0g (sat 0g, mono 0g, poly 0g); PROTEIN 0g; CARB 1.3g; FIBER 0g; CHOL 0mg; IRON 0mg; SODIUM 0mg; CALC 0mg

DO YOU OVERPOUR ALCOHOL?

Portion control is important when it comes to alcohol. Moderate drinking means no more than one drink per day for women and two drinks for men. Try to have two or three glasses of water for every alcoholic drink.

1 drink =

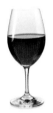

Wine: 5 fluid ounces *(130 calories)* Keep wine pours prudent by using smaller glasses instead of oversized, bowl-like ones.

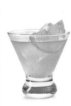

Spirits: 1.5 fluid ounces *(225 calories)* For liquor, spirits, or liqueurs, a shot-sized serving is a perfectly portioned nightcap. The calories in cocktails can vary dramatically depending on the mixer.

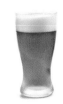

Beer: 12 fluid ounces *(150 calories)* Servings add up quickly with premium beers that come in pint-sized (16-ounce) bottles.

Add Soups to the Mix

THE LARGE AMOUNT OF LIQUID in soups makes them particularly satisfying and filling. So find more ways to work soup—especially broth-based vegetable kinds—into your weekly menu rotation.

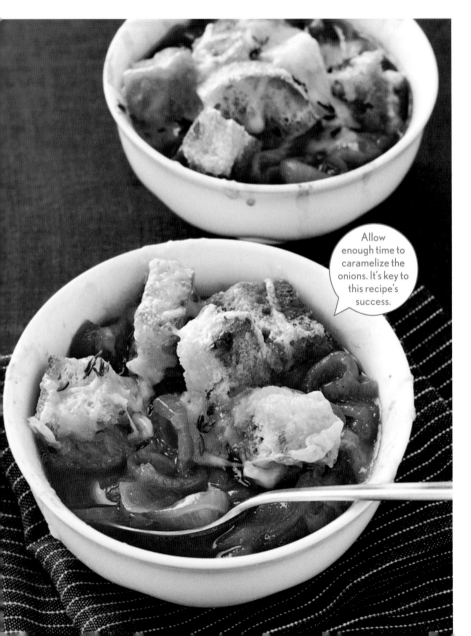

Allow enough time to caramelize the onions. It's key to this recipe's success.

French Onion and Apple Soup

TravelChickie on CookingLight.com said, "Wow. Not only the best French onion soup I've ever had, but one of the most fabulous *Cooking Light* recipes I've ever used!"

3 tablespoons unsalted butter
15 cups sliced yellow onion (about 4 pounds)
¾ teaspoon black pepper
3 thyme sprigs
2 bay leaves
1 Honeycrisp or Pink Lady apple, peeled, quartered, and cut into julienne strips
½ cup Madeira wine or dry sherry
6 cups lower-sodium beef broth
½ cup apple cider
1 tablespoon sherry vinegar
10 (½-ounce) slices sourdough bread, cut into 1-inch cubes
2 cups (8 ounces) grated Gruyère or Swiss cheese
Thyme leaves (optional)

1. Melt butter in a Dutch oven over medium heat. Add onion to pan; cook 5 minutes, stirring frequently. Continue cooking 50 minutes or until deep golden brown, stirring occasionally. Add pepper, thyme sprigs, bay leaves, and apple; cook 3

minutes or until apple softens. Add wine; cook 2 minutes, scraping pan to loosen browned bits. Add broth and cider; bring to a boil. Reduce heat, and simmer 45 minutes. Discard bay leaves; stir in vinegar.

2. Preheat broiler.

3. Arrange bread cubes in a single layer on a jelly-roll pan; broil 2 minutes or until toasted, turning after 1 minute.

4. Preheat oven to 500°.

5. Ladle 1 cup soup into each of 10 ovenproof soup bowls. Divide croutons evenly among bowls, and top each serving with about 3 tablespoons cheese. Place bowls on a jelly-roll pan. Bake at 500° for 8 minutes or until cheese melts. Garnish with thyme leaves, if desired. Serves 10.

CALORIES 254; FAT 11g (sat 6.4g, mono 3.1g, poly 0.7g); PROTEIN 11.1g; CARB 29.2g; FIBER 4.1g; CHOL 33mg; IRON 1.1mg; SODIUM 426mg; CALC 278mg

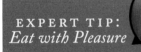

EXPERT TIP:
Eat with Pleasure

"Popular diets tend to demonize certain foods like potatoes, pasta, cheese, and even fruit, yet the reality is no food is fattening unless you overconsume it. Food is not the problem, your portions are. I think it's important to eat with pleasure and without guilt. Just keep sight of how much you're eating."

—*Manuel Villacorta, MS, RD, blogger,* The Huffington Post, *and author of* Eating Free

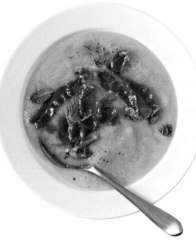

Melon Gazpacho with Frizzled Prosciutto

5 cups cubed peeled cantaloupe (about 3½ pounds)
4 cups chopped ripe peaches (about 4 large)
½ cup water
2 tablespoons minced shallots
2 tablespoons fresh lemon juice
1 tablespoon sherry vinegar
⅜ teaspoon kosher salt
2 teaspoons olive oil
4 ounces thinly sliced prosciutto, cut into ribbons
4 teaspoons chopped fresh mint
¼ teaspoon freshly ground black pepper

1. Place first 7 ingredients in a blender; process until smooth (process in batches, if necessary). Place in freezer to chill while prosciutto cooks.

2. Heat a large skillet over medium heat. Add oil to pan; swirl to coat. Add prosciutto; cook 10 minutes or until crisp, stirring occasionally. Drain on paper towels.

3. Spoon soup into bowls; top with prosciutto, mint, and pepper. Serves 4 (serving size: about 1¼ cups soup, about 1 ounce prosciutto, 1 teaspoon mint, and a dash of pepper).

CALORIES 206; FAT 5.6g (sat 1.3g, mono 3g, poly 0.9g); PROTEIN 9.7g; CARB 32.7g; FIBER 4g; CHOL 17mg; IRON 1.3mg; SODIUM 638mg; CALC 34mg

Fresh Green Pea Gazpacho

2½ cups shelled fresh English peas
2¼ cups ice water
1½ cups chopped peeled English cucumber
1 cup (½-inch) cubes French bread
2 tablespoons extra-virgin olive oil
1½ tablespoons sherry vinegar
2 garlic cloves
½ teaspoon kosher salt
½ teaspoon freshly ground black pepper
Fresh pea shoots
1 tablespoon small fresh mint leaves
1½ teaspoons extra-virgin olive oil

1. Cook English peas in boiling water 4 minutes. Drain and rinse with cold water until cool. Set aside ½ cup peas. Place remaining peas, 2¼ cups ice water, and next 5 ingredients in a blender; process until smooth. Stir in salt and pepper. Ladle 1 cup soup into each of 6 bowls. Garnish with reserved peas, fresh pea shoots, mint leaves, and 1½ teaspoons oil. Serves 6.

CALORIES 128; FAT 6.1g (sat 0.9g, mono 4.2g, poly 0.9g); PROTEIN 4.5g; CARB 14g; FIBER 3g; CHOL 0mg; IRON 1.1mg; SODIUM 222mg; CALC 12mg

Bring Your Own Lunch

WHEN YOU BYOL TO WORK, you get to control the portion size and exactly what's in it. A little pre-planning on the weekend will help you avoid super-sized restaurant meals and all-you-can-eat buffets. Be sure to stash some healthy snacks at your desk, so you won't be tempted by vending machine treats.

Tabbouleh with Chicken and Red Bell Pepper

1/2 cup uncooked bulgur
1/2 cup boiling water
1 1/2 cups diced plum tomato
3/4 cup shredded cooked chicken breast
3/4 cup minced fresh flat-leaf parsley
1/2 cup finely chopped red bell pepper
1/2 cup diced English cucumber
1/4 cup minced fresh mint
1 1/2 tablespoons fresh lemon juice
1 tablespoon extra-virgin olive oil
1/2 teaspoon salt
1/4 teaspoon freshly ground black pepper

1. Combine bulgur and 1/2 cup boiling water in a large bowl. Cover and let stand 15 minutes or until bulgur is tender. Drain well; return bulgur to bowl. Cool. Add tomato and remaining ingredients; toss well. Serves 4 (serving size: 1 1/4 cups).

CALORIES 150; FAT 4.7g (sat 0.8g, mono 2.9g, poly 0.7g); PROTEIN 11.2g; CARB 16.9g; FIBER 4.5g; CHOL 22mg; IRON 1.6mg; SODIUM 326mg; CALC 33mg

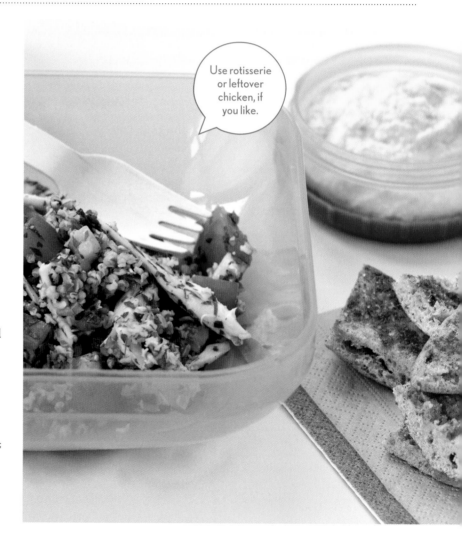

Use rotisserie or leftover chicken, if you like.

Southwestern White Bean Pita Pockets

1½ tablespoons lime juice, divided
4 teaspoons extra-virgin olive oil, divided
½ teaspoon ground cumin
¼ teaspoon salt, divided
¼ teaspoon ground red pepper
2 (15-ounce) cans organic white beans, rinsed, drained, and divided
½ cup diced plum tomato
¼ cup diced red bell pepper
¼ cup diced seeded peeled cucumber
3 tablespoons diced red onion
1 tablespoon chopped fresh cilantro
1 small jalapeño pepper, seeded and minced
2 (6-inch) pitas, cut in half
4 Boston lettuce leaves
½ cup crumbled queso fresco
4 lime wedges

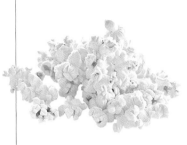

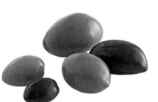

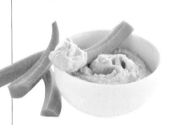

BUILD YOUR OWN PORTABLE 100-CALORIE SNACKS

Portion-controlled snack packs can help you eat less, but pay attention to what's inside that wrapper. Few are nutritional powerhouses. If you want something that satisfies, saves money, and offers a nutritional boost, make your own pre-portioned snacks.

3½ cups 94% fat-free microwave popcorn
Benefit: One of your three servings of whole grains.

1⅓ ounces pitted olives
Benefit: This fruit satisfies a salty craving and supplies a decent amount of heart-healthy fats.

¼ cup hummus with 4 carrot sticks
Benefit: Five grams of filling fiber means you won't feel hungry for a while.

1. Place 1 tablespoon lime juice, 2 teaspoons oil, cumin, ⅛ teaspoon salt, red pepper, and 1 cup beans in a food processor; process until smooth, scraping sides of bowl as needed.
2. Place remaining 1½ teaspoons lime juice, remaining 2 teaspoons olive oil, remaining ⅛ teaspoon salt, remaining beans, tomato, bell pepper, cucumber, red onion, cilantro, and jalapeño in a bowl; toss well to combine.
3. Spread about 3½ tablespoons processed bean mixture inside each pita half. Place 1 lettuce leaf, about ¾ cup tomato mixture, and 2 tablespoons cheese inside each pita half. Serve with lime wedges. Serves 4 (serving size: 1 pita half and 1 lime wedge).

CALORIES 363; FAT 9g (sat 2.6g, mono 4.1g, poly 0.9g); PROTEIN 16g; CARB 54.9g; FIBER 7.6g; CHOL 10mg; IRON 4mg; SODIUM 546mg; CALC 196mg

Enjoy a Little Something Sweet

S OMETIMES ALL YOU NEED is a small bite of something sweet to eat. A little treat built into your day will keep you from feeling deprived. You may find when you savor these mini sweets that one is all you want.

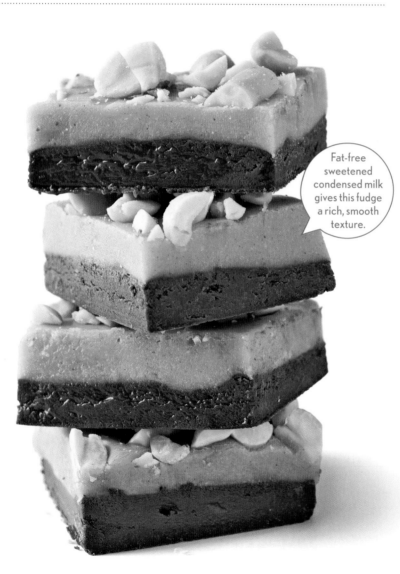

Fat-free sweetened condensed milk gives this fudge a rich, smooth texture.

Peanut Butter and Dark Chocolate Fudge

1 (14-ounce) can fat-free sweetened condensed milk, divided
¾ cup semisweet chocolate chips
2 tablespoons unsweetened dark cocoa powder
¼ teaspoon instant coffee granules
1 teaspoon vanilla extract, divided
¾ cup peanut butter chips
1 tablespoon peanut butter
¼ cup salted, dry-roasted peanuts, coarsely chopped

1. Line an 8-inch square glass or ceramic baking dish with wax paper. Place 9 tablespoons milk in a microwave-safe bowl. Add chocolate chips, cocoa, and coffee. Microwave at HIGH 1 minute or until melted. Stir in ½ teaspoon vanilla. Spread into prepared pan.
2. Combine remaining milk, peanut butter chips, and peanut butter in a microwave-safe bowl. Microwave at HIGH 1 minute or until melted. Stir in remaining ½ teaspoon vanilla. Spread evenly over chocolate layer, and sprinkle with peanuts. Cover and chill 2 hours. Serves 25 (serving size: 1 square).

CALORIES 123; FAT 4.7g (sat 3.1g, mono 0.7g, poly 0.1g); PROTEIN 3.5g; CARB 17g; FIBER 0.6g; CHOL 2mg; IRON 0.3mg; SODIUM 47mg; CALC 43mg

For an adult version, use chilled Champagne in place of the sparkling grape juice.

Slow down when you snack; you'll likely eat less. A study in *Appetite* found that people who snacked on in-shell pistachios ate 41% fewer calories than those who munched on the shelled nuts. Stopping to remove the shells helped the snackers eat less, yet they reported feeling equally satisfied.

Quick Dessert

Date and Almond Truffles

Place 2½ cups whole pitted dates, 2 cups toasted slivered blanched almonds, 1 tablespoon honey, ½ teaspoon ground cinnamon, and ⅛ teaspoon kosher salt in a food processor. Process 45 seconds, scraping down sides as needed, or until mixture forms a thick paste. Place 1 cup toasted flaked unsweetened coconut in a shallow bowl. Shape almond mixture into 36 (1-inch) balls. Roll balls in toasted coconut. Serves 18 (serving size: 2 truffles).

CALORIES 158; FAT 9.1g (sat 3g, mono 4g, poly 1.6g); PROTEIN 3.3g; CARB 19g; FIBER 3.6g; CHOL 0mg; IRON 0.8mg; SODIUM 15mg; CALC 47mg

Sparkling Strawberry Pops

Combine ¾ cup sugar and ¼ cup water in a microwave-safe bowl; microwave at HIGH 3 minutes or until boiling. Stir until sugar dissolves, and cool. Place 6 cups sliced fresh strawberries (about 2 pounds), 2 tablespoons fresh lemon juice, and 2 teaspoons light-colored corn syrup in a food processor; process until smooth. Strain through a sieve over a bowl, pressing to extract juices; discard solids. Combine sugar syrup, strawberry mixture, and 1¼ cups chilled nonalcoholic sparkling grape juice. Divide mixture among 8 (4-ounce) ice-pop molds. Top with lid; insert craft sticks. Freeze 4 hours or until thoroughly frozen. Serves 8 (serving size: 1 pop).

CALORIES 139; FAT 0.4g (sat 0g, mono 0.1g, poly 0.2g); PROTEIN 0.9g; CARB 35.5g; FIBER 2.5g; CHOL 0mg; IRON 0.5mg; SODIUM 9mg; CALC 21mg

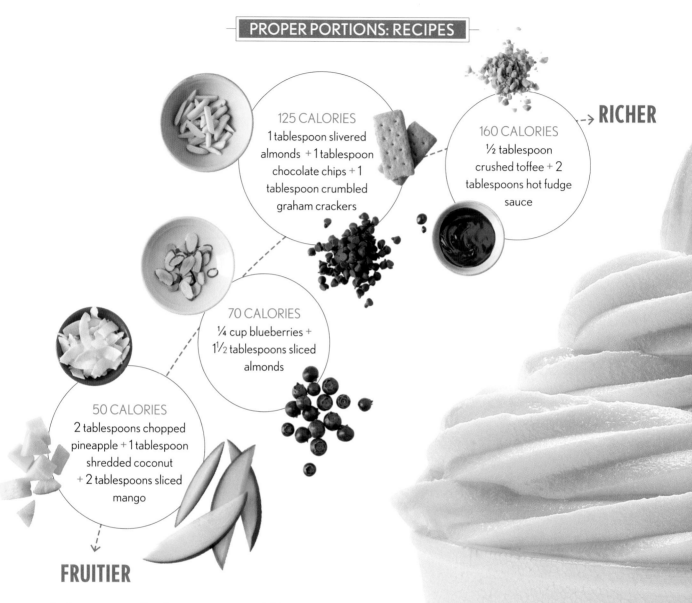

RICHER

125 CALORIES
1 tablespoon slivered almonds + 1 tablespoon chocolate chips + 1 tablespoon crumbled graham crackers

160 CALORIES
½ tablespoon crushed toffee + 2 tablespoons hot fudge sauce

70 CALORIES
¼ cup blueberries + 1½ tablespoons sliced almonds

50 CALORIES
2 tablespoons chopped pineapple + 1 tablespoon shredded coconut + 2 tablespoons sliced mango

FRUITIER

Keep Yogurt Toppers in Check

FROZEN YOGURT IS LIGHTER than ice cream and some even supply good-for-you probiotic bacteria, but it's easy to go overboard with large portions and excess toppings. The trick to keeping it all in check: Start with ½ cup (about 3.5 ounces), which will yield 80 to 120 calories, depending on your flavor choice. Top it off with some of these tasty topping combinations.

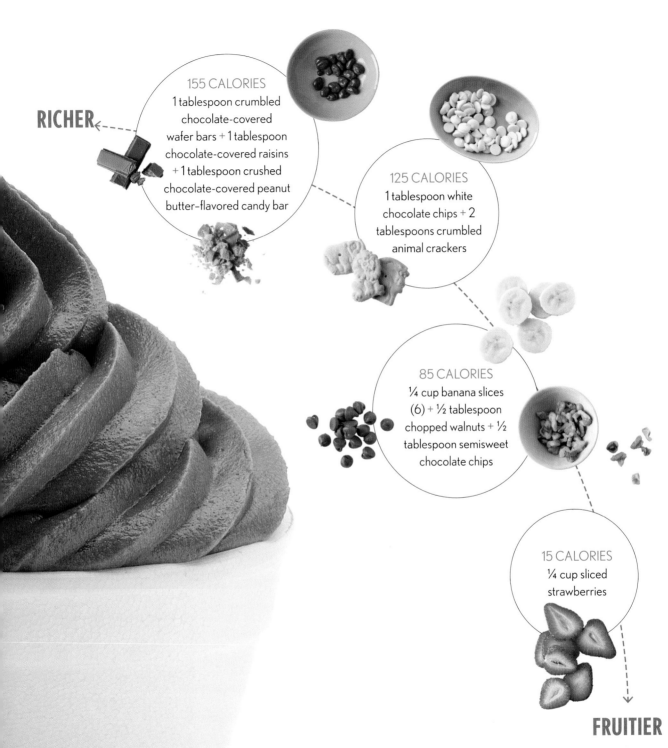

RICHER

155 CALORIES
1 tablespoon crumbled chocolate-covered wafer bars + 1 tablespoon chocolate-covered raisins + 1 tablespoon crushed chocolate-covered peanut butter–flavored candy bar

125 CALORIES
1 tablespoon white chocolate chips + 2 tablespoons crumbled animal crackers

85 CALORIES
¼ cup banana slices (6) + ½ tablespoon chopped walnuts + ½ tablespoon semisweet chocolate chips

15 CALORIES
¼ cup sliced strawberries

FRUITIER

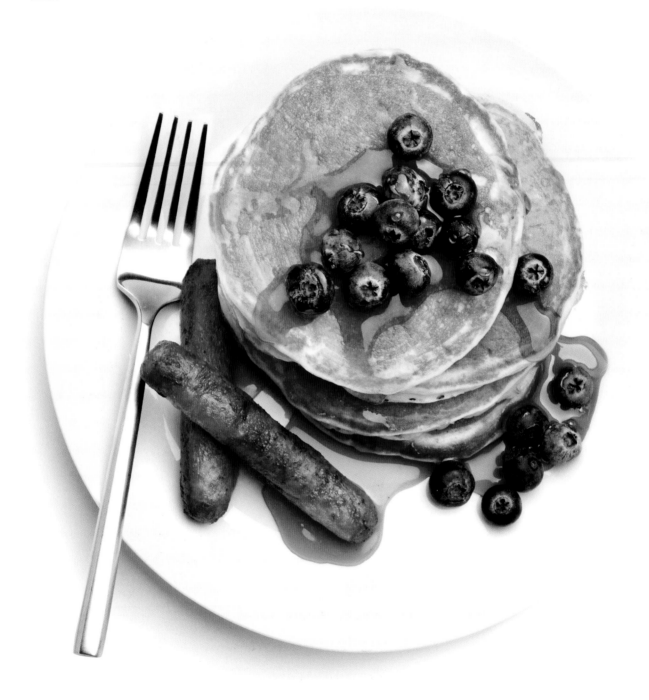

EAT MINDFULLY

TAKE YOUR TIME AND ENJOY.

IMAGINE ENJOYING EVERYTHING YOU EAT—really savoring the tastes and textures of food. Imagine a menu where food is abundant, nothing is off limits, and you make your choices without judgment or guilt and eat until you are truly satisfied.

This doesn't have to be fantasy—this can truly be your reality. Mindful eating is to eat with pleasure, without fear or regret. It's about eating for joy's sake and not constantly worrying about losing control. Instead, you trust yourself to enjoy all foods, and to recognize when you've had enough.

Mindful eating is an ancient concept that has been practiced for thousands of years, yet it's never been more relevant. Mindful eating is part of a rapidly growing non-diet movement that rejects restrictive regimens and embraces the idea of healthy habits, not diets—which is exactly what this book is all about.

While many of our other healthy habits have focused on what to eat, this habit is more about how you eat. It's about keeping your mind on your meals. It's about eating without distractions and concentrating completely on the food in front of you, which may take some practice. Yet this focus helps ensure that your mind is in tune with your body, allowing you to feel the subtle messages that you're getting full.

This chapter will help you understand the basic principles of mindful eating. You'll learn to abandon your past beliefs about diets, avoid eating on autopilot, and seek out the joy in food. Most importantly, once you master the concept of mindful eating, you'll find yourself naturally making long-term changes so all 12 healthy habits will stick.

YOUR GOAL

Be mindful, purposeful, and joyful each time you eat.

The 12 Healthy Habits

| · 01 · GET COOKING | · 02 · BREAKFAST DAILY | · 03 · WHOLE GRAINS | · 04 · GET MOVING | · 05 · VEGGIE UP | · 06 · MORE SEAFOOD | · 07 · HEALTHY FATS | · 08 · GO MEATLESS | · 09 · GET STRONGER | · 10 · LESS SALT | · 11 · BE PORTION-AWARE | · 12 · EAT MINDFULLY |

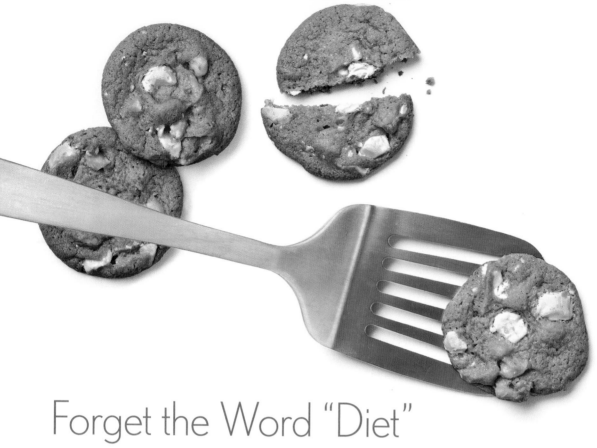

Forget the Word "Diet"

M INDFUL EATING ISN'T A DIET that you go on and off. It's about creating your own goals for healthy eating and physical activity that you can stick with for life. Take these five rules to heart:

1. ALL FOOD IS GOOD.
When you label certain foods as "bad" you'll feel bad about yourself when you eat them, which can cause you to overeat.

2. NO FOODS ARE FORBIDDEN.
"Knowing that you can eat what you want with attunement will help you avoid feelings of deprivation, which often leads to uncontrollable cravings and 'Last Supper' overeating, then overwhelming guilt," says Evelyn Tribole, MS, RD, co-author of *Intuitive Eating*.

3. SAY GOODBYE TO GUILT.
If you judge food, it makes it hard to fully enjoy certain foods because of the guilt associated with eating them. It's this guilt that often leads to more overeating, not less.

4. DON'T PUNISH YOURSELF IF YOU OVEREAT.
Instead, remember what it feels like to be overly full, and work on new strategies to decrease the likelihood that you'll eat more than you intended next time.

5. HOME IN ON YOUR OWN HUNGER.
Forget following the rigid rules set by the latest fad diet. Your body is the best barometer for how much food you need to consume to stay at a healthy weight. Mindful eating expert Michelle May, MD, suggests using a 1-to-10 scale to determine how hungry you really are (1 is ravenous, 10 is stuffed). Ideally, you want to end each meal at around a 5 or a 6 so you feel comfortable at the end of your meal.

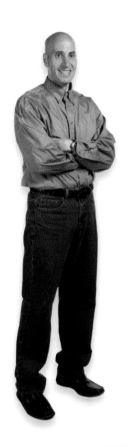

The Classic Yo-Yo Dieter

"I had a hard time giving up my favorite foods."

ATHAN PERAHORITIS
Hospital Phone Room Technician

➤ **MINDFUL CHALLENGE:** Athan has gained and lost over 50 pounds on various diets over the years. His problem? Following a too-strict diet that dictated seven mini-meals a day with a long list of restricted foods. Now, Athan has been able to lose 60 pounds eating the foods he loves. His success strategies:

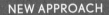 **NEW APPROACH** ▪ **Don't restrict yourself.** Athan has welcomed back previously forbidden foods and said the freedom to eat these foods when he wants has helped him avoid overeating. "I learned to listen to my body and what I wanted," he said. "Since the labels were taken off of food ('good' or 'bad'), I was free to eat what I really wanted for that meal. Now when we go out I don't have to worry about what to eat. I do not have to stress over what people are going to serve or where we are going to eat. I just look for the food that looks best to me."

▪ **Listen to your body.** Athan has learned to distinguish between physical hunger and the other reasons he was eating, such as stress or fatigue. Even though weight loss is not the primary goal of mindful eating (the emphasis is on health, happiness, and vitality), Athan has lost 60 pounds eating the foods he loves. He's now going through training to become a mindful eating facilitator for the "Am I Hungry?" workshops that were so helpful to him.

 Expert Chatter on Mindful Eating

@JessicaO_RD: Eat at a table and take time to eat...stop checking email or watching TV or whatever else...just concentrate on the food.

@tobyamidor: Mindful eating is being conscious of food you buy, what you eat, when you eat...putting thought into food you put in your body.

@anndunawayteh: Slow down, enjoy your food and enjoy your dining companions. Put your fork down between bites—still working on this myself.

Turn Off the Autopilot

I F YOU EAT QUICKLY OR WHILE WATCHING TV, working on the computer, or talking on the telephone, you won't be giving your food or your body's satiety signals your full attention. These distractions make it easy to overeat.

EAT SLOWLY.

It takes about 20 minutes for your stomach to send the stop-eating signals to your brain, so by the time those chemical messengers reach their destination, you may be on your way to overeating. In fact, chewing your food 40 times (instead of the average 15 times) can help you eat about 12% less food, according to a Chinese study published in the *American Journal of Clinical Nutrition.*

TAKE A CUE FROM THE JAPANESE.

Practice the concept of *hara hachi bu.* This cultural habit involves eating until you're only 80% full. That way you can give your brain a chance to register that you've had enough, and you'll stop before you feel stuffed.

ALWAYS SIT AT A TABLE TO EAT.

This tells your brain that you're having a meal (something that doesn't happen when you're hovering over the sink or standing in front of the fridge). Aim to make eating an event of its own.

TURN OFF THE TELEVISION.

The vast wasteland of TV can lead to vast waists: One University of Massachusetts study found that people who watched TV during a meal consumed 288 more calories on average than those who didn't.

AVOID ANY SORT OF MULTITASKING.

Shut off your computer, power off your smartphone, and focus on the task at hand: enjoying your meal. A UK study found that people who played a computer game during lunch ate faster, couldn't remember everything they ate, and felt less full compared to the non-distracted group.

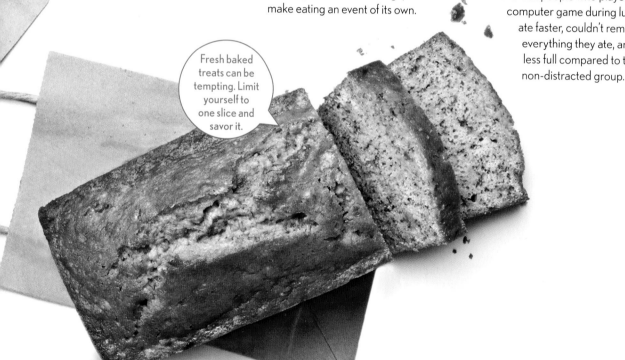

Fresh baked treats can be tempting. Limit yourself to one slice and savor it.

Seek Out the Joy

IF YOU'RE CONSTANTLY EATING ON THE RUN or turning to food for reasons other than hunger, chances are you're not allowing yourself to enjoy the true taste of your meal. The true testament to the power of food is the feelings of unity, love, friendship, and family it often evokes. Martha Beck, PhD, life coach and author of *The Four Day Win: End Your Diet War and Achieve Thinner Peace*, offers advice on how to make every eating occasion an enjoyable one.

1. INHALE AND EXHALE.

"Slow, deep, even breathing tells the brain stem to put the entire brain into a state of calm," says Beck. Take five deep in-and-out breaths after you sit down at the table and before you lift your fork.

2. GIVE THANKS.

"If you're focused on gratitude, the stress can't take over," says Beck. "Gratitude stops addictive patterns in the brain." After your five deep breaths, allow yourself a moment of gratitude, silent reflection, or prayer for the food you are about to eat.

3. REPLAY FRUSTRATING SITUATIONS.

When you do find yourself mindlessly eating, forgive yourself and move on. "Because we tend to remember what we did wrong, it helps to replay it in your mind with a different outcome," Beck says. "It's a way of rehearsing that behavior so it replicates more easily." For example, you're unhappy that you went overboard with the cheese board at a cocktail party. Replay the scenario, only this time you're taking a bite or sip, enjoying it slowly, and truly savoring every flavor.

4. ENJOY WHAT'S ON YOUR PLATE.

"Never eat anything you don't enjoy, and truly enjoy everything you eat," says Beck. Take the first four bites of your meals slowly and with full attention on the food: Savor the flavors and textures so that you can begin to understand what mindful eating feels like.

COACHING SESSION
with JANET HELM, MS, RD

LOVING FOOD IS A GOOD THING

One of the main principles of mindful eating is loving food. There are so many reasons why it's good to be a food lover.

■ When you love food, you take your time with it. You don't rush through your meal so fast that you barely notice the taste after the first few bites. Savoring every mouthful will help you slow down so you'll enjoy what you're eating and won't miss the signals that you're getting full.

■ If you love food, you'll give your meal undivided attention and won't be tempted to work, read, watch TV, or surf the Internet while you're eating.

Splitting your focus means you're not allowing yourself to fully enjoy what you're eating, and you'll likely eat more without even noticing.

■ Loving food means you want to associate it with pleasure, not discomfort or pain as a result of overeating. Why ruin a positive culinary experience by eating to the point of feeling uncomfortably full? A food lover fearlessly enjoys the eating experience from start to finish without guilt or regret.

Get Inspired by Stories of Gratitude

THE NATURAL BY-PRODUCT OF A THANKFUL ATTITUDE toward food is a desire to share it with others. Below are the inspiring stories of three women who used food as a way to give back to their communities.

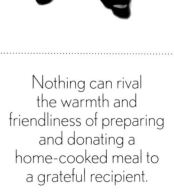

While her son serves in Iraq, she serves up home-cooked meals to returning soldiers.

SUSAN VOSMIK
USO Volunteer

➤ **TWENTY-NINE YEARS AGO,** Susan Vosmik met her husband, Roger, in the mess hall when they were volunteers with the Illinois National Guard. Their son Christopher is a medical lab technician who served in a combat support hospital in Iraq. "I got started with the USO because they were very good to my son," says Susan, who, along with Roger, helps bake everything from blueberry pancakes and sausage breakfasts to Russian apple cake—all of which she serves to the many soldiers in transit or in waiting at one of the USO facilities in Chicago's O'Hare International Airport. "It's so nice to see the troops, thank them personally, and help get them on their way," she says. "For some of them it's the first homemade food they've had since basic training. They're so polite and awesome, and they say 'thank you' constantly. I couldn't be prouder to do it."

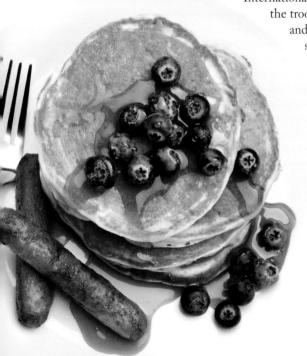

Nothing can rival the warmth and friendliness of preparing and donating a home-cooked meal to a grateful recipient.

She turned her love for entertaining into charitable fund-raising success.

JULIE EVARTS
Silent Auction Charity Dinner Hostess

➤ **JULIE IS A WORKING MOM** with a passion for cooking, entertaining, and creating scenic tables to set the stage for her events—all skills she attributes to a childhood of watching her mother work magic in the kitchen. Four years ago, it struck her that her knack for entertaining could be used outside her home to help others—she could donate her talents to a local silent auction that raises money for several charities. Julie's annual contribution: a four- or five-course dinner and cocktails for six that includes a beautifully set table. "Whatever people bid, it all goes to charity," she says. "It's fun for them, and I enjoy it. I love entertaining and am great about talking, so most end up in the kitchen with me."

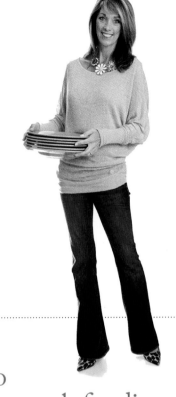

A mom turns grief into public awareness and research funding, one cookie at a time.

GRETCHEN HOLT WITT
Founder of Cookies for Kids' Cancer

➤ **GRETCHEN FIRST HAD THE IDEA** to bake cookies as a way to raise money for children's cancer research in 2007, after her then-3-year-old son Liam had finished his own cancer treatments. "I wanted to come up with something that was so easy anybody could do it anywhere—something so innocent and warm and friendly and inviting that people couldn't turn away." In the beginning, Gretchen and 250 volunteers baked 96,000 cookies and raised $420,000 for pediatric cancer research. Today, this grassroots organization (cookiesforkidscancer.org) helps people set up bake sales across the country, sending 100% of profits to fund the fight against pediatric cancer. "Something magical happens every time people have a bake sale," says Gretchen. "It's this power of being a good cookie, the affirmation of moving in the right direction." The empowerment of doing something is also what helps keep Gretchen going. "The awful twist is that we started this when Liam was cancer-free, and then we lost him. So as much as I would like to curl up in a ball and cry, I have to do it for him," she says.

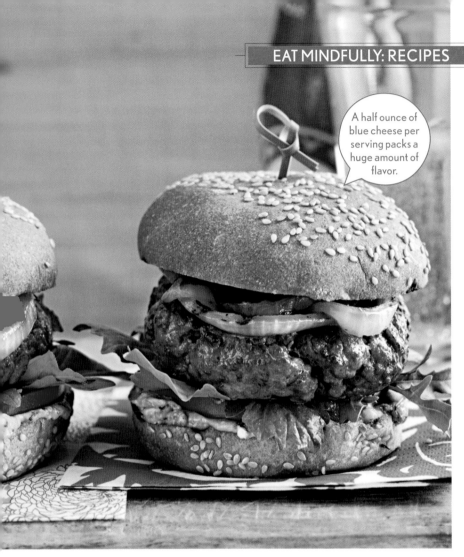

A half ounce of blue cheese per serving packs a huge amount of flavor.

Burgers with Blue Cheese Mayo and Sherry Vidalia Onions

"This is by far the best burger I have ever had that was cooked at home," said Sraede on CookingLight.com. Flowerpot916 said, "Hands down, best blue cheese burger yet!"

½ cup (2 ounces) crumbled blue cheese
¼ cup canola mayonnaise
2 teaspoons chopped fresh thyme, divided
¼ teaspoon hot pepper sauce
1 pound lean ground sirloin
1 teaspoon black pepper, divided
⅛ teaspoon kosher salt
½ teaspoon extra-virgin olive oil
4 (¼-inch-thick) slices Vidalia or
   other sweet onion
Cooking spray
2 teaspoons sherry vinegar
4 (1½-ounce) whole-wheat hamburger
   buns, toasted
4 (¼-inch-thick) slices tomato
2 cups loosely packed arugula

1. Preheat grill to medium-high heat.
2. Combine cheese, mayonnaise, 1 teaspoon thyme, and hot pepper sauce in a small bowl; stir well.
3. Divide beef into 4 equal portions, gently shaping each into a ½-inch-thick patty. Press a nickel-sized indentation in center of each patty; sprinkle patties evenly with ½ teaspoon black pepper and salt.
4. Brush oil evenly over both sides of onion slices; sprinkle with remaining ½ teaspoon pepper. Place patties and onions on grill rack coated with cooking spray; cover and grill 3 minutes on each side. Set patties aside; keep warm. Place onion slices

Prepare a Better Burger

Mindful eating means you can find a way to enjoy all foods, including a juicy, delicious, and satisfying burger, if that's what you're really in the mood for. These ground sirloin burgers are big on flavor but aren't super-sized, so you can feel good about firing up the grill.

in a zip-top plastic bag; seal. Let stand 5 minutes; toss with remaining 1 teaspoon thyme and vinegar.
5. Spread cut sides of buns evenly with mayonnaise mixture. Place 1 tomato slice on bottom half of each bun; top with ½ cup arugula, 1 patty, 1 onion slice, and top half of bun. Serves 4 (serving size: 1 burger).

CALORIES 420; FAT 21.8g (sat 5.1g, mono 10.6g, poly 5.2g); PROTEIN 31.5g; CARB 26.7g; FIBER 4.2g; CHOL 76mg; IRON 3.2mg; SODIUM 623mg; CALC 149mg

Out-N-In California Burger

"The sauce is delicious and I even tried it with a hot dog. I think that this will be one of our everyday burger favorites in the future," said Mtblke40 on CookingLight.com.

3 tablespoons ketchup
2 tablespoons canola mayonnaise
2 teaspoons sweet pickle relish
1 teaspoon Dijon mustard
1 pound ground sirloin
⅛ teaspoon salt
⅛ teaspoon black pepper
Cooking spray
4 (1-ounce) slices reduced-fat, reduced-sodium Swiss cheese
4 green leaf lettuce leaves
4 (1½-ounce) hamburger buns
4 (¼-inch-thick) slices red onion
8 (¼-inch-thick) slices tomato
½ ripe peeled avocado, cut into ⅛-inch-thick slices
8 bread-and-butter pickle chips

1. Combine first 4 ingredients in a small bowl.
2. Divide beef into 4 equal portions, gently shaping each into a ½-inch-thick patty. Press a nickel-sized indentation in center of each patty; sprinkle patties evenly with salt and pepper. Heat a large skillet or grill pan over medium-high heat. Coat pan with cooking spray. Add patties to pan; cook 3 minutes on each side. Top each patty with 1 cheese slice; cook 2 minutes or until cheese melts and patties are desired degree of doneness.
3. Place 1 lettuce leaf on bottom half of each hamburger bun; top with 1 patty, 1 onion slice, 2 tomato slices, about 2 avocado slices, 2 pickle chips,

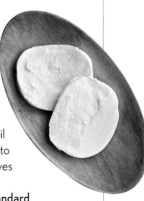

about 1½ tablespoons sauce, and top half of bun. Serves 4 (serving size: 1 burger).

CALORIES 417; FAT 19.5g (sat 5.6g, mono 5.3g, poly 4.3g); PROTEIN 38g; CARB 34.6g; FIBER 2.8g; CHOL 73mg; IRON 3.2mg; SODIUM 802mg; CALC 272mg

100-CALORIE BURGER TOPPERS

A quarter-pound of lean ground sirloin and a hearty whole-grain bun start you out at 250 calories. Try finishing it off with one of these 100-calorie combinations:

The Poached Egger
1 large poached egg + 1 tablespoon fresh salsa + ¼ cup green leaf lettuce + 1 tablespoon queso fresco

Beefy Caprese
1 ounce fresh buffalo mozzarella + ½ teaspoon extra-virgin olive oil + 2 heirloom tomato slices + 6 basil leaves

The American Standard
2 teaspoons ketchup + 3 dill pickle chips + 1 thin slice sharp cheddar cheese + green leaf lettuce + 1 heirloom tomato slice

Savor the Comfort

COMFORT FOODS NOURISH the body and soul, and there may not be a more nostalgic dish than mac 'n' cheese. Here are a couple of family-friendly versions that will surely put a smile on your face:

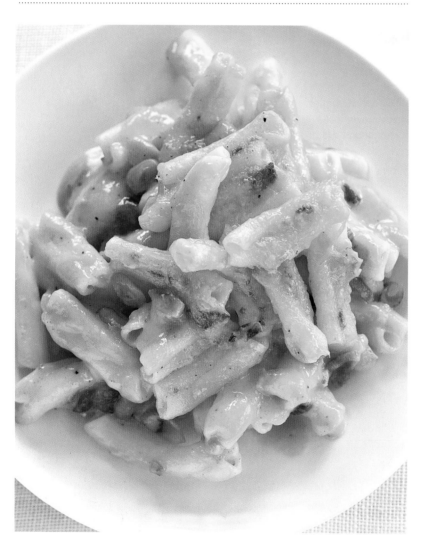

Bacon Mac

6 quarts water
3¼ teaspoons salt, divided
12 ounces strozzapreti or penne pasta
1½ cups fat-free milk
4 teaspoons all-purpose flour
2 cups finely shredded sharp cheddar cheese, divided
¼ cup sliced green onions
1 teaspoon hot sauce
¼ teaspoon freshly ground black pepper
2 center-cut bacon slices, cooked and crumbled
Cooking spray

1. Preheat broiler.
2. Bring 6 quarts water and 1 tablespoon salt to a boil. Add pasta; cook 8 minutes or until al dente. Drain.
3. Combine ½ cup milk and flour in a saucepan over medium heat. Gradually add remaining 1 cup milk; bring to a boil. Cook 1 minute, stirring constantly. Remove from heat; let stand 4 minutes or until mixture cools to 155°. Stir in 1½ cups cheese. Add remaining ¼ teaspoon salt, onions, hot sauce, pepper, and bacon; stir. Add pasta; toss. Spoon into a 2-quart broiler-safe dish coated with cooking spray; top with remaining ½ cup cheese. Broil 7 minutes. Serves 6 (serving size: about 1 cup).

CALORIES 399; FAT 13.8g (sat 8.5g, mono 4g, poly 0.8g); PROTEIN 20g; CARB 48.7g; FIBER 2g; CHOL 44mg; IRON 2.1mg; SODIUM 544mg; CALC 358mg

Creamy, Light Macaroni and Cheese

3 cups cubed peeled butternut squash (about 1 [1-pound] squash)
1¼ cups fat-free, lower-sodium chicken broth
1½ cups fat-free milk
2 garlic cloves
2 tablespoons plain fat-free Greek yogurt
1 teaspoon kosher salt
½ teaspoon black pepper
1¼ cups (5 ounces) shredded Gruyère cheese
1 cup (4 ounces) grated fresh pecorino Romano cheese
¼ cup (1 ounce) finely grated fresh Parmigiano-Reggiano cheese, divided
1 pound uncooked cavatappi
Cooking spray
1 teaspoon olive oil
½ cup panko (Japanese breadcrumbs)
2 tablespoons chopped fresh parsley

1. Preheat oven to 375°.
2. Combine first 4 ingredients in a medium saucepan; bring to a boil over medium-high heat. Reduce heat to medium, and simmer until squash is tender when pierced with a fork (about 25 minutes). Remove from heat.

INSTEAD OF THE TRADITIONAL buttery, heavy sauce, butternut squash stands in to help squash out half the calories and three-fourths of the sat fat.

3. Place hot squash mixture in a blender. Add Greek yogurt, salt, and pepper. Remove center piece of blender lid (to allow steam to escape); secure blender lid on blender. Place a clean towel over opening in blender lid (to avoid splatters). Blend until smooth. Place blended squash mixture in a bowl; stir in Gruyère, pecorino Romano, and 2 tablespoons Parmigiano-Reggiano. Stir until combined.
4. Cook pasta according to package directions, omitting salt and fat; drain well. Add pasta to squash mixture, and stir until combined. Spread mixture evenly into a 13 x 9–inch glass or ceramic baking dish coated with cooking spray.
5. Heat a medium skillet over medium heat. Add oil to pan; swirl to coat. Add panko, and cook 2 minutes or until golden brown.

Remove from heat; stir in remaining 2 tablespoons Parmigiano-Reggiano cheese. Sprinkle evenly over hot pasta mixture. Lightly coat topping with cooking spray.
6. Bake at 375° for 25 minutes or until bubbly. Sprinkle with parsley, and serve immediately. Serves 8 (serving size: 1⅓ cups).

CALORIES 390; FAT 10.9g (sat 6.1g, mono 2.1g, poly 0.4mg); PROTEIN 19.1g; CARB 53.9g; FIBER 3.2g; CHOL 31mg; IRON 2.4mg; SODIUM 589mg; CALC 403mg

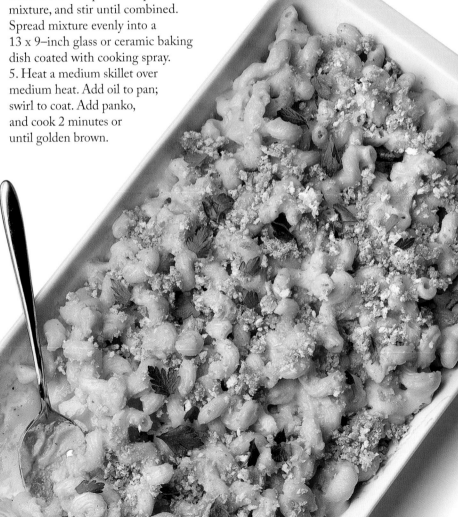

Celebrate Your Meal

A MEAL SHARED WITH FRIENDS AND FAMILY goes beyond any sensory gratification to the feelings of love and togetherness it elicits. Yet, it's easy to overlook the deeper pleasures of the table amid our hectic lives. These festive entrées can help you slow down and truly celebrate special occasions with family and friends.

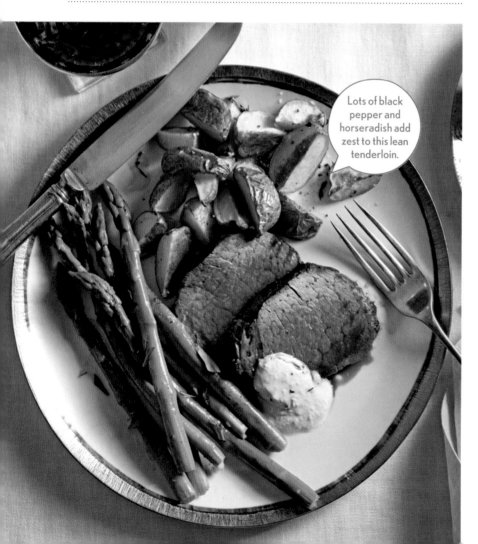

Lots of black pepper and horseradish add zest to this lean tenderloin.

Beef Tenderloin with Horseradish-Chive Sauce

"Easy to make, easy to serve, impressive, and delicious. What more could you ask for?" said HouseofGee on CookingLight.com.

1 (2-pound) beef tenderloin, trimmed
1 tablespoon olive oil
1½ teaspoons coarsely ground black pepper
¾ teaspoon kosher salt
⅔ cup light sour cream
2 tablespoons chopped fresh chives
3 tablespoons prepared horseradish
1 teaspoon fresh lemon juice
1 teaspoon Dijon mustard
⅛ teaspoon kosher salt

1. Preheat oven to 450°.
2. Heat a large skillet over medium-high heat. Rub beef with oil; coat on all sides with pepper and ¾ teaspoon salt. Add beef to pan; cook 3 minutes, browning on all sides.
3. Place beef on a broiler pan. Bake at 450° for 25 minutes or until a thermometer registers 125°. Remove from oven; let stand 10 minutes before slicing. Combine sour cream and remaining ingredients; serve with beef. Serves 8 (serving size: 3 ounces beef and about 1½ tablespoons sauce).

CALORIES 210; FAT 10.1g (sat 4.1g, mono 3.9g, poly 0.5g); PROTEIN 25.7g; CARB 2.4g; FIBER 0.3g; CHOL 67mg; IRON 1.7mg; SODIUM 310mg; CALC 21mg

Roast Pork Tenderloin with Plum Barbecue Sauce

Asian spices give this barbecue sauce a complex flavor, which enhances the sweet-tart flavor of the plums.

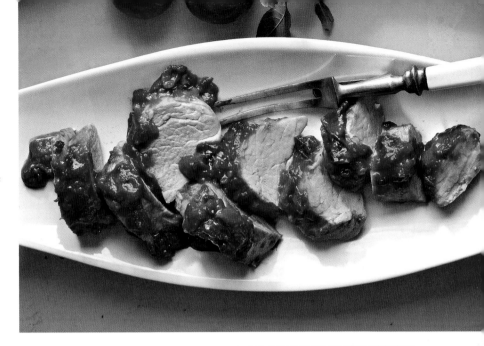

Sauce:
2 tablespoons canola oil
1 cup chopped onion
2 garlic cloves, finely chopped
¼ cup packed brown sugar
¼ cup rice wine vinegar
¼ cup ketchup
2 tablespoons lower-sodium soy sauce
2 teaspoons dry mustard
1 teaspoon ground ginger
½ teaspoon black pepper
⅛ teaspoon crushed red pepper
2 whole cloves
1½ pounds black plums, quartered and pitted
1 star anise

Pork:
2 tablespoons canola oil
2 (1-pound) pork tenderloins, trimmed
½ teaspoon salt
½ teaspoon freshly ground black pepper

1. To prepare sauce, heat a large saucepan over medium-high heat. Add 2 tablespoons canola oil to pan; swirl to coat. Add onion and garlic; sauté 5 minutes, stirring constantly. Add sugar and next 10 ingredients; bring to a boil. Reduce heat, and simmer, partially covered, 30 minutes or until plums break down and sauce thickens, stirring occasionally. Discard cloves and anise.

2. Preheat oven to 450°.
3. To prepare pork, heat a large skillet over medium-high heat. Add 2 tablespoons oil to pan; swirl to coat. Sprinkle pork evenly with ½ teaspoon salt and ½ teaspoon black pepper. Add pork to pan; sauté 7 minutes, turning to brown on all sides.
4. Transfer pork to a foil-lined jelly-roll pan; coat with ½ cup plum sauce. Roast pork at 450° for 15 minutes. Remove pork from oven. Turn pork over; coat with an additional ½ cup plum sauce. Roast 7 minutes or until a thermometer inserted in thickest portion of pork registers 145°. Remove from pan; let stand 10 minutes. Slice crosswise. Serve with remaining plum sauce. Serves 8 (serving size: 3 ounces pork and about ⅓ cup sauce).

CALORIES 378; FAT 10.3g (sat 1.6g, mono 5.6g, poly 2.4g); PROTEIN 25.2g; CARB 50.7g; FIBER 4.7g; CHOL 62mg; IRON 2mg; SODIUM 417mg; CALC 22mg

EXPERT TIP:
You Are in Charge

"Mindful eating means your body is in charge. You make choices that help you feel good, eating what you want, when you want. You don't fight or resist your environment. Instead, you have natural brakes in place to make sure that you don't eat out of control. Sure, you see delicious food around you, but if you're not hungry, you're not as tempted by it. And you don't feel deprived by not eating it."

—*Linda Bacon, PhD, nutrition professor at City College of San Francisco and author of* Health at Every Size: The Surprising Truth About Your Weight

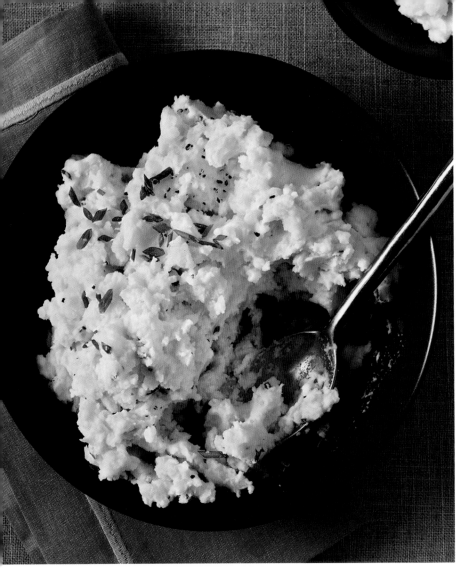

Microwave Smashed Potatoes

4 (6-ounce) baking potatoes, peeled
   and cut into 1-inch pieces
½ cup reduced-fat sour cream
½ cup 1% low-fat milk
2 tablespoons minced fresh chives
½ teaspoon salt
½ teaspoon freshly ground black
   pepper

1. Place potato pieces in a large
microwave-safe bowl. Cover bowl
with plastic wrap; cut a 1-inch slit
in center of plastic wrap. Microwave at HIGH 10 minutes. Let
stand 2 minutes. Add sour cream
and remaining ingredients to bowl;
mash with a potato masher. Serves
4 (serving size: about 1 cup).

CALORIES 225; FAT 4.1g (sat 2.5g, mono 1.1g, poly 0.2g);
PROTEIN 5.6g; CARB 42.6g; FIBER 2.8g; CHOL 13mg;
IRON 0.8mg; SODIUM 333mg; CALC 78mg

Southwest Variation:

Omit sour cream and chives;
decrease milk to 2 tablespoons
and salt to ¼ teaspoon. Add ¾ cup
plain low-fat yogurt; 1 tablespoon
chopped chipotle chile, canned
in adobo sauce; and ¼ teaspoon
ground cumin. Serves 4 (serving
size: about 1 cup).

CALORIES 206; FAT 1g (sat 0.6g, mono 0.2g, poly 0.1g);
PROTEIN 6.3g; CARB 43.9g; FIBER 3.2g; CHOL 3mg;
IRON 0.9mg; SODIUM 236mg; CALC 104mg

Don't Disown Potatoes

POTATOES ARE OFTEN DEMONIZED as a starchy
carb and thrown into the forbidden category for
dieters. Yet, mindful eating makes room for all foods.
If you've been eliminating potatoes from your menu
rotation, here are some easy, praise-worthy ways to bring
them back.

The potato is the humble star of the comfort-food pantry. Fresh herbs, reduced-fat sour cream, and reasonable portions of high-flavor cheeses amp up the flavor.

Roasted Garlic Variation:

You can find roasted garlic cloves at the salad bar in many grocery stores. Omit sour cream and chives; increase milk to ¾ cup. Add ¼ cup coarsely chopped roasted garlic cloves and 1 tablespoon chopped fresh sage. Serves 4 (serving size: about 1 cup).

CALORIES 203; FAT 0.7g (sat 0.3g, mono 0.1g, poly 0.1g); PROTEIN 5.7g; CARB 44.9g; FIBER 3g; CHOL 2mg; IRON 0.9mg; SODIUM 329mg; CALC 82mg

Bacon and Cheddar Variation:

Decrease salt to ¼ teaspoon. Add ¼ cup (1 ounce) reduced-fat shredded extra-sharp cheddar cheese and 1 center-cut bacon slice, cooked and crumbled; mash with a potato masher to desired consistency. Serves 4 (serving size: about 1 cup).

CALORIES 254; FAT 6.1g (sat 3.7g, mono 1.1g, poly 0.2g); PROTEIN 7.8g; CARB 42.9g; FIBER 2.8g; CHOL 20mg; IRON 0.8mg; SODIUM 280mg; CALC 129mg

Spinach Baked Potato

"Another winner," said SDanielson1973 on CookingLight.com. "My daughter loved this. We used goat cheese instead of feta and threw a couple of cherry tomatoes in with the spinach while it was wilting."

4 (6-ounce) Yukon gold potatoes
1½ tablespoons extra-virgin olive oil
1 tablespoon white wine vinegar
½ teaspoon Dijon mustard
¼ teaspoon freshly ground black pepper
⅛ teaspoon salt
¼ cup vertically sliced red onion
3 garlic cloves, thinly sliced
1 (9-ounce) package fresh spinach
½ cup crumbled feta cheese

1. Pierce each potato several times with a fork. Microwave at HIGH 13 minutes or until tender, turning after 7 minutes.
2. Combine oil and next 4 ingredients in a bowl, stirring well with a whisk. Heat vinaigrette in a large skillet over medium-high heat. Add onion and garlic; sauté 2 minutes. Gradually add spinach; toss until wilted. Divide spinach among potatoes. Top each with 2 tablespoons crumbled feta cheese. Serves 4 (serving size: 1 topped potato).

CALORIES 255; FAT 8.1g (sat 2.8g, mono 4.4g, poly 0.6g); PROTEIN 7.7g; CARB 39g; FIBER 5.2g; CHOL 13mg; IRON 3.7mg; SODIUM 358mg; CALC 121mg

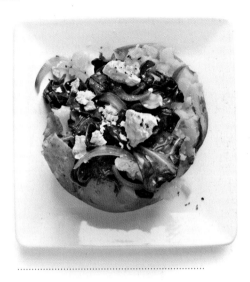

EXPERT TIP:
Get to the Root of Your Habit

"Dieting is like weeding your garden with nail clippers; it's a difficult, endless, futile chore that will never get to the root of the problem. Until you know the real answers to why you're eating when you're not hungry or why you continue the eat-repent-repeat cycle, you're doomed to repeat those behaviors again and again. Mindful eating allows you to put away your nail clippers so you can get to the root of your issues and cultivate the habits you really want."

—*Michelle May, MD, author of* Eat What You Love, Love What You Eat *and founder of amihungry.com*

Enjoy Your Chocolate

CHOCOLATE IS ONE of those intensely loved and also intensely feared foods. But it's OK to love chocolate. If you ban it, your cravings will only intensify. Knowing that you can eat chocolate means you'll likely eat less. These delectable desserts are the perfect reminder of why you're so passionate about cacao, the food of the gods.

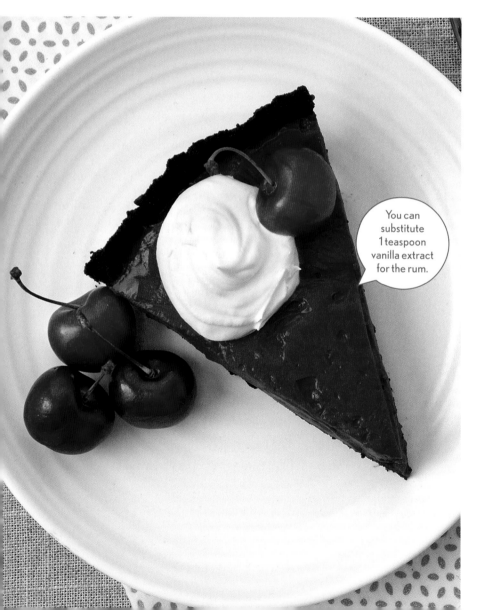

You can substitute 1 teaspoon vanilla extract for the rum.

Rich Chocolate Pudding Pie

"The crust is amazing and goes incredibly well with the filling, whipped cream, and berries," said Lifeisgood on CookingLight.com. "Although I like an Oreo crust, it can't even compare to this one!"

Crust:
30 chocolate wafers
3 ounces bittersweet chocolate, melted
1 tablespoon canola oil

Filling:
¾ cup sugar
¼ cup cornstarch
¼ cup unsweetened cocoa
¼ teaspoon salt
1 ¾ cups 1% low-fat milk
2 large egg yolks
4 ounces bittersweet chocolate, finely chopped
1 tablespoon white rum
¾ cup fresh cherries
10 tablespoons fat-free frozen whipped topping, thawed

1. To prepare crust, place wafers in a food processor; process until finely ground. Add 3 ounces melted chocolate and oil; process until blended.

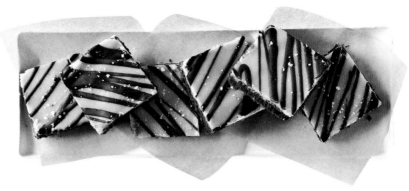

Press into bottom and up sides of a 9-inch pie plate. Freeze 15 minutes or until set.

2. To prepare filling, combine sugar, cornstarch, cocoa, and salt in a large saucepan; stir with a whisk. Add half of milk and yolks; stir with a whisk until smooth. Stir in remaining milk. Cook over medium heat 5 minutes or until thick and bubbly, stirring constantly. Remove from heat. Add 4 ounces chocolate, and stir until smooth. Stir in rum. Pour filling into prepared crust. Cover with plastic wrap; chill 4 hours or until set. Serve with cherries and whipped topping. Serves 10 (serving size: 1 pie slice, about 1 tablespoon cherries, and 1 tablespoon whipped topping).

CALORIES 320; FAT 14.2g (sat 5.9g, mono 5.3g, poly 1.8g); PROTEIN 5.5g; CARB 49.5g; FIBER 3.2g; CHOL 44mg; IRON 1.7mg; SODIUM 193mg; CALC 77mg

EXPERT TIP:
Forget "Forbidden"

"If you give up the idea that certain foods are forbidden, you may find that you don't want them as much as you thought you did. You may also discover that you're satisfied with smaller amounts when you do eat them."

—*Marsha Hudnall, MS, RD, blogger, A Weight Lifted*

Salted Caramel Brownies

"These are amazing!" said Suelatham on CookingLight.com. "I made them for a neighborhood get-together and they were a big hit. Everyone wanted the recipe! It's a keeper!"

Brownies:
3.38 ounces all-purpose flour (about ¾ cup)
1 cup granulated sugar
¾ cup unsweetened cocoa
½ cup packed brown sugar
½ teaspoon baking powder
6 tablespoons butter, melted
2 large eggs
1 teaspoon vanilla extract
Cooking spray

Topping:
¼ cup butter
¼ cup packed brown sugar
3 ½ tablespoons evaporated fat-free milk, divided
½ cup powdered sugar
¼ teaspoon vanilla extract
1 ounce bittersweet chocolate, coarsely chopped
⅛ teaspoon coarse sea salt

1. Preheat oven to 350°.
2. To prepare brownies, weigh or lightly spoon flour into dry measuring cups; level with a knife. Combine flour and next 4 ingredients in a large bowl, stirring well with a whisk. Combine 6 tablespoons butter, eggs, and 1 teaspoon vanilla. Add butter mixture to flour mixture; stir to combine. Scrape batter into a 9-inch square metal baking pan lightly coated with cooking spray. Bake at 350° for 19 minutes or until a wooden pick inserted in center comes out with moist crumbs clinging. Cool in pan on a wire rack.
3. To prepare topping, melt ¼ cup butter in a saucepan over medium heat. Add ¼ cup brown sugar and 1½ tablespoons milk; cook 2 minutes. Remove from heat. Add powdered sugar and vanilla; stir with a whisk until smooth. Spread mixture evenly over cooled brownies. Let stand 20 minutes or until set.
4. Combine remaining 2 tablespoons milk and chocolate in a microwave-safe bowl; microwave at HIGH 45 seconds or until melted, stirring after 20 seconds. Stir just until smooth; drizzle over caramel. Sprinkle with sea salt; let stand until set. Cut into squares. Serves 20.

CALORIES 180; FAT 7.2g (sat 4.1g, mono 1.7g, poly 0.3g); PROTEIN 2.1g; CARB 27.8g; FIBER 0.8g; CHOL 37mg; IRON 0.9mg; SODIUM 76mg; CALC 26mg

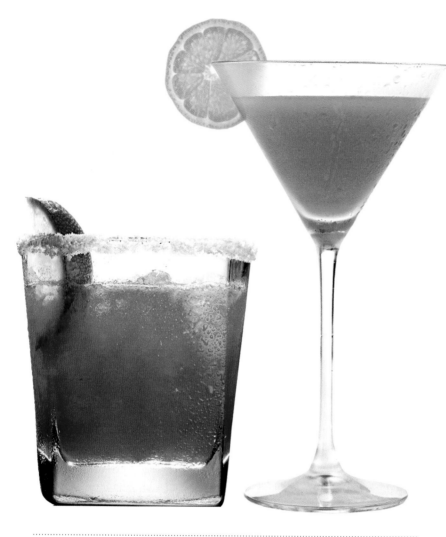

Blackberry Margaritas

1½ tablespoons sugar
½ teaspoon kosher salt
1 lime
1¼ cups water
½ cup sugar
1 cup 100% agave blanco tequila
⅔ cup fresh lime juice
½ cup Grand Marnier (orange-
  flavored liqueur)
12 ounces fresh blackberries

1. Combine 1½ tablespoons sugar and salt in a dish. Cut lime into 9 wedges; rub rims of 8 glasses with 1 lime wedge. Dip rims of glasses in salt mixture.
2. Combine 1¼ cups water and ½ cup sugar in a microwave-safe glass measuring cup. Microwave at HIGH 2½ minutes, stirring to dissolve sugar; cool. Place syrup, tequila, fresh lime juice, Grand Marnier, and blackberries in a blender; process until smooth. Strain mixture through a cheesecloth-lined sieve over a pitcher; discard solids. Serve over ice. Garnish with remaining lime wedges. Serves 8 (serving size: about ½ cup and 1 lime wedge).

CALORIES 179; FAT 0.2g (sat 0g, mono 0g, poly 0.1g); PROTEIN 0.5g; CARB 23.1g; FIBER 1.6g; CHOL 0mg; IRON 0.2mg; SODIUM 121mg; CALC 11mg

Drink Mindfully

MINDFULNESS IS SOMETHING you can apply to drinking, too. While research shows having one glass of wine or beer with your evening meal is unlikely to affect your total calories, more than that can add calories and prime your appetite. The key to mindful drinking is taking your time, tasting every sip so you're less tempted to overdo it. Here are some festive ways to say cheers to moderation.

Satsuma Vodka-Tini

1 cup fresh cranberries
1 cup vodka
½ cup sugar
4 satsumas, peeled
¾ cup Grand Marnier
¼ cup fresh lime juice
½ cup crushed ice

1. Place first 4 ingredients in a food processor; process until pureed. Refrigerate 8 hours or overnight. Strain mixture through a cheesecloth-lined sieve over a bowl, pressing to extract juice. Discard solids. Stir in Grand Marnier and lime juice. Place 1 cup satsuma mixture in a martini shaker with ½ cup crushed ice; shake. Strain mixture into 2 martini glasses. Repeat procedure to yield 10 cocktails. Serves 10.

CALORIES 156; FAT 0g (sat 0g, mono 0g, poly 0g); PROTEIN 0.1g; CARB 18.8g; FIBER 0.1g; CHOL 0mg; IRON 0.1mg; SODIUM 2mg; CALC 7mg

Apricot-Ginger Bellinis

Sugar syrup:
¾ cup water
¾ cup sugar
1 (2-inch) piece peeled fresh ginger, halved

Remaining ingredients:
1 teaspoon grated lime rind
1 teaspoon fresh lime juice
1 (15-ounce) can apricot halves in light syrup, drained
1 (750-milliliter) bottle prosecco or other sparkling white wine
Fresh lime slices (optional)

1. To prepare sugar syrup, combine ¾ cup water and sugar in a small saucepan. Bring to a boil; cook 2 minutes or until sugar dissolves. Add ginger. Remove from heat; cool. Chill 4 hours.
2. Strain sugar syrup through a colander into a bowl; discard ginger. Place ⅓ cup sugar syrup in a blender; reserve remaining syrup for another use. Add rind, juice, and apricots to blender; process until smooth. Spoon 2 tablespoons apricot puree into each of 8 glasses. Top each with ⅓ cup prosecco; stir gently. Garnish with lime slices, if desired. Serves 8.

CALORIES 112; FAT 0g (sat 0g, mono 0g, poly 0g); PROTEIN 0.2g; CARB 13.1g; FIBER 0.5g; CHOL 0mg; IRON 0.1mg; SODIUM 1mg; CALC 4mg

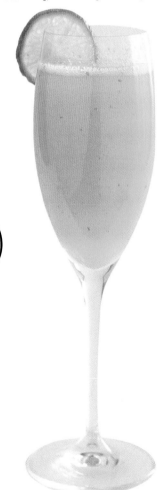

EXPERT TIP: *Learn the Art of Stopping*

"There is a Zen story about a man riding a horse that's galloping. A bystander asks, 'Where are you going in such a hurry?' and the rider replies, 'I don't know, ask the horse!' This is how many people lead their lives. They're riding a horse, but don't know where they're going and can't stop. The horse is our 'habit energy,' the relentless force of habit that pulls us along. Being mindful means learning the art of stopping—stopping your running so you can be present and conscious when you eat. Only until you are fully aware of what's going on in your daily life can you begin to change."

—*Lilian Cheung, DSc, RD, lecturer, Harvard School of Public Health*

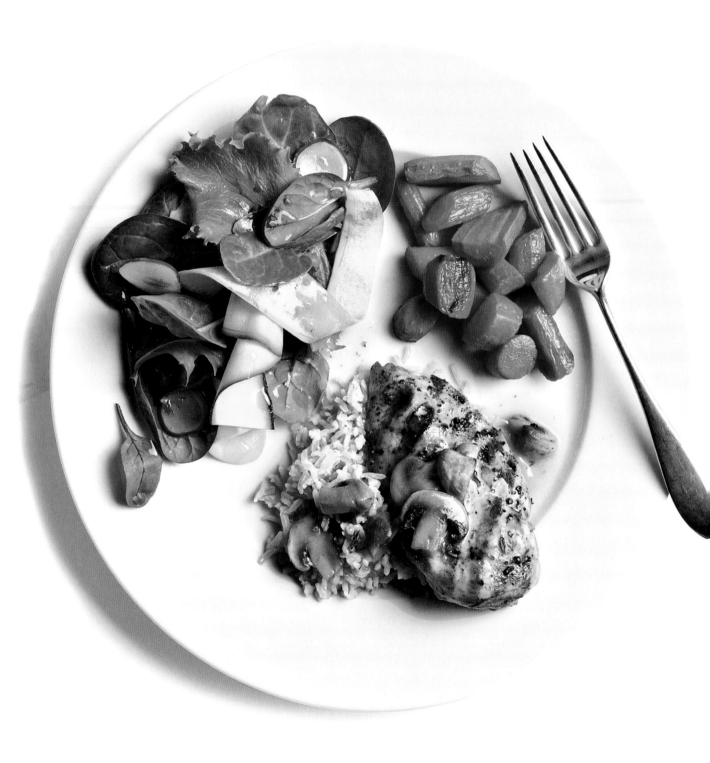

6-WEEK PLAN

NOW IT'S TIME TO BRING EVERYTHING TOGETHER. This 6-week action plan can help you jump-start your healthy habits, giving you a structure so you can adopt all 12. Each week focuses on two habits—featuring sample meals and snacks that will help you meet the daily and weekly goals outlined in each chapter. By the end of six weeks, you'll be well on your way to making these 12 habits part of your routine. After all, habits are all about making daily decisions that eventually become automatic. Soon enough, you'll start eating healthier and exercising more often without even thinking about it.

Committing your good intentions to paper and tracking your progress—including planning your menus in advance and scheduling your workouts—are proven ways to change habits. Get started by keeping your kitchen well stocked and doing some advanced prep on the weekends (or whenever you can). Recipes representing each habit are included in the meal plan, but you can easily swap them out for others in that chapter that better suit your schedule and your taste buds. The idea is to get you cooking at home more often, which is the first step to helping you eat more vegetables, fruits, whole grains, healthy fats, seafood, and breakfast, and is a vital part of slashing salt, reducing unhealthy fats, and controlling portions.

The menus are based on an average of 2,000 calories per day and include the following daily food group targets: 2½ cups vegetables, 2 cups fruits, 6 ounces grains, 3 cups dairy, 5½ ounces protein, and 6 teaspoons oils. This MyPlate meal pattern also includes about 250 extra calories that can be spent on alcoholic beverages or sweet treats. You can adjust this total calorie level based on your own needs. But keep in mind, simply focusing on "eating less" is really not the answer. It's difficult to keep up a restrictive regimen that severely limits the amount you eat. That's why two of the habits involve physical activity. Being active and practicing mindful eating are what allows you to enjoy all the sumptuous food featured throughout this book. Maintaining the pleasures of the table is how you're going to make these healthy habits stick. You can reach your goals one delicious meal, one healthy habit at a time.

	MONDAY	TUESDAY	WEDNESDAY
BREAKFAST	**Rise and Shine Oatmeal, page 60,** 1 serving Banana, 1 medium Fat-free milk, 1 cup	**Quick Garden Omelet, page 72,** 1 serving Whole-grain toast, 1 slice Butter, 1 teaspoon Orange, 1 medium Latte (made with 1 cup fat-free milk)	**Greek Yogurt Parfaits, page 70,** 1 serving Orange juice, 1 cup
LUNCH	**Tuna and White Bean Salad, page 201,** 1 serving	**Herbed Chicken Salad Sandwiches,* page 130,** 1 serving Celery, 3 medium stalks Light ranch dressing, 1½ tablespoons Apple, 1 medium *Make with your leftover roasted chicken or pick up a rotisserie chicken.	**Southwestern Salad, page 146,** 1 serving Whole-grain crackers, 5 Fat-free milk, 1 cup
SNACK	**Traditional Hummus, page 162,** ¼ cup Red bell pepper strips, ½ cup	Low-fat vanilla yogurt, 1 (6-ounce) carton Diced peaches, ½ cup	Almonds, 12 Dried apricots, 3 Chai tea with fat-free milk, 1 cup
DINNER	**Classic Roast Chicken, page 36,** 1 serving **Sautéed Carrots with Sage, page 153,** 1 serving Brown rice, ½ cup Whole-grain baguette, 2-inch piece Butter, 1 teaspoon Vanilla frozen yogurt, 1 cup Strawberries, 1 cup	**Smoky Pan-Grilled Pork Chops, page 47,** 1 serving **Simple Steamed Broccoli, page 150,** 1 serving Mashed potatoes with caramelized onions, ½ cup Mixed salad greens, 2 cups (with ⅓ cup grape tomatoes + 1½ ounces Gorgonzola cheese + 1 tablespoon **Easy Herb Vinaigrette, page 223**)	**Shrimp Pad Thai, page 29,** 1 serving **Steamed Sugar Snap Peas, page 150,** 1 serving **Asian Caramelized Pineapple, page 167,** 1 serving

Cook your favorite Asian takeout dishes in your own kitchen (pages 28–29).

6-WEEK PLAN WEEK 1

YOUR GOALS

Cook at least three more meals per week.

Eat a healthy breakfast every day of the week.

THURSDAY	FRIDAY	SATURDAY	SUNDAY	
Blueberry Oatmeal Muffins, page 66, 1 serving Hard-cooked egg, 1 large Fat-free milk, 1 cup	**Banana Breakfast Smoothie, page 125,** 1 serving Whole-grain toast, 1 slice Peanut butter, 2 teaspoons *Prepare two loaves and freeze one for later.*	**Peanut Butter Banana Bread, page 68,** 1 serving Light cream cheese, 1 tablespoon Strawberry jam, 1 teaspoon Apple slices, 1 medium apple Fat-free milk, 1 cup	**Whole-Wheat Buttermilk Pancakes, page 64,** 1 serving Cantaloupe chunks, 1 cup Fat-free milk, 1 cup	**BREAKAST**
Chicken breast–topped salad, page 147, 1 serving Rye crispbreads, 2 Cashew butter, 1 tablespoon Pomegranate spritzer (1 cup sparkling water + ½ cup pomegranate juice) *Learn to make your own nut butters (page 265).*	**Roasted Butternut Squash Soup,* page 157,** 1 serving **Goat Cheese Toasts, page 157,** 1 serving Pear, 1 medium *Freeze extra servings of soup in zip-top plastic freezer bags to store for quick meals later.	**Open-Faced Hummus Sandwiches,* page 131,** 1 serving Baby carrots and cucumber slices, 1 cup Low-fat yogurt, 1 (6-ounce) carton *You can use Traditional Hummus, page 162, if you like.	**Greek Salad, page 147,** 1 serving Whole-wheat breadsticks, 2	**LUNCH**
Air-popped popcorn, 3 cups (mixed with 1 tablespoon dried cranberries + 1 tablespoon pumpkinseed kernels)	**Traditional Hummus, page 162,** ¼ cup Red bell pepper strips, ½ cup	Red grapes, ½ cup String cheese, 1 ounce	Low-fat cottage cheese, 1 cup Fresh pineapple chunks, ½ cup	**SNACK**
Black Bean Fiesta Tacos, page 32, 2 tacos **Cabbage Slaw, page 33,** 1 serving Raspberries, ½ cup (topped with 2 tablespoons plain 2% reduced-fat Greek yogurt + 1 teaspoon honey)	**Farmers' Market Pizza, page 31,** 1 slice Mixed salad greens, 2 cups **Champagne Vinaigrette, page 223,** 1 tablespoon Mango sorbet, ½ cup *Skip delivery and make your own pizza piled with veggies.*	Flank steak, 4 ounces cooked **Roasted Potatoes with Thyme and Garlic, page 148,** 1 serving **Steamed Green Beans with Tomato-Garlic Vinaigrette, page 151,** 1 serving Whole-grain baguette, 2-inch piece Butter, 1 teaspoon	**Chickpea Chili,* page 42,** 1 serving Whole-wheat pita, 1 Vanilla pudding, 1 cup *Freeze individual portions of the chili to take to work for lunch or reheat for dinner on a busy night.	**DINNER**

6-WEEK PLAN WEEK 2

YOUR GOALS

Eat three servings of whole grains each day.

Be active for 30 minutes a day, three times a week.

	MONDAY	TUESDAY	WEDNESDAY
BREAKFAST	Bacon, egg, and cheese sandwich (1 whole-grain English muffin, toasted + 1 scrambled egg + 1 center-cut bacon slice + 1 slice cheddar cheese) Orange juice, 1 cup	Whole-grain cereal, 1 cup Blueberries, ½ cup Fat-free milk, 1 cup *Be sure you're buying a real whole grain and not an imposter (page 84).*	**Simple Baked Eggs, page 72,** 1 serving Mini whole-grain bagel, 1 Butter, 1 teaspoon Grapefruit, ½ medium Latte (made with 1 cup fat-free milk)
LUNCH	Toasted Millet and Confetti Vegetable Salad with Sesame and Soy Dressing, page 108, 1 serving Whole-grain crackers, 5 Mixed berries, 1 cup	**Tuscan Tuna Sandwiches, page 131,** 1 serving Whole-grain baked tortilla chips, 10 Green grapes, 1 cup *Fit in a 30-minute walk at lunch if you can.	**Roasted Butternut Squash Soup, page 157,** 1 serving Whole-grain baguette, 2-inch piece Butter, 1 teaspoon Plum, 1 medium *This lunch reheats quickly, leaving you plenty of time for a mid-day workout or walk.*
SNACK	Whole-wheat fig bars, 2 Fat-free milk, 1 cup	**Spicy Red Pepper Hummus, page 163,** ¼ cup Baby carrots, ½ cup *Popcorn is a whole grain!*	Air-popped popcorn, 3 cups (topped with 1 tablespoon grated fresh Parmesan cheese + pinch of cayenne pepper)
DINNER	Whole-Wheat Pasta with Edamame, Arugula, and Herbs, page 97, 1 serving Mixed salad greens, 2 cups **Mustard Seed–Chive Vinaigrette, page 223,** 1 tablespoon *Switch to whole-grain pastas; they're tastier than you may think.* *Prepare **Spicy Red Pepper Hummus, page 163,** tonight for a week of healthy snacks.	Grilled salmon, 4 ounces **Multigrain Pilaf with Sunflower Seeds, page 104,** 1 serving **Roasted Asparagus with Browned Butter, page 149,** 1 serving	**Grilled shrimp with Ponzu, page 25,** 4 ounces shrimp, 2 tablespoons sauce **Bulgur with Dried Cranberries, page 104,** 1 serving Steamed green beans, 1 cup Low-fat vanilla yogurt, 1 (6-ounce) carton Mixed berries, ½ cup *Roast the grapes for tomorrow's breakfast while you're preparing dinner.

THURSDAY	FRIDAY	SATURDAY	SUNDAY	

BREAKFAST

Slow-Roasted Grape and Yogurt Parfaits, page 71, 1 serving
Whole-grain toast, 1 slice
Almond butter, 1 tablespoon

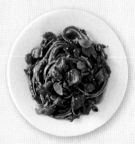

Breakfast burrito (2 scrambled eggs + 2 tablespoons shredded cheddar cheese + 1 tablespoon salsa or pico de gallo + 1 [6-inch] whole-grain tortilla)
Orange juice, 1 cup

Oatmeal Pancakes, page 65, 1 serving
Maple syrup, 1 tablespoon
Butter, 1½ teaspoons
Honeydew melon chunks, 1 cup
Steamed fat-free milk (with ¼ teaspoon almond extract + ⅛ teaspoon ground cinnamon)

Quinoa, ⅔ cup cooked (topped with ¼ cup blueberries + 1 tablespoon chopped toasted walnuts + 2 teaspoons brown sugar + ¼ teaspoon ground cinnamon)
Latte (made with 1 cup fat-free milk)

LUNCH

Wheat Berry Salad with Raisins and Pistachios, page 107, 1 serving
Whole-grain breadsticks, 2
Fat-free milk, 1 cup

Pork and Wild Rice Soup, page 102, 1 serving
Baby carrots and cucumber slices, 1 cup
Whole-wheat Melba toast crackers, 2
Herbed goat cheese, 1 ounce

Quinoa and Parsley Salad, page 109, 1 serving
Fat-free milk, 1 cup

> Make an extra batch of quinoa to have for breakfast the next day.

Meyer Lemon Chicken Piccata, page 39, 1 serving
Multigrain Pilaf with Sunflower Seeds, page 104, 1 serving
Sautéed spinach, ½ cup

SNACK

Whole-grain biscotti, 1
Chocolate milk (1 cup fat-free milk + 2 teaspoons dark chocolate syrup)

Pear, 1 medium
Cashew butter, 1 tablespoon
Fat-free milk, 1 cup

Plain 2% reduced-fat Greek yogurt, 1 (6-ounce) carton (topped with ½ cup blackberries + ½ ounce shaved dark chocolate)

Spicy Red Pepper Hummus, page 163, ¼ cup
Steamed sugar snap peas, 1 cup

DINNER

Beef-Broccoli Stir-Fry, page 45, 1 serving
Mixed salad greens, 2 cups
Sesame Vinaigrette, page 223, 1 tablespoon

*Find a way to fit in 30 minutes of activity today.

Mushroom–Brown Rice Risotto, page 101, 1 serving
Spinach-Strawberry Salad, page 167, 1 serving

Grilled skirt steak, 4 ounces
Brown rice, ½ cup
Broccoli Rabe with Onions and Pine Nuts, page 153, 1 serving
Whole-grain baguette, 2-inch piece

*Be active today for 30 minutes.

Eggplant Bolognese, page 98, 1 serving
Chocolate frozen yogurt, 1 cup
Raspberries, ½ cup

YOUR GOALS

Eat three more servings of vegetables each day.

Make seafood the centerpiece of two meals a week.

	MONDAY	TUESDAY	WEDNESDAY
BREAKFAST	Vegetable omelet (2 eggs + 1 cup diced red bell pepper, onions, and mushrooms + 2 tablespoons shredded sharp cheddar cheese) Whole-grain toast, 1 slice Butter, 1 teaspoon Fat-free milk, 1 cup	Rise and Shine Oatmeal, **page 60**, 1 serving Grapefruit, ½ medium Fat-free milk, 1 cup	Blueberry-Orange Parfaits, **page 71**, 1 serving Latte (made with 1 cup fat-free milk)
LUNCH	Broiled Tilapia Gyros, **page 189**, 1 serving Red grapes, 1 cup	Tuna and White Bean Salad, **page 201**, 1 serving Plum, 1 medium *Keep canned or jarred tuna stashed in your pantry for topping salads.*	Cajun Salmon Cakes with Lemon-Garlic Aioli,* **page 200**, 1 serving Cabbage Slaw, **page 33**, 1 serving Mango chunks, 1 cup *Make the salmon cakes the day before and heat up at work, or add canned salmon to a pasta-veggie salad.
SNACK	Low-fat vanilla yogurt, 1 (6-ounce) carton Mixed berries, ½ cup	Greek-Style Tzatziki, **page 259**, 2 tablespoons Zucchini sticks, 1 cup *Other good dippers: carrots, celery, cucumber slices, red bell pepper strips*	Provolone cheese, 1 ounce Whole-grain crackers, 5 Low-sodium vegetable juice, 1 cup
DINNER	Baked chicken, 4 ounces cooked Smoky Asparagus and Mushroom Sauté, **page 152**, 1 serving Roasted red potatoes, ½ cup Whole-grain baguette, 2-inch piece Olive oil for dipping, 1 tablespoon *Get in 30 minutes of activity today.	Arctic Char with Blistered Cherry Tomatoes, **page 182**, 1 serving Mixed salad greens, 2 cups (with 1 ounce shredded cheese and ½ cup cherry tomatoes) Easy Herb Vinaigrette, **page 223**, 1 tablespoon	Turkey Tenders, page 41, 1 serving Sautéed Brussels Sprouts with Bacon, **page 154**, 1 serving Brown rice, ½ cup *Do two 15-minute bouts of exercise today to reach your 30-minute goal.

THURSDAY	FRIDAY	SATURDAY	SUNDAY	
Breakfast burrito (2 scrambled eggs + ¼ avocado, sliced + 2 tablespoons diced red bell pepper + 1 tablespoon fresh salsa + 1 [6-inch] whole-grain tortilla) Fat-free milk, 1 cup	Whole-grain English muffin, 1 Peanut butter, 2 tablespoons Honeydew melon chunks, 1 cup Latte (made with 1 cup fat-free milk)	Overnight Honey-Almond Multigrain Cereal, page 61, 1 serving Banana, 1 medium Fat-free milk, 1 cup 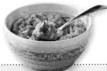	Summer Vegetable Frittata, page 74, 1 serving Mini whole-grain bagel, 1 Strawberry jam, 1 teaspoon Latte (made with 1 cup fat-free milk) Add a little smoked salmon to the frittata if you're not eating fish for dinner.	BREAKFAST
Shrimp-topped Protein-Packed Salad, page 146, 1 serving Whole-grain breadsticks, 2	Veggie pita (⅓ cup hummus + ½ cup shredded carrot + ½ cup chopped cucumber + ½ cup baby spinach + ½ whole-grain pita) Fat-free milk, 1 cup	Herbed Chicken Salad Sandwiches, page 130, 1 serving Celery sticks, 3 medium stalks Green grapes, 1 cup Canned tuna and salmon are easy swaps for the chicken.	Indian-Spiced Roasted Squash Soup, page 159, 1 serving Whole-grain baguette, 2-inch piece Apple, 1 medium	LUNCH
Air-popped popcorn, 3 cups Chocolate milk (1 cup fat-free milk + 2 teaspoons dark chocolate syrup)	Low-fat vanilla yogurt, 1 (6-ounce) carton Blueberries, 1 cup	Whole-grain pretzels, 1 ounce Honey mustard, 2 tablespoons	Vanilla frozen yogurt, 1 cup Strawberries, 1 cup	SNACK
Grilled beef tenderloin, 4 ounces cooked **Curried Cauliflower with Capers, page 155,** 1 serving Tomato and cucumber salad, 1 cup (with 1 ounce feta cheese + 1 tablespoon balsamic vinaigrette) Blackberries, 1 cup	**Maple-Glazed Salmon, page 186,** 1 serving **Scallion Couscous, page 45,** 1 serving Grilled zucchini slices, 1 cup Mixed salad greens, 2 cups (topped with 1 tablespoon walnuts + 1 tablespoon Gorgonzola cheese + 1 tablespoon balsamic vinaigrette) *Make sure you get in 30 minutes of activity.	**Peppery Pasta with Arugula and Shrimp, page 192,** 1 serving **Spinach-Strawberry Salad, page 167,** 1 serving Chocolate frozen yogurt, ½ cup 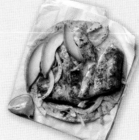	**Blackened Tilapia Baja Tacos, page 190,** 1 serving Baked tortilla chips, 5 **Pico de Gallo, page 277,** 1 serving Fresh pineapple chunks, 1 cup Keep tilapia in your freezer for easy fish taco prep.	DINNER

YOUR GOALS

Increase healthy fats and decrease unhealthy fats every day.

Go meatless one day a week.

	MONDAY	**TUESDAY**	**WEDNESDAY**
BREAKFAST	Oatmeal, 1 cup (topped with 1 tablespoon chopped walnuts + 2 teaspoons honey) Fat-free milk, 1 cup	Whole-grain toast, 2 slices (topped with ¼ cup mashed avocado + 4 slices tomato) Orange juice, 1 cup	Whole-grain English muffin, 1 Cashew butter, 2 tablespoons Grapefruit, ½ medium Fat-free milk, 1 cup
LUNCH	Roasted Corn and Radish Salad with Avocado-Herb Dressing, page 218, 1 serving Nectarine, 1 medium *Take a 30-minute break for some activity.	Salmon Burgers, page 188, 1 serving Baby carrots and cucumbers, 1 cup Fat-free milk, 1 cup	Perfect Pear-Up Salad, page 147, 1 serving Whole-grain crackers, 5 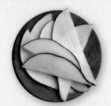
SNACK	Apple, 1 medium Peanut butter, 1 tablespoon Fat-free milk, 1 cup	White Bean and Roasted Garlic Hummus, page 162, ¼ cup Baby carrots and cucumber slices, 1 cup	Rosemary Roasted Almonds, page 213, 1 serving Fat-free milk, 1 cup
DINNER	Baked Vegetable Lasagna, page 234, 1 serving Mixed salad greens, 2 cups (topped with 1 tablespoon pepitas + 1 tablespoon balsamic vinaigrette)	Apricot, Plum, and Chicken Tagine with Olives, page 221, 1 serving Arugula salad, 2 cups (topped with 1 tablespoon grated fresh Parmesan cheese + 1 tablespoon toasted pine nuts + 1 tablespoon **Champagne Vinaigrette, page 223**)	Black Bean Burgers with Mango Salsa, page 236, 1 serving Sweet potato fries, 1 medium potato Chocolate frozen yogurt, 1 cup Raspberries, ½ cup

> Adding avocado to your toast is a tasty, satisfying way to boost healthy fats.

> Skip the creamy bottled dressings and make your own vinaigrettes (pages 222–223).

	THURSDAY	FRIDAY	SATURDAY	SUNDAY
BREAKFAST	**Peanut Butter Banana Bread, page 68,** 1 serving Light cream cheese, 1 tablespoon Fat-free milk, 1 cup	Scrambled egg sandwich (1 scrambled egg + whole-grain English muffin + 1 tomato slice + ¼ cup arugula leaves) Cantaloupe chunks, 1 cup Latte (made with 1 cup fat-free milk)	**Greek Yogurt Parfaits, page 70,** 1 serving Latte (made with 1 cup fat-free milk)	**Open-Faced Sandwiches with Ricotta, Arugula, and Fried Egg, page 75,** 1 serving Low-sodium tomato juice, 1 cup
LUNCH	**Baked Falafel Sandwiches with Yogurt-Tahini Sauce, page 237,** 1 serving Red grapes, 1 cup	**Avocado Corn Chowder with Grilled Chicken, page 219,** 1 serving Whole-grain baguette, 2-inch piece Olive oil for dipping, 1 tablespoon *Olive oil offers a rich alternative to butter.*	**Shrimp, Avocado, and Grapefruit Salad, page 145,** 1 serving *Go outdoors for your cardio today.	**Moroccan Chickpea Stew, page 239,** 1 serving Whole-grain pita, ½ pita Plum, 1 medium
SNACK	Part-skim mozzarella string cheese, 1 ounce Whole-grain crackers, 5	Pear, 1 medium Cashew butter, 2 tablespoons Fat-free milk, 1 cup	**White Bean and Roasted Garlic Hummus, page 162,** ¼ cup Baby carrots, 1 cup *Nuts are healthy-fat power players; find our A-Z guide (pages 210–211).*	Almonds, 12 Dried apricots, 3 Fat-free milk, 1 cup
DINNER	**Three-Bean Vegetarian Chili, page 235,** 1 serving Corn bread, 2-inch square Mixed salad greens, 2 cups (topped with 1 tablespoon slivered almonds + 1 tablespoon grated fresh Parmesan cheese) Mixed berries with kiwi, 1 cup *Try a new exercise class or DVD to get in your 30-minute workout.	**Salmon with Hoisin Glaze, page 187,** 1 serving **Garlicky-Spicy Snow Peas, page 187,** 1 serving Brown rice, ½ cup 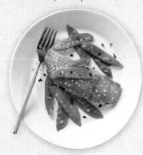	**Linguine with Two-Olive Marinara, page 220,** 1 serving Mixed green salad, 2 cups (topped with 1 tablespoon slivered almonds + 1 tablespoon **Sesame Vinaigrette, page 223**)	**Tempeh and Green Bean Stir-Fry with Peanut Sauce, page 247,** 1 serving Vanilla yogurt, 1 (6-ounce) carton Mixed berries, 1 cup *Wash and cut veggies for the week ahead, and keep at eye level in your fridge for easy snacking.

6-WEEK PLAN WEEK 5

	MONDAY	TUESDAY	WEDNESDAY
BREAKFAST	Rise and Shine Oatmeal, **page 60**, 1 serving Banana, 1 medium Fat-free milk, 1 cup	Scrambled eggs, 2 large Sriracha sauce, 1 teaspoon Whole-grain toast, 1 slice Watermelon chunks, 1 cup Latte (made with 1 cup fat-free milk)	Whole-grain cereal, 1 cup Blueberries, ½ cup Fat-free milk, ½ cup Latte (made with 1 cup fat-free milk)
LUNCH	Turkey and Bean Chili, **page 280**, 1 serving Low-sodium whole-grain crackers, 5 Pear, 1 medium	Peanut Butter Plus Sandwiches, **page 264**, 1 sandwich Red and yellow bell pepper strips, 1 cup Fat-free milk, 1 cup	Baked sweet potato, 1 medium (topped with 2 tablespoons shredded cheddar cheese + 2 tablespoons **Pico de Gallo, page 277**) Apple, 1 medium Almond butter, 2 tablespoons
SNACK	Greek-Style Tzatziki, **page 259**, 2 tablespoons Sugar-snap peas, 1 cup	Sweet Chipotle Snack Mix, **page 282**, 1 serving	Sweet Spiced Almonds, **page 212**, 1 serving Fat-free milk, 1 cup
DINNER	Whole-wheat penne, 1 cup cooked (with ½ cup **Basic Marinara, page 278** + 1 ounce shaved fresh Parmesan cheese) Mixed salad greens, 2 cups **Easy Herb Vinaigrette, page 223**, 1 tablespoon *Start small, incorporating strength training into your existing cardio routine. Three sets of 12 reps for each exercise is a good starting point.	Pan-Grilled Thai Tuna Salad, **page 199**, 1 serving Mixed berries, 1 cup (topped with ½ cup 2% reduced-fat Greek yogurt + 1 tablespoon honey)	Flank steak, 3 ounces cooked **Smoky Three-Bean Bake, page 261**, 1 serving Steamed green beans, ½ cup *Cardio today!

Adding some heat to your eggs will lessen the need for salt.

Make your own sauces to add a ton of flavor with just a touch of salt (pages 276–277).

YOUR GOALS

Include strength training in your fitness regimen at least two times per week.

Reduce the amount of sodium you eat every day.

THURSDAY	FRIDAY	SATURDAY	SUNDAY	
Plain 2% reduced-fat Greek yogurt, 1 cup (with 1 cup blueberries + 1 cup orange sections + 1 tablespoon honey) Latte (made with 1 cup fat-free milk)	Quick Garden Omelet, page 72, 1 serving Whole-grain toast, 1 slice Butter, 1 teaspoon Orange, 1 medium Fat-free milk, 1 cup	Whole-Wheat Buttermilk Pancakes, page 64, 1 serving Latte (made with 1 cup fat-free milk)	Muesli with Cranberries and Flaxseed, page 61, 1 serving Plain 2% reduced-fat Greek yogurt, ½ cup Orange juice, 1 cup	BREAKFAST
Classic Caprese Salad, page 147, 1 serving Peach, 1 medium	Double Tomato Soup, page 281, 1 serving Grilled cheese sandwich (2 slices whole-grain bread + 1 slice cheddar cheese + 1 slice tomato) Apple, 1 medium	Chicken breast–topped Southwestern Salad, page 147, 1 serving Dried apricots, 3 *Cardio for 30 minutes + strength training. Make sure you work opposing muscle groups for a complete strength session.	Shanghai-Inspired Fish Stew, page 195, 1 serving Whole-grain pita, ½ pita *Buy lower-sodium chicken broth and soy sauce instead of the regular.*	LUNCH
Unsalted, dry-roasted peanuts, 1 ounce Dried cranberries, 2 tablespoons Fat-free milk, 1 cup	Maple-Chile Popcorn, page 283, 1 serving Steamed milk (1 cup fat-free milk + ½ teaspoon vanilla extract + ¼ teaspoon ground nutmeg)	Four-Herb Green Goddess Dressing, page 259, 2½ tablespoons Celery and carrot sticks, 1 cup	Baked Mozzarella Bites, page 284, 1 serving	SNACK
Baked tilapia, 4 ounces cooked Sicilian Pesto, page 276, 1 serving Simple Steamed Broccoli, page 150, 1 serving Brown rice, ½ cup	Arctic Char and Vegetables in Parchment Hearts, page 197, 1 serving Arugula salad, 2 cups Champagne Vinaigrette, page 223, 1 tablespoon *Cooking fish in packets results in flavorful, moist fish that doesn't rely on a lot of salt.*	Grilled flank steak, 4 ounces cooked Zingy Chimichurri, page 276, 1 serving Truffled Roasted Potatoes, page 285, 1 serving Roasted asparagus, 5 spears Vanilla frozen yogurt, 1 cup Blueberries, ½ cup	Grilled pork chop, 4 ounces cooked Tangy Coffee Barbecue Sauce, page 277, 1 serving Sautéed spinach, 1 cup Wild rice, ½ cup Baked apples (1 medium apple + 2 tablespoons raisins + ½ teaspoon ground cinnamon + 1 teaspoon maple syrup)	DINNER

YOUR GOALS

Find strategies to help you eat a little less.

....

Be mindful, purposeful, and joyful each time you eat.

	MONDAY	TUESDAY	WEDNESDAY
BREAKFAST	Pistachio-Chai Muffins, **page 67,** 1 serving Cheddar cheese, 1 ounce Latte (made with 1 cup fat-free milk)	Overnight Honey-Almond Multigrain Cereal, page 61, 1 serving Banana, 1 medium Fat-free milk, 1 cup	Simple Baked Eggs, **page 72,** 1 serving Whole-grain toast, 1 slice Butter, 1 teaspoon Cantaloupe chunks, 1 cup Fat-free milk, 1 cup
LUNCH	French Onion and Apple Soup, **page 300,** 1 serving Whole-grain baguette, 2-inch piece Butter, 1 teaspoon Pear, 1 medium *Take a break for 30 minutes of cardio.	Chicken Tabbouleh with Tahini Drizzle, **page 106,** 1 serving Mixed berries, 1 cup	Spinach Baked Potato, **page 323,** 1 serving Mixed berries, 1 cup Vanilla yogurt, 1 (6-ounce) carton
SNACK	Salted Caramel Brownies, **page 325,** 1 serving Fat-free milk, 1 cup *If you ban chocolate, your cravings will only intensify. Savor every bite.*	Whole-grain fig bars, 2 Fat-free milk, 1 cup	Unshelled pistachios, ½ cup String cheese, 1 ounce
DINNER	Creamy, Light Macaroni and Cheese, **page 319,** 1 serving Steamed Broccolini, 1 cup Mixed salad greens, 2 cups (with 2 tablespoons grated carrot + ¼ cup cherry tomatoes + 1 tablespoon balsamic vinaigrette) *Prep your overnight oats tonight so they'll be ready in the morning.	Cheesy Meat Loaf Minis, **page 40,** 1 serving Steamed green beans, 1 cup Mashed potatoes, ½ cup Apple slices, ½ cup	Baked Shrimp with Tomatoes, **page 297,** 1 serving Roasted asparagus, 1 cup *Add cardio and strength training to your to-do list today. *By using individual gratin dishes, you're creating built-in portion control.*

	THURSDAY	FRIDAY	SATURDAY	SUNDAY
BREAKFAST	Rise and Shine Oatmeal, **page 60,** 1 serving Banana, 1 medium Fat-free milk, 1 cup *Do not be tempted to skip breakfast to save calories; it will backfire.*	Fig, Applesauce, and Almond Breakfast Loaf, **page 69,** 1 serving Cream cheese, 1 tablespoon Strawberry jam, 1 teaspoon Fat-free milk, 1 cup	Breakfast BLT (2 slices whole-grain bread, toasted + 1 tomato slice + 1 green lettuce leaf + 2 center-cut bacon slices + 1 tablespoon canola mayonnaise) Grapefruit, ½ medium Fat-free milk, 1 cup	Banana-Chocolate French Toast, **page 65,** 1 serving Strawberries, 1 cup Fat-free milk, 1 cup *Go ahead and enjoy your chocolate—even for breakfast.*
LUNCH	Southwestern White Bean Pita Pockets, **page 303,** 1 serving Plum, 1 medium	Roasted Butternut Squash Soup, **page 157,** 1 serving Whole-grain baguette, 2-inch piece Butter, 1 teaspoon Clementines, 2 *Soup is a proven way to feel full faster and help you eat less.*	Chicken Fried Rice, **page 28,** 1 serving Orange, 1 medium *Cardio + strength training	Open-Faced Hummus Sandwiches, **page 131,** 1 serving Baby carrots and cucumber slices, 1 cup
SNACK	Rye crispbreads, 2 Soft herbed cheese, 1 ounce Green grapes, 1 cup	Greek-Style Tzatziki, **page 259,** 1 serving Baby carrots and cucumber slices, 1 cup	Air-popped popcorn, 3 cups (mixed with 1 tablespoon grated fresh Parmesan cheese)	Date and Almond Truffles, **page 305,** 1 serving
DINNER	Grilled chicken kebabs with **Ponzu, page 25,** 4 ounces cooked chicken, 2 tablespoons sauce Whole-wheat couscous, ½ cup Mixed salad greens, 2 cups (topped with ¼ avocado, sliced + 1 ounce crumbled feta cheese + ¼ cup cherry tomatoes + 1 tablespoon balsamic vinaigrette)	Burgers with Blue Cheese Mayo and Sherry Vidalia Onions, **page 316,** 1 serving Baked sweet potato fries, 1 medium potato Ketchup, 2 tablespoons Chocolate frozen yogurt, 1 cup *Mindful eating means finding a way to enjoy all foods, even a juicy, sumptuous burger.*	Roast Pork Tenderloin with Plum Barbecue Sauce, **page 321,** 1 serving **Roasted Pumpkin and Sweet Potato Pilaf, page 158,** 1 serving Sautéed green beans, 1 cup	Beef Tenderloin with Horseradish Chive Sauce, **page 320,** 1 serving **Microwave Smashed Potatoes, page 322,** 1 serving Steamed asparagus, 5 spears Mixed salad greens, 2 cups (with 1 ounce feta cheese + ¼ cup cherry tomatoes + 1 tablespoon **Champagne Vinaigrette, page 223**)

Nutritional Analysis

What the Numbers Mean For You

To interpret the nutritional analysis in *Cooking Light The Food Lover's Healthy Habits Cookbook,* use the figures below as a daily reference guide. One size doesn't fit all, so take lifestyle, age, and circumstances into consideration. For example, pregnant or breast-feeding women need more protein, calories, and calcium. Go to choosemyplate.gov for your own individualized plan.

IN OUR NUTRITIONAL ANALYSIS, WE USE THESE ABBREVIATIONS

sat	saturated fat	**CHOL**	cholesterol
mono	monounsaturated fat	**CALC**	calcium
poly	polyunsaturated fat	**g**	gram
CARB	carbohydrates	**mg**	milligram

Daily Nutrition Guide

	WOMEN ages 25 to 50	WOMEN over 50	MEN ages 25 to 50	MEN over 50
CALORIES	2,000	2,000*	2,700	2,500
PROTEIN	50g	50g	63g	60g
FAT	65g*	65g*	88g*	83g*
SATURATED FAT	20g*	20g*	27g*	25g*
CARBOHYDRATES	304g	304g	410g	375g
FIBER	25g to 35g	25g to 35g	25g to 35g	25g to 35g
CHOLESTEROL	300mg*	300mg*	300mg*	300mg*
IRON	18mg	8mg	8mg	8mg
SODIUM	2,300mg*	1,500mg*	2,300mg*	1,500mg*
CALCIUM	1,000mg	1,200mg	1,000mg	1,000mg

NUTRITIONAL VALUES USED IN OUR CALCULATIONS EITHER COME FROM THE FOOD PROCESSOR, VERSION 10.4 (ESHA RESEARCH) OR ARE PROVIDED BY FOOD MANUFACTURERS.

*Or less, for optimum health.

Metric Equivalents

The information in the following charts is provided to help cooks outside the United States successfully use the recipes in this book. All equivalents are approximate.

Cooking/Oven Temperatures

	Fahrenheit	Celsius	Gas Mark
Freeze Water	32° F	0° C	
Room Temp.	68° F	20° C	
Boil Water	212° F	100° C	
Bake	325° F	160° C	3
	350° F	180° C	4
	375° F	190° C	5
	400° F	200° C	6
	425° F	220° C	7
	450° F	230° C	8
Broil			Grill

Liquid Ingredients by Volume

¼ tsp	=					1 ml	
½ tsp	=					2 ml	
1 tsp	=					5 ml	
3 tsp	=	1 tbl	=	½ fl oz	=	15 ml	
2 tbls	=	⅛ cup	=	1 fl oz	=	30 ml	
4 tbls	=	¼ cup	=	2 fl oz	=	60 ml	
5⅓ tbls	=	⅓ cup	=	3 fl oz	=	80 ml	
8 tbls	=	½ cup	=	4 fl oz	=	120 ml	
10⅔ tbls	=	⅔ cup	=	5 fl oz	=	160 ml	
12 tbls	=	¾ cup	=	6 fl oz	=	180 ml	
16 tbls	=	1 cup	=	8 fl oz	=	240 ml	
1 pt	=	2 cups	=	16 fl oz	=	480 ml	
1 qt	=	4 cups	=	32 fl oz	=	960 ml	
				33 fl oz	=	1000 ml	= 1 l

Dry Ingredients by Weight

(To convert ounces to grams, multiply the number of ounces by 30.)

1 oz	=	¹⁄₁₆ lb	=	30g
4 oz	=	¼ lb	=	120g
8 oz	=	½ lb	=	240g
12 oz	=	¾ lb	=	360g
16 oz	=	1 lb	=	480g

Length

(To convert inches to centimeters, multiply the number of inches by 2.5.)

1 in	=				2.5 cm	
6 in	=	½ ft		=	15 cm	
12 in	=	1 ft		=	30 cm	
36 in	=	3 ft	=	1yd =	90 cm	
40 in	=				100 cm	= 1m

Equivalents for Different Types of Ingredients

Standard Cup	Fine Powder (ex. flour)	Grain (ex. rice)	Granular (ex. sugar)	Liquid Solids (ex. butter)	Liquid (ex. milk)
1	140g	150g	190g	200g	240 ml
¾	105g	113g	143g	150g	180 ml
⅔	93g	100g	125g	133g	160 ml
½	70g	75g	95g	100g	120 ml
⅓	47g	50g	63g	67g	80 ml
¼	35g	38g	48g	50g	60 ml
⅛	18g	19g	24g	25g	30 ml

References

Introduction

Buettner D. *The Blue Zones: Lessons for Living Longer From the People Who've Lived the Longest.* Washington, DC: National Geographic Society, 2008. www.bluezones.com

Covey SR. *The 7 Habits of Highly Effective People: Powerful Lessons in Personal Change.* New York: Free Press, 2004.

Housman J, Dorman S. The Alameda County study: A systematic, chronological review. *American Journal of Health Education.* 2005; 36: 302-308.

Knäuper B, McCollam A, Rosen-Brown A, Lacaille J, Kelso E, Roseman M. Fruitful plans: Adding targeted mental imagery to implementation intentions increases fruit consumption. *Psychology and Health.* 2011; 26: 601-617.

Lally P, van Jaarsveld CHM, Potts HWW, Wardle J. How are habits formed: Modelling habit formation in the real world. *European Journal of Social Psychology.* 2010; 40: 998-1009.

Lally P, Chipperfield A, Wardle J. Healthy habits: Efficacy of simple advice on weight control based on a habit-formation model. *International Journal of Obesity.* 2008; 32: 700-707.

Nelson M, Ackerman J. *The Social Network Diet: Change Yourself, Change the World.* Campbell, CA: FastPencil Premiere, 2011.

Pachucki MA, Jacques PF, Christakis NA. Social network concordance in food choice among spouses, friends, and siblings. *American Journal of Public Health.* 2011; 101: 2170-2177.

U.S. Department of Agriculture and U.S. Department of Health and Human Services. *Dietary Guidelines for Americans 2010.* 7th edition. Washington, DC: U.S. Government Printing Office, December 2010. www.cnpp.usda.gov/dietaryguidelines.htm

U.S. Department of Agriculture. MyPlate. www.ChooseMyPlate.gov

U.S. Department of Health and Human Services. National Heart, Lung and Blood Institute. Guide to Behavior Change. www.nhlbi.nih.gov

Get Cooking

Chen RCY, Lee MS, Chang YH, Wahlqvist ML. Cooking frequency may enhance survival in Taiwanese elderly. *Public Health Nutrition.* 2012; 15: 1142-1149.

Cutler DM, Glaeser EL, Shapiro JM. Why have Americans become more obese? *Journal of Economic Perspective.* 2003; 17: 93-118.

Lichtenstein AH, Ludwig DS. Bring back home economics education. *Journal of the American Medical Association.* 2010; 303: 1857-1858.

Poti JM, Popkin BM. Trends in energy intake among US children by eating location and food source, 1977-2006. *Journal of the American Dietetic Association.* 2011; 111: 1156-1164.

Todd JE, Mancino L, Lin BH. The impact of food away from home on adult diet quality. *Advances in Nutrition.* 2011; 2: 442-443.

Breakfast Daily

Barton BA, Eldridge AL, Thompson D, Affenito SG, Striegel-Moore RH, Franko DL, Albertson AM, Crockett SJ. The relationship of breakfast and cereal consumption to nutrient intake and body mass index: The National Heart, Lung, and Blood Institute Growth and Health Study. *Journal of the American Dietetic Association.* 2005; 105: 1383-1389.

Berkey CS, Rockett HR, Gillman MW, Field AE, Colditz GA: Longitudinal study of skipping breakfast and weight change in adolescents. *International Journal of Obesity and Related Metabolic Disorders.* 2003; 27: 1258-1266.

Blom WA, Lluch A, Stafleu A, Vinoy S, Holst JJ, Schaafsma G, Hendriks HF. Effect of a high-protein breakfast on the postprandial ghrelin response. *American Journal of Clinical Nutrition.* 2006; 83: 211-220.

Cho S, Dietrich M, Brown CJ, Clark CA, Block G. The effect of breakfast type on total daily energy intake and body mass index: Results from the Third National Health and Nutrition Examination Survey (NHANES III). *Journal of the American College of Nutrition.* 2003; 22: 296-302.

Deshmukh-Taskar PR, Nicklas TA, O'Neil CE, Keast DR, Dadcliffe JD, Cho S. The relationship of breakfast skipping and type of breakfast consumption with nutrient intake and weight status in children and adolescents: The National Health and Nutrition Examination Survey 1999-2006. *Journal of the American Dietetic Association.* 2010; 110: 869-878.

Huang CJ, Hu HT, Fan YC, Liao YM, Tsai PS. Associations of breakfast skipping with obesity and health-related quality of life: Evidence from a national survey in Taiwan. *International Journal of Obesity.* 2010; 34: 720-725.

Jakubowicz D, Froy O, Wainstein J, Boaz M. Meal timing and composition influence ghrelin levels, appetite scores and weight loss maintenance in overweight and obese adults. *Steroids,* 2012; 77: 323-331.

Ma Y, Bertone ER, Stanek EJ, Reed GW, Hebert JR, Cohen NL, Merriam PA, Ockene IS. Association between eating patterns and obesity in a free-living US adult population. *American Journal of Epidemiology.* 2003; 158: 85-92.

National Weight Control Registry. http://www.nwcr.ws

Rampersaud GC, Pereira MA, Girard BL, Adams J, Metzl JD. Breakfast habits, nutritional status, body weight, and academic performance in children and adolescents. *Journal of the American Dietetic Association.* 2005; 105: 743-760.

Ratliff J, Leite JO, de Ogburn R, Puglisi MJ, VanHeest J, Fernandez ML. Consuming eggs for breakfast influences plasma glucose and ghrelin, while reducing energy intake during the next 24 hours in adult men. *Nutrition Research.* 2010; 30: 96-103.

Smith KJ, Gall SL, McNaughton SA, Blizzard L, Dwyer T, Venn AJ. Skipping breakfast: Longitudinal associations with cardiometabolic risk factors in the Childhood Determinants of Adult Health Study. *American Journal of Clinical Nutrition.* 2010; 92: 1316-1325.

Song WO, Chun OK, Obayashi S, Cho S, Chung CE. Is consumption of breakfast associated with body mass index in US adults? *Journal of the American Dietetic Association.* 2005; 105: 1373-1382.

Vander Wal JS, Gupta A, Khosla P, Dhurandhar NV. Egg breakfast enhances weight loss. *International Journal of Obesity.* 2008; 32: 1545-1551.

Wyatt HR. Long-term weight loss and breakfast in subjects of the National Weight Control Registry. *Obesity Research.* 2002; 10: 78-82.

Go For Whole Grains

Aune D, Chan DS, Lau R, Vieira R, Greenwood DC, Kampman E, Norat T. Dietary fibre, whole grains, and risk of colorectal cancer: Systematic review and dose-response meta-analysis of prospective studies. *British Medical Journal.* 2011; 343: d6617.

Cleveland LE, Moshfegh AJ, Albertson AM, Goldman JD. Dietary intake of whole grains. *Journal of the American College of Nutrition.* 2000; 19: 331S-338S.

de Munter JS, Hu FB, Spiegelman D, Franz M, van Dam RM. Whole grain, bran, and germ intake and risk of type 2 diabetes: A prospective cohort study and systematic review. *PLoS Medicine.* 2007; 4: e261.

Giacco R, Della Pepa G, Luongo D, Riccardi G. Whole grain intake in relation to body weight: From epidemiological evidence to clinical trials. *Nutrition, Metabolism and Cardiovascular Diseases.* 2011; 21: 901-908.

Jonnalagadda SS, Harnack L, Liu RH, McKeown N, Seal C, Liu S, Fahey GC. Putting the whole grain puzzle together: Health benefits associated with whole grains. *Journal of Nutrition.* 2011; 141: 1011S-1022S.

Mancino L, Kuchler F, Leibtag E. Getting consumers to eat more whole-grains: The role of policy, information, and food manufacturers. *Food Policy.* 2008; 33: 489-496.

Mellen PB, Walsh TF, Herrington DM. Whole grain intake and cardiovascular disease: A meta-analysis. *Nutrition, Metabolism and Cardiovascular Diseases.* 2008; 18: 283-290.

O'Neil CE, Nicklas TA, Zanovec M, Cho S. Whole-grain consumption is associated with diet quality and nutrient intake in adults: The National Health and Nutrition Examination Survey, 1999-2004. *Journal of the American Dietetic Association.* 2010; 110: 1461-1468.

Whole Grains Council. www.wholegrainscouncil.org

Get Moving

Beers EA, Roemmich JN, Epstein LH, Horvath PJ. Increasing passive energy expenditure during clerical work. *European Journal of Applied Physiology.* 2008; 103: 353-360.

Belloc N, Breslow L. Relationship of physical health status and health practices. *Preventive Medicine.* 1972; 1: 409-421.

Black CD, Herring MP, Hurley DJ, O'Connor PJ. Ginger (zingiber officinale) reduces muscle pain caused by eccentric exercise. *Journal of Pain.* 2010; 11: 894-903.

Bravata DM, Smith-Spangler C, Sundaram V, Gienger A, Lin ND, Lewis R, Stave CD, Olkin I, Sirard JR. Using pedometers to increase physical activity and improve health: A systematic review. *Journal of the American Medical Association.* 2007; 298: 2296-2304.

Breslow L, Enstrom J. Persistence of health habits and their relationship to mortality. *Preventive Medicine.* 1980; 9: 469-483.

Eichenberger E, Colombani PC, Mettler S. Effects of 3-week consumption of green tea extracts on whole-body metabolism during cycling exercise in endurance-trained men. *International Journal for Vitamin and Nutrition Research.* 2009; 79: 24-33.

Fu J. Effect on antioxidative capacity of California almond supplementation in elite Chinese cycling. *Medicine & Science in Sports & Exercise.* 2009; 41: 2.

Holthusen J, Porcari J, Foster C, Doberstein S, Anders M. Effective hooping: Workout or child's play? American Council on Exercise. www.acefitness.org

Hulmi JJ, Lockwood CM, Stout JR. Effect of protein/essential amino acids and resistance training on skeletal muscle hypertrophy: A case for whey protein. *Nutrition & Metabolism.* 2010; 7: 51.

Kammer L, Ding Z, Wang B, Hara D, Liao YH, Ivy JL. Cereal and nonfat milk support muscle recovery following exercise. *Journal of the International Society of Sports Nutrition.* 2009; 6: 11.

Karfonta KE, Lunn WR, Colletto MR, Anderson JH, Rodriguez NR. Chocolate milk enhances glycogen replenishment after endurance exercise in moderately trained males. *Medicine and Science in Sports and Exercise.* 2006; 42: S64.

Karp JH, Johnston JD, Tecklenburg S, Mickleborough TD, Fly AD, Stager JM. Chocolate milk as a post-exercise recovery aid. *International Journal of Sport Nutrition and Exercise Metabolism.* 2006; 16: 78-91.

Kuehl KS, Perrier ET, Elliot DL, Chesnutt JC. Efficacy of tart cherry juice in reducing muscle pain during running: A randomized controlled trial. *Journal of the International Society of Sports Nutrition.* 2010; 7: 17.

Patel AV, Bernstein L, Deka A, Feigelson HS, Campbell PT, Gapstur SM, Colditz GA, Thun MJ. Leisure time spent sitting in relation to total mortality in a prospective cohort of US adults. *American Journal of Epidemiology.* 2010; 172: 419-429.

Saat M, Singh R, Sirisinghe RG, Nawawi M. Rehydration after exercise with fresh young coconut water, carbohydrate-electrolyte beverage and plain water. *Journal of Physiological Anthropology and Applied Human Science.* 2002; 21: 93-104.

U.S. Department of Health and Human Services. *2008 Physical Activity Guidelines for Americans.* www.health.gov/PAGuidelines

Zahour K, Porcari J. Casual and comfortable clothing workdays promote increased physical activity. American Council on Exercise. www.acefitness.org

Veggie Up

Environmental Working Group 2012 Shopper's Guide to Pesticides in Produce. http://www.ewg.org/foodnews/summary/

He FJ, Nowson CA, Lucas M, MacGregor GA. Increased consumption of fruit and vegetables is related to reduced risk of coronary heart disease: Meta-analysis of cohort studies. *Journal of Human Hypertension.* 2007; 21: 717-728.

He FJ, Nowson CA, MacGregor GA. Fruit and vegetable consumption and stroke: Meta-analysis of cohort studies. *Lancet.* 2006; 367: 320-326.

Hyson DA. *Fruits, Vegetables, and Health: A Scientific Overview, 2011.* Produce for Better Health Foundation, 2011. www.pbhfoundation.org

Key T. Fruit and vegetables and cancer risk. *British Journal of Cancer.* 2011; 104: 6-11.

State of the Plate: 2010 Study on America's Consumption of Fruits and Vegetables, 2010. Produce for Better Health Foundation. www.pbhfoundation.org

U.S. Department of Agriculture. MyPlate. www.ChooseMyPlate.gov

Zeinstra GG, Koelen MA, Kok FJ, de Graaf C. The influence of preparation method on children's liking for vegetables. *Food Quality and Preference.* 2010; 21: 906-914.

Eat More Fish

American Heart Association. Fish 101. www.heart.org

Belin RJ, Greenland P, Martin L, Oberman A, Tinker L, Robinson J, Larson J, Van Horn L, Lloyd-Jones D. Fish intake and the risk of incident heart failure: The Women's Health Initiative. *Circulation.* 2011; 110. 960450.

Blue Ocean Institute. www.blueocean.org

Danaei G, Ding EL, Mozaffarian D, Taylor B, Rehm J, Murray CJ, Ezzati M. The preventable causes of death in the United States: Comparative risk assessment of dietary, lifestyle, and metabolic risk factors. *PLoS Medicine.* 2009; 6: e1000058.

De-coding Seafood Eco-labels: Why We Need Public Standards. Washington, DC: Food & Water Watch, 2010. www.foodandwaterwatch.org

Friend of the Sea. www.friendofthesea.org

Institute of Medicine, Food and Nutrition Board. *Dietary Reference Intakes: Energy, Carbohydrates, Fiber, Fat, Fatty Acids, Cholesterol, Protein, and Amino Acids.* Washington, DC: National Academies Press, 2002.

Kris-Etherton PM, Harris WS, Appel LJ. AHA Scientific Statement: Fish consumption, fish oil, omega-3 fatty acids, and cardiovascular disease. *Circulation.* 2002; 106: 2747-2757.

Marine Stewardship Council. www.msc.org

Monterey Bay Aquarium Seafood Watch. www.seafoodwatch.org

Mozaffarian D, Rimm EB. Fish intake, contaminants, and human health: Evaluating the risks and the benefits. *Journal of the American Medical Association.* 2006; 296: 1885-1899.

Nahab F, Le A, Judd S, Frankel MR, Ard J, Newby PK, Howard VJ. Racial and geographic differences in fish consumption. The Regards Study. *Neurology.* 2011; 76: 154-158.

National Marine Fisheries Service, National Oceanic and Atmospheric Administration. Fish Watch. www.nmfs.noaa.gov/fishwatch

Dietary Guidelines for Americans, 2010. www.dietaryguidelines.gov

Eat More Healthy Fats

American Heart Association. Know Your Fats. www.heart.org

Akbaraly TN, Ferrie JE, Berr C, Brunner EJ, Head J, Marmot MG, Singh-Manoux A, Ritchie K, Shipley MJ, Kivimaki M. Alternative Healthy Eating Index and mortality over 18 y of follow-up: Results from the Whitehall II cohort. *American Journal of Clinical Nutrition.* 2011; 94: 247-253.

Banel DK, Hu FB. Effects of walnut consumption on blood lipids and other cardiovascular risk factors: A meta-analysis and systematic review. *American Journal of Clinical Nutrition.* 2009; 90: 1-8.

Brown MJ, Ferruzzi MG, Nguyen ML, Cooper DA, Eldridge AL, Schwartz SJ, White WS. Carotenoid bioavailability is higher from salads ingested with full-fat than with fat-reduced salad dressings as measured with electrochemical detection. *American Journal of Clinical Nutrition.* 2004; 80: 396-403.

Gillingham LG, Harris-Janz S, Jones PJ. Dietary monounsaturated fatty acids are protective against metabolic syndrome and cardiovascular disease risk factors. *Lipids.* 2011; 46: 209-228.

Hu FB, Manson JE, Willett WC. Types of dietary fat and risk of coronary heart disease: A critical review. *Journal of the American College of Nutrition.* 2001; 20: 5-19.

Institute of Medicine, Food and Nutrition Board. *Dietary Reference Intakes: Energy, Carbohydrates, Fiber, Fat, Fatty Acids, Cholesterol, Protein, and Amino Acids.* Washington, DC: National Academies Press, 2002.

Kris-Etherton PM, Hu FB, Ros E, Sabaté J. The role of tree nuts and peanuts in the prevention of coronary heart disease: Multiple potential mechanisms. *Journal of Nutrition.* 2008; 138: 1746S-1751S.

Sabate J. Ang Y. Nuts and health outcomes: New epidemiologic evidence. *American Journal of Clinical Nutrition.* 2009; 89: 1643S-1648S.

Unlu NZ, Bohn T, Clinton SK, Schwartz SJ. Carotenoid absorption from salad and salsa by humans is enhanced by the addition of avocado or avocado oil. *Journal of Nutrition.* 2005; 135: 431-436.

U.S. Department of Agriculture, U.S. Department of Health and Human Services. Report of the Dietary Guidelines Advisory Committee on the Dietary Guidelines for Americans, 2010. www.dietaryguidelines.gov

Go Meatless

Bernstein AM, Sun Q, Hu FB, Stampfer MJ, Manson JE, Willet WC. Major dietary protein sources and risk of coronary heart disease in women. *Circulation.* 2010; 122: 876-883.

Blatner DJ. *The Flexitarian Diet.* New York: McGraw Hill, 2009.

Craig WJ, Mangels AR, American Dietetic Association. Position of the American Dietetic Association: Vegetarian diets. *Journal of the American Dietetic Association.* 2009; 109: 1266-1282.

Farmer B, Larson BT, Fulgoni VL, Rainville AJ, Liepa GU. A vegetarian dietary pattern as a nutrient-dense approach to weight management: An analysis of the National Health and Nutrition Examination Survey 1999-2004. *Journal of the American Dietetic Association.* 2011; 111: 819-827.

Lea EJ, Crawford D, Worsley A. Public views of the benefits and barriers to the consumption of a plant-based diet. *European Journal of Nutrition.* 2006; 60: 828-837.

Meatless Monday. www.meatlessmonday.com

Sabaté J. The contribution of vegetarian diets to health and disease. A paradigm shift? *American Journal of Clinical Nutrition.* 2003; 78: 502S-507S.

Schösler H, Boer JD, Boersema JJ. Can we cut out the meat of the dish? Constructing consumer-oriented pathways towards meat substitution. *Appetite.* 2011; 58: 39-47.

U.S. Department of Agriculture. MyPlate. www.ChooseMyPlate.gov

Get Stronger

American College of Sports Medicine, American Dietetic Association, Dietitians of Canada. Joint position statement: Nutrition and athletic performance. *Medicine and Science in Sports and Exercise.* 2009; 41: 709-731. www.acsm.org

Ciccolo JT, Dunsiger SI, Williams DM, Bartholomew JB, Jennings EG, Ussher MH, Kraemer WJ, Marcus BH. Resistance training as an aid to standard smoking cessation treatment: A pilot study. *Nicotine and Tobacco Research.* 2011; 13: 756-760.

Glass SC. Effect of a learning trial on self-selected resistance training load. *Journal of Strength and Conditioning.* 2008; 22-1025-1029.

Glass SC, Stanton DR. Self-selected resistance training intensity in novice weightlifters. *Journal of Strength and Conditioning.* 2004; 18: 324-7.

Institute of Medicine, Food and Nutrition Board. *Dietary Reference Intakes: Energy, Carbohydrates, Fiber, Fat, Fatty Acids, Cholesterol, Protein, and Amino Acids.* Washington, DC: National Academies Press, 2002.

Nelson M. *Strong Women Stay Young.* New York: Bantam Books, 2000. www.strongwomen.com

Nielsen survey. Research proves power of group fitness. www.lesmills.com

Porcari J, Hendrickson K, Foster C, Anders M. Drop and give me 20! American Council on Exercise. www.acefitness.org

Schnettler C, Porcari J, Foster C, Anders M. Kettlebells: Twice the results in half the time? American Council on Exercise. www.acefitness.org

U.S. Department of Health and Human Services. *2008 Physical Activity Guidelines for Americans.* www.health.gov/PAGuidelines

Eat Less Salt

Appel LJ, Brands MW, Daniels SR, Karanja N, Elmer PJ, Sacks FM. Dietary approaches to prevent and treat hypertension: A scientific statement from the American Heart Association. *Hypertension.* 2006; 47: 296-308.

Appel LJ, Frohlich ED, Hall JE, Pearson TA, Sacco RL, Seals DR, Sacks FM, Smith SC, Vafiadis DK, Van Horn L. The importance of population-wide sodium reduction as a means to prevent cardiovascular disease and stroke: A call to action from the American Heart Association. *Circulation.* 2011; 123: 1138-1143.

Appel LJ, Moore TJ, Obarzanek E, Vollmer WM, Svetkey LP, Sacks FM, Bray GA, Vogt TM, Cutler JA, Windhauser MM, Lin PH, Karanja N, Simons-Morton D, McCullough M, Swain J, Steele P, Evans MA, Miller ER, Harsha DW for the DASH Collaborative Research Group. A clinical trial of the effects of dietary patterns on blood pressure. *New England Journal of Medicine.* 1997; 336: 1117-1124.

Centers for Disease Control and Prevention, Morbidity and Mortality Weekly Report. Sodium Intake Among Adults—United States, 2005–2006. *Journal of the American Medical Association.* 2010; 304: 738-740.

Duyff RL, Mount JR, Jones JB. Sodium reduction in canned beans after draining, rinsing. *Journal of Culinary Science and Technology.* 2011; 9: 106-112.

Graudal NA, Hubeck-Graudal T, Jurgens G. Effects of a low-sodium diet vs. high-sodium diet on blood pressure, renin, aldosterone, catecholamines, cholesterol, and triglyceride (Cochrane review). *American Journal of Hypertension.* 2012; 25: 1-15.

He FJ, MacGregor GA. Salt reduction lowers cardiovascular risk: Meta-analysis of outcome trials. *Lancet.* 2011; 378: 380-382.

Institute of Medicine, Food and Nutrition Board. *Strategies to Reduce Sodium Intake in the United States.* Washington, DC: National Academies Press, 2010.

Institute of Medicine, Food and Nutrition Board. *Dietary Reference Intakes: Water, Potassium, Sodium, Chloride, and Sulfate.* Washington, DC: National Academies Press, 2004.

Stolarz-Skrzypek K, Kuznetsova T, Thijs L, Tikhonoff V, Seidlerova J, Richart T, Jin Y, Olszanecka A, Malyutina S, Casiglia E, Filipovsky J, Kawecka-Jaszcz K, Nikitin Y, Staessen JA. Fatal and nonfatal outcomes, incidence of hypertension, and blood pressure changes in relation to urinary sodium excretion. *Journal of the American Medical Association.* 2011; 305: 1777-1785.

Yang Q, Liu T, Kuklina EV, Flanders WD, Hong Y, Gillespie C, Chang MH, Gwinn M, Dowling N, Khoury MJ, Hu FB. Sodium and potassium intake and mortality among US adults: Prospective data from the Third National Health and Nutrition Examination Survey. *Archives of Internal Medicine.* 2011; 171: 1183-1191.

Be Portion-Aware

Duffey KJ, Popkin BM. Energy density, portion size, and eating occasions: Contributions to increased energy intake in the United States, 1977-2006. *PLoS Medicine.* 2011; 8: e1001050.

Ello-Martin JA, Ledikwe JH, Rolls BJ. The influence of food portion size and energy density on energy intake: Implications for weight management. *American Journal of Clinical Nutrition.* 2005; 82: 236S-241S.

Flood JE, Rolls BJ. Soup preloads in a variety of forms reduce meal energy intake. *Appetite.* 2007; 49: 626-634.

Hill JO, Peters JC, Wyatt HR. Using the energy gap to address obesity: A commentary. *Journal of the American Dietetic Association.* 2009; 109: 1848-1853.

Honselman CS, Painter JE, Kennedy-Hagan KJ, Halvorson A, Rhodes K, Brooks TL, Skwir K. In-shell pistachio nuts reduce caloric intake compared to shelled nuts. *Appetite.* 2011; 57: 414-417.

Rolls B, Hermann M. *The Ultimate Volumetrics Diet.* New York: HarperCollins, 2012.

Wansink B. *Mindless Eating: Why We Eat More Than We Think.* New York: Bantam Books, 2006.

Wansink B. From mindless eating to mindlessly eating better. *Physiology and Behavior.* 2010; 100: 454-463.

Wansink B, van Ittersum K. Portion size me: Downsizing our consumption norms. *Journal of the American Dietetic Association.* 2007; 107: 1103-1106.

Wansink B. Environmental factors that increase the food intake and consumption volume of unknowing consumers. *Annual Review of Nutrition.* 2004; 24: 455-479.

Young LR. *The Portion Teller Plan.* New York: Morgan Road Books, 2005.

Eat Mindfully

Am I Hungry? www.amihungry.com

Bacon L. *Health at Every Size: The Surprising Truth About Your Weight.* Dallas: Benbella Books, 2008.

Beck M. *The Four-Day Win: End Your Diet War and Achieve Thinner Peace.* New York: Rodale, 2007.

Blass EM, Anderson DR, Kirkorian HL, Pempek TA, Price I, Koleni MF. On the road to obesity: Television viewing increases intake of high-density foods. *Physiology and Behavior.* 2006; 88: 597-604.

Center for Mindful Eating. www.tcme.org

Hanh TN, Cheung L. *Savor: Mindful Eating, Mindful Life.* New York: HarperOne, 2010.

Li J, Zhang N, Hu L, Li Z, Li R, Li C, Wang S. Improvement in chewing activity reduces energy intake in one meal and modulates plasma gut hormone concentrations in obese and lean young Chinese men. *American Journal of Clinical Nutrition.* 2011; 94: 709-716.

May M. *Eat What You Love, Love What You Eat: How to Break Your Eat-Repent-Repeat Cycle.* Austin: Greenleaf Book Group Press, 2010.

Oldham-Cooper RE, Hardman CA, Nicoll CE, Rogers PJ, Brunstrom JM. Playing a computer game during lunch affects fullness, memory for lunch, and later snack intake. *American Journal of Clinical Nutrition.* 2011; 93: 308-313.

Scisco JL, Muth ER, Dong Y, Hoover AW. Slowing bite-rate reduces energy intake: An application of the bite counter. *Journal of the American Dietetic Association.* 2011; 111: 1231-1235.

Tribole E, Resch E. *Intuitive Eating: A Revolutionary Program That Works.* New York: St. Martin's Press, 2012.

Subject Index

Beans, 16, 260
  Best-in-Nutrient-Class Beans, 160
Blogger Tips
  Consider a Buying Club, 99
  Let Go of "All or Nothing," 119
  Make a Grain Salad, 107
  Step Outside Your Comfort Zone, 109
  Whole-Grain Meal Ideas, 98
breakfast, 19, 50-75, 134
  Avoid the Over-Pour, 59
  dinner for breakfast, 53, 56, 59
  Fast Food Breakfast Options, 55
  Follow the Balanced Breakfast Rules, 52
  skipping, 51, 56, 58, 59

Cereal, 58, 60, 78
  Avoid the Over-Pour, 59
Coaching Session
  with Allison Fishman
    Don't Fear Fats, 221
    Gain Fish-Cooking Confidence, 172
    Less Salt Doesn't Mean Less Flavor, 271
    Sharpen Your Knife Skills, 137
  with Ann Pittman
    Simple Dinner Solutions: "What I Made This Week," 26
  with Janet Helm, MS, RD
    Combating the Mindless Margin, 295
    Loving Food Is a Good Thing, 313
    "Yes, You Can Do It!," 118
  with Myatt Murphy, CSCS
    Cardio Blast Workout, 120
    Fitness Made Faster, 256

Eggs, 17, 57, 59, 72, 233
  Decoding Egg Cartons, 74
  How to Make a Great Omelet, 73
  Perfecting the Hard-Cooked Egg, 75
  White vs. Brown Eggs, 74
exercise, 111-123. *See also* strength training.
  Blogger Tip: Let Go of "All or Nothing," 119
  Cardio Blast Workout, 120-121
  equipment, 112, 114-115, 119
  Expert Tips
    Adopt Healthy Hobbies, 121
    Give Exercise Meaning, 129
    Powering Through a Tough Workout, 115
    Reclaim Yourself, 262
    Schedule Shorter Sessions, 250
    Stay Hydrated, 113
  when traveling, 263
Expert Tips
  Add a Vinaigrette to Your Veggies, 151
  Adopt Healthy Hobbies, 121
  Appearance Is Important, 189
  Avoiding "Oops" in the Kitchen, 22
  Be a Veggie Role Model, 140
  Build in a Stopping Place, 293
  Consider the Catch of the Day, 195

  Create a Midpoint in Your Meal, 289
  Eat with Pleasure, 301
  Fats Have Staying Power, 213
  Forget "Forbidden," 325
  Forgo Faux, 233
  Get Started Early, 78
  Get to Know the Nuances of Olive Oil, 205
  Get to the Root of Your Habit, 323
  Give Exercise Meaning, 129
  Go Slow Once a Week, 43
  Incorporate the Unfamiliar, 135
  Learn the Art of Stopping, 327
  Make a Grain Salad, 86
  One Isn't Always One, 294
  Open with Salad, 145
  Outside Your Comfort Zone, 109
  Perfect Meatless Pasta Formula, A, 243
  Powering Through a Tough Workout, 115
  Preventing Whole-Grain Boredom, 97
  Put Kids in Charge, 41
  Put Some Soup On, 159
  Read the Fine Print, 85
  Reclaim Yourself, 262
  Rethink Your Cereal Bowl, 93
  Schedule Shorter Sessions, 250
  Set a Baking Goal, 69
  Stay Hydrated, 113
  Women Need to Build Muscle, 254
  You Are in Charge, 321

Fats, 202-223
  Don't Fear Fats, 221
  Expert Tips
    Fats Have Staying Power, 213
    Get to Know the Nuances of Olive Oil, 205
  Oops! The Biggest Fat Mistakes, 214
  Reader Tips
    Make Your Own Nut Butter, 207
    Switch Up Stir-Fries, 214
  Seek Out Seeds, 217
  Smart Swaps, 205
  What's a Serving?, 206
fish, 168-201. *See also* Omega-3s; Sustainable Seafood.
  buying, Handle with Care, 174
  Expert Tips
    Appearance Is Important, 189
    Consider the Catch of the Day, 195
  Fishing for Flavors, flavor pairings for salmon, 187
  Gain Fish-Cooking Confidence, 172
  How to Cook Fish in a Packet, 197
  Menu Navigator, 173
  The Super Green List, 180
  What About Mercury?, 177
Follow Up: Make Healthy Options Convenient, 58
food labels, 77, 82, 83, 85, 175, 201, 206, 207, 215, 273, 287
  for sustainable seafood, 178
  Read the Label (sodium amounts), 269
  The Fuzzy Math of Food Labels, 289

fruits, 58, 133, 135, 166, 270
  Expert Tip: Incorporate the Unfamiliar, 135
  Reader Tip: Try Freeze-Dried Fruit, 167

How to
  Buy Organic, 143
  Cook Fish in a Packet, 197
  Cook Pasta, 127
  Easily Slice Beef into Strips, 45
  Make a Great Omelet, 73
  Mix a Basic Vinaigrette, 222
  Pan-Fry Chicken 39
  Prep Pumpkin, 158
  Roast a Whole Chicken, 36

Ingredients
  Asian staples, 28
  10 all-star for meatless meals, 232
  20 all-star essential, 16-17

Meatless, 224-247
  Expert Tips
    Forgo Faux, 233
    A Perfect Meatless Pasta Formula, 243
    A New View of Protein, 229
    A Quick Tofu Tutorial, 247
    Blogger Tip: Step Outside Your Comfort Zone, 245
    Utilize 10 All-Star Ingredients for Meatless Meals, 232
mindful eating, 308-327
  Expert Tips
    Forget "Forbidden," 325
    Get to the Root of Your Habit, 323
    Learn the Art of Stopping, 327
    You Are in Charge, 321
  five rules for, 310
  Forget the Word "Diet," 310
  Loving Food Is a Good Thing, 313
muffins, 19, 53
  Five Tips for Perfect Muffins, 67

Nut butter, 269
  Explore a New Nut Butter, 265
  Reader Tip: Make Your Own Nut Butter, 207
nuts, 54, 212, 264
  An A-Z Guide, 210-211

Oats, Know Your Oat Options, 60
omega-3s, 169, 180
  Know Your Omega-3s, 176-177
organic, 16
  How to Buy Organic, 143

Pizza, delivery, 31
popcorn, 79, 209
portion-aware, 286-307
  Build Your Own Portable 100-Calorie Snacks, 303
  Do You Overpour Alcohol?, 299
  Expert Tips
    Build in a Stopping Place, 293

portion-aware *(continued)*
    Create a Midpoint in Your Meal, 289
    Eat with Pleasure, 301
    One Isn't Always One, 294
    The Fuzzy Math of Food Labels, 289
    "portion size" and "serving size," 287
    visual cues, 290
potassium, The Power of Potassium, 270
profiles
    Busy Mom, The, 138
    Busy Young Mom, The, 87
    Classic Yo-Yo Dieter, The, 311
    Clean-Plate Champion, The, 294
    Country Midwife, The, 251
    Disinterested Exerciser, The, 123
    Embattled Dad, The, 140
    Empty-Stomach Warrior, The, 53
    Fish-on-a-Budget Challenge, The, 175
    Healthy Habits Graduate, 93
    Healthy Habits Success Story, 21
    Injured Athlete, The, 113
    Lapsed Solo Cook, The, 19
    No-Time-Whatsoever Working Mom, The, 253
    No Way, No How, No Fish!, 171
    Raised-on-Butter Cook, The, 208
    Really, No Meat?, 227
    Restaurant-Goer, The, 139
    Saving-My-Calories-for-Later Mom, The, 58
    Show Me the Flavor, 273
    Show Me the Menu, 233
    Snack-Happy Family, The, 209
    Sodium-Clueless Mom, The, 275
    Time-Pressed Professional, The, 117
    Whole-Grain Newbie, The, 81
    Whole-Grain Seeker on a Budget, The, 83
    Woman Who Fears Fat, The, 215
    "You call that a portion?," 293
protein, 52, 77, 82, 128, 135, 147, 225, 260
    A New View of Protein, 229
    A Primer, 258

Reader Tips
    Change Your Method, 95
    Consider Canned, 165
    Count on Leftovers, 37
    Keep Healthy Snacks on Hand, 54
    Make Breakfast Ahead, 61
    Make Your Own Nut Butter, 207
    Perfect Your Knife Skills, 149
    Prepping Veggies, 156
    Switch-It-Up Solution, The, 257
    Switch Up Stir-Fries, 214
    Try Freeze-Dried Fruit, 167

Salads
    before the entrée, 292
    How to Mix a Basic Vinaigrette, 222
    Make It a Meal, 147
    100-calorie toppers for, 146-147
salt, 266-285. *See also* sodium.
    Drain and Rinse Canned Foods, 281
    How to Read Salt Labels, 272
    Less Salt Doesn't Mean Less Flavor, 271
    Marinara Basics, 278

Read the Label, 269
Salty Add-Ons, 268
Salty Snack Smackdown, 283
A Spud Spectrum, 285
sandwiches, Go Beyond Sliced Bread, 49
seafood. *See* fish; Sustainable Seafood.
seeds, Seek Out Seeds, 217
shrimp, The Scoop on Shrimp, 193
snacks, 209, 229
    Build Your Own Portable 100-Calorie Snacks, 303
    dividing into individual containers, 288
    Salty Snack Smackdown, 283
Social media
    Are you going meatless one day a week?, 241
    Expert Chatter: Advice to Inspire More Cooking at
      Home, 47
    Expert Chatter on Meatless Meals, 235
    Expert Chatter on Mindful Eating, What does eating
      mindfully mean to you?, 311
    Expert Chatter: Talking Fish, 199
    How are you incorporating more fish?, 191
    How are you overcoming your exercise habit
      hurdles?, 117
    How do you fit in two days of strength training?, 261
    How do you stay motivated to do strength training?, 255
    What are your a.m. solutions?, 59
    What are your tips for eating more vegetables and
      fruits?, 164
    What are your tricks for keeping your portions in
      check?, 297
    What are your tricks for staying active?, 131
    What tricks have you found for cutting back on
      salt?, 269
sodium, 15, 29, 170. *See also* salt.
    foods naturally low in, 270
    kids' intake of, 274
strength training, 248-257. *See also* exercise.
    equipment, 250, 251, 252, 254
    Expert Tips
      Reclaim Yourself, 262
      Schedule Shorter Sessions, 250
      Women Need to Build Muscle, 254
    Oops! five biggest mistakes, 252
    Reader Tip: The Switch-It-Up Solution, 257
    20-minute routine, 256-257
Sustainable Seafood, 178-179
    Three Reasons You Should Go Sustainable, interview
      with Barton Seaver, 179

Tofu, 228, 246
    A Quick Tofu Tutorial, 247
The 12 Healthy Habits
    1. Get Cooking, 14-49
    2. Eat Breakfast Daily, 50-75
    3. Go for Whole Grains, 76-109
    4. Get Moving, 110-131
    5. Veggie Up, 132-167
    6. Eat More Fish, 168-201
    7. Eat More Healthy Fats, 202-223
    8. Go Meatless One Day a Week, 224-247
    9. Get Stronger, 248-265
    10. Eat Less Salt, 266-285
    11. Be Portion-Aware, 286-307
    12. Eat Mindfully, 308-327

Umami Factor, 230
U.S. Department of Agriculture, 135
    MyPlate, 135

Vegetables, 132-167, 270
    Cruciferous Veggies (list), 154
    Expert Tips
      Add a Vinaigrette to Your Veggies, 151
      Be a Veggie Role Model, 140
      Incorporate the Unfamiliar, 135
      Open with Salad, 145
      Put Some Soup On, 159
    How to Buy Organic, 143
    Purchase Produce in Season, 142-143
    Reader Tips
      Consider Canned, 165
      Perfect Your Knife Skills, 149
      Prepping Veggies, 156
    Roast 1-2-3, 148
    Sauté 1-2-3, 152
    Steaming 1-2-3, 150
vegetarian, 169, 225
    Expert Tip: Forgo Faux, 233
    making adjustments to go, 226, 233
    A New View of Protein, 229
    A Quick Tofu Tutorial, 247
    and the Umami Factor, 230
    Utilize 10 All-Star Ingredients for Meatless
      Meals, 232
    What Is a Serving?, 231
volunteer, 116
    Gretchen Holt Witt, Founder of Cookies for Kids'
      Cancer, 315
    Julie Evarts, Silent Auction Charity Dinner
      Hostess, 315
    Susan Vosmik, USO Volunteer, 314

What Is a Serving?, 86, 206, 231, 291
    A Day's Worth, 291
whole grains, 51, 58, 64, 76-109, 135, 228
    and food labels, 78, 82, 83, 85
    A-Z guide, 88-91
    Blogger Tips
      Consider a Buying Club, 99
      Make a Grain Salad, 107
      Whole-Grain Meal Ideas, 98
    buying and storing, 92
    cooking, 92
    Expert Tips
      Get Started Early, 78
      Make a Grain Salad, 86
      Preventing Whole-Grain Boredom, 97
      Read the Fine Print, 85
      Rethink Your Cereal Bowl, 93
      Step Outside Your Comfort Zone, 109
    Reader Tip: Change Your Method, 95
    risottos, 228
    What Is a Serving?, 86
    What Isn't a Whole Grain, 84-85
    Whole Grains Council stamp, 83

Yogurt, 58, 70, 80, 306-307
    Things to Know About Yogurt, 259

Recipe Index

Almonds
    Cereal, Overnight Honey-Almond Multigrain, 61
    Roasted Almonds, Rosemary, 213
    Snack Mix, Sweet Chipotle, 282
    Sweet Spiced Almonds, 212
Appetizers. *See also* Snacks.
    Beef Teriyaki Crisps with Wasabi Mayonnaise, 298
    Chickpeas and Spinach with Smoky Paprika, 260
    Dips
        Artichoke, Spinach, and White Bean Dip, 165
        Guacamole with Fish Sauce, 207
        Hummus, Traditional, 162
        Hummus variation, Feta-Baked, 162
        Hummus variation, Spicy Red Pepper, 163
        Hummus variation, White Bean and Roasted
            Garlic, 162
        Muhammara with Crudites, 217
        Raita, Indian-Style, 259
        Tzatziki, Greek-Style, 259
    Mozzarella Bites, Baked, 284
    Smoked Salmon and Cheese Mini Twice-Baked
        Potatoes, 299
Apples
    Salad with Steel-Cut Oats, Waldorf, 107
    Slaw, Green Apple, 166
Apricot, Plum, and Chicken Tagine with Olives, 221
Artichoke, Spinach, and White Bean Dip, 165
Asparagus and Mushroom Sauté, Smoky, 152
Asparagus with Browned Butter, Roasted, 149
Avocados
    Chowder with Grilled Chicken, Avocado Corn, 219
    Dressing, Avocado-Herb, 218
    Guacamole with Fish Sauce, 207
    Salad, Shrimp, Avocado, and Grapefruit, 145

Bacon Mac, 318
    Bacon, Sautéed Brussels Sprouts with, 154
Bananas
    Bread, Peanut Butter Banana, 68
    French Toast, Banana-Chocolate, 65
    Smoothie, Banana Breakfast, 125
Beans. *See also* Lentils.
    Bake, Smoky Three-Bean, 261
    Black Bean Burgers with Mango Salsa, 236
    Black Bean Fiesta taco topping, 32
    Casserole, Mexican, 241
    Chickpeas
        Chili, Chickpea, 42
        Crispy Chickpea Salad with Grilled
            Prawns, 198
        Falafel Sandwiches with Yogurt-Tahini Sauce,
            Baked, 237
        Spinach with Smoky Paprika, Chickpeas
            and, 260
        Stew, Moroccan Chickpea, 239
        Stew with Brown Rice Pilaf, Curried
            Chickpea, 103
    Chili, Three-Bean Vegetarian, 235

Chili, Turkey and Bean, 280
Green Bean Stir-Fry with Peanut Sauce, Tempeh
    and, 247
Green Beans with Tomato-Garlic Vinaigrette,
    Steamed, 151
Salad, Zesty Three-Bean and Roasted Corn, 160
White
    Fish Stew with White Beans, Saffron, 194
    Pita Pockets, Southwestern White Bean, 303
    Salad, Tuna and White Bean, 201
Beef. *See also* Beef, Ground.
    Provençal Beef Daube, 43
    Steaks
        Crisp Steak Bits, Edamame Salad with, 128
        Fajita-Style Steak taco filling, 33
        Stir-Fry, Beef-Broccoli, 45
        Teriyaki Crisps with Wasabi Mayonnaise,
            Beef, 298
    Tagine with Butternut Squash, Beef, 44
    Tenderloin with Horseradish Chive Sauce, Beef, 320
Beef, Ground
    Burgers
        Blue Cheese Mayo and Sherry Vidalia Onions,
            Burgers with, 316
        100-calorie burger toppers, 317
        Out-N-In California Burger, 317
    Classic taco filling, 32
    Meat Loaf Minis, Cheesy, 40
Beverages
    Alcoholic
        Bellinis, Apricot-Ginger, 327
        Cocktail, Sparkling Pear, 299
        Margaritas, Blackberry, 326
        Tini, Satsuma Vodka-, 327
    Refresher, Carrot, Apple, and Ginger, 125
    Smoothies
        Banana Breakfast Smoothie, 125
        Peach-Mango Smoothie, 125
        Strawberry-Guava Smoothie, 125
    Virgin Mary, 134
Blueberry Oatmeal Muffins, 66
Blueberry-Orange Parfaits, 71
Bok Choy with Soy-Ginger Drizzle, Steamed Baby, 155
Breads. *See also* Muffins.
    Fig, Applesauce, and Almond Breakfast Loaf, 69
    Peanut Butter Banana Bread, 68
    Pudding, Fontina and Parmesan Mushroom
        Bread, 95
    Toasts, Goat Cheese, 157
Broccoli
    Noodles with Broccoli, Sesame, 97
    Steamed Broccoli, Simple, 150
    Stir-Fry, Beef-Broccoli, 45
Broccolini and Spicy Tofu, Udon Noodle
    Salad with, 246
Broccoli Rabe with Onions and Pine Nuts, 153
Brussels Sprouts with Bacon, Sautéed, 154
Bulgur with Dried Cranberries, 104

Candies
    Fudge, Peanut Butter and Dark Chocolate, 304
    Truffles, Date and Almond, 305
Caramel Brownies, Salted, 325
Carrots and Lentils, Turkish, 262
Carrots with Sage, Sautéed, 153
Casseroles
    Lasagna, Baked Vegetable, 234
    Macaroni and Cheese, Creamy, Light, 319
    Mexican Casserole, 241
    Moussaka, Vegetarian, 240
Cauliflower with Capers, Curried, 155
Cereal
    Muesli with Cranberries and Flaxseed, 61
    Overnight Honey-Almond Multigrain Cereal, 61
Cheese
    Bacon Mac, 318
    Bread Pudding, Fontina and Parmesan Mushroom, 95
    Casserole, Mexican, 241
    Macaroni and Cheese, Creamy, Light, 319
    Meat Loaf Minis, Cheesy, 40
    Mozzarella Bites, Baked, 284
    Toasts, Goat Cheese, 157
Cherry-Wheat Germ Muffins, 66
Chicken
    BBQ Yardbird pizza topping, The, 31
    Fried Rice, Chicken, 28
    Grilled Chicken, Avocado Corn Chowder with, 219
    Pesto Party pizza topping, The Chicken, 30
    Piccata, Meyer Lemon Chicken, 39
    Roast Chicken, Classic, 36
    Salads
        Sandwiches, Herbed Chicken Salad, 130
        Tabbouleh with Chicken and Red Bell
            Pepper, 302
        Tabbouleh with Tahini Drizzle, Chicken, 106
    Shawarma, Spicy Chicken, 35
    Stock, Roasted Chicken, 279
    Tagine with Olives, Apricot, Plum, and Chicken, 221
    Tandoori-Spiced Chicken, 38
Chili
    Chickpea Chili, 42
    Turkey and Bean Chili, 280
    Vegetarian Chili, Three-Bean, 235
Chips, Zucchini Oven, 141
Chocolate
    Brownies, Salted Caramel, 325
    French Toast, Banana-Chocolate, 65
    Fudge, Peanut Butter and Dark Chocolate, 304
    Pie, Rich Chocolate Pudding, 324
Chowder with Grilled Chicken, Avocado Corn, 219
Clams, Paella with Poblanos, Corn, and, 184
Clams, Pasta with Fresh Tomato Sauce and, 98
Coconut Mussels, Curried, 183
Corn
    Chowder with Grilled Chicken, Avocado
        Corn, 219
    Paella with Poblanos, Corn, and Clams, 184

Corn (continued)
Salad with Avocado-Herb Dressing, Roasted Corn and Radish, 218
Salad, Zesty Three-Bean and Roasted Corn, 160
Couscous, Scallion, 45
Cranberries and Flaxseed, Muesli with, 61
Cranberries, Bulgur with Dried, 104
Cucumbers
Gazpacho with Shrimp Relish, Cucumber, 258
Raita, Indian-Style, 259
Tzatziki, 25
Tzatziki, Greek-Style, 259

Date and Almond Truffles, 305
Desserts. See also Candies.
Brownies, Salted Caramel, 325
Pie, Rich Chocolate Pudding, 324
Pops, Sparkling Strawberry, 305

Edamame
Country Captain, Vegetarian, 238
Pasta with Edamame, Arugula, and Herbs, Whole-Wheat, 97
Salad with Crisp Steak Bits, Edamame, 128
Succotash, Edamame, 161
Eggplant
Bolognese, Eggplant, 98
Grilled Eggplant Pita Sandwiches with Yogurt-Garlic Spread, 49
Moussaka, Vegetarian, 240
Eggs
Baked Eggs, Simple, 72
Fried Egg, Open-Faced Sandwiches with Ricotta, Arugula, and, 75
Frittata, Summer Vegetable, 74
Mug It Up, 134
Omelet, Quick Garden, 72

Falafel Sandwiches with Yogurt-Tahini Sauce, Baked, 237
Farro Risotto with Mushrooms, 100
Fig, Applesauce, and Almond Breakfast Loaf, 69
Fish. See also Salmon, Tuna.
Arctic Char and Vegetables in Parchment Hearts, 197
Arctic Char with Blistered Cherry Tomatoes, 182
Gulf Fish en Papillote, 196
Halibut Tacos, Chimichurri, 190
Mahi & Mango taco filling, 32
Stew, Shanghai-Inspired Fish, 195
Stew with White Beans, Saffron Fish, 194
Sticks, Fancy Fish, 41
Tilapia Baja Tacos, Blackened, 190
Tilapia Gyros, Broiled, 189
Tilapia Tacos with Grilled Peppers and Onions, Sautéed, 191
Trout with Tomato-Basil Sauté, Pan-Fried, 181
French Toast, Banana-Chocolate, 65
Frittata, Summer Vegetable, 74

Glaze, Acorn Squash Wedges with Maple-Harissa, 156
Glaze, Salmon with Hoisin, 187
Grape and Yogurt Parfaits, Slow-Roasted, 71

Grilled
Chicken, Avocado Corn Chowder with Grilled, 219
Eggplant Pita Sandwiches with Yogurt-Garlic Spread, Grilled, 49
Fish and Shellfish
Halibut Tacos, Chimichurri, 190
King Salmon with Tomato-Peach Salsa, Grilled, 187
Prawns, Crispy Chickpea Salad with Grilled, 198
Salmon Burgers, 188
Tilapia Tacos with Grilled Peppers and Onions, Sautéed, 191
Guacamole with Fish Sauce, 207

Hummus
Sandwiches, Open-Faced Hummus, 131
Traditional Hummus, 162
Feta-Baked Hummus variation, 162
Spicy Red Pepper Hummus variation, 163
White Bean and Roasted Garlic Hummus variation, 162

Kale, Caramelized Onions, and Parsnips, Pasta with Black, 242

Lamb
Meatballs with Spiced Yogurt Sauce, Kibbeh, 34
Shepherd's Pie, Moroccan, 296
Sloppy Lentils in Pita, 263
Lasagna, Baked Vegetable, 234
Lemon Chicken Piccata, Meyer, 39
Lentils in Pita, Sloppy, 263
Lentils, Turkish Carrots and, 262
Lime Salsa, Tomatillo-, 277
Linguine with Shrimp and Veggies, Creamy, 127
Linguine with Two-Olive Marinara, 220
Lunch ideas for kids
Beefy Sandwich, 274
Chicken Salad, 274
For the Rabbits, 274
Whole-Wheat PB&J, 274

Mango Salsa, Black Bean Burgers with, 236
Mango taco filling, Mahi &, 32
Mayo and Sherry Vidalia Onions, Burgers with Blue Cheese, 316
Mayonnaise, Beef Teriyaki Crisps with Wasabi, 298
Meatballs with Spiced Yogurt Sauce, Kibbeh, 34
Meatless crumbles
Casserole, Mexican, 241
Meat Loaf Minis, Cheesy, 40
Melon Gazpacho with Frizzled Prosciutto, 301
Millet and Confetti Vegetable Salad with Sesame and Soy Dressing, Toasted, 108
Muesli with Cranberries and Flaxseed, 61
Muffins
Blueberry Oatmeal Muffins, 66
Cherry-Wheat Germ Muffins, 66
Pistachio-Chai Muffins, 67

Mushrooms
Bread Pudding, Fontina and Parmesan Mushroom, 95
Risotto, Mushroom–Brown Rice, 101
Risotto with Mushrooms, Farro, 100
Sauce, Mushroom, 25
Sauté, Smoky Asparagus and Mushroom, 152
Stock, Mushroom, 101
Tuna, Sesame Albacore, 180
Mussels, Curried Coconut, 183

Noodles
Pad Thai, Shrimp, 29
Sesame Noodles with Broccoli, 97
Udon Noodle Salad with Broccolini and Spicy Tofu, 246

Oatmeal
Muffins, Blueberry Oatmeal, 66
Pancakes, Oatmeal, 65
Rise and Shine Oatmeal, 60
Toppings
Adventurous, 63
Chewy, 62
Crunchy, 63
Fruity, 63
Savory, 63
Sweet, 62
Olive Marinara, Linguine with Two-, 220
Onions
Broccoli Rabe with Onions and Pine Nuts, 153
Caramelized Onions, and Parsnips, Pasta with Black Kale, 242
Chimichurri, Zingy, 276
Farfalle with Roasted Peppers, Onions, Feta, and Mint, Mini, 126
Grilled Peppers and Onions, Sautéed Tilapia Tacos with, 191
Scallion Couscous, 45
Soup, French Onion and Apple, 300
Vidalia Onions, Burgers with Blue Cheese Mayo and Sherry, 316
Orange Chipotle Spiced Pecan Mix, 213
Oysters with Garlic-Buttered Breadcrumbs, Broiled, 183

Paella with Poblanos, Corn, and Clams, 184
Pancakes, Oatmeal, 65
Pancakes, Whole-Wheat Buttermilk, 64
Pasta. See also Noodles.
Bacon Mac, 318
Black Kale, Caramelized Onions, and Parsnips, Pasta with, 242
Farfalle with Roasted Peppers, Onions, Feta, and Mint, Mini, 126
Macaroni and Cheese, Creamy, Light, 319
Peppery Pasta with Arugula and Shrimp, 192
Puttanesca, Pasta, 193
Tomato Sauce and Clams, Pasta with Fresh, 98
Whole-Wheat Pasta with Edamame, Arugula, and Herbs, 97
Peanut Butter
Bread, Peanut Butter Banana, 68

Fudge, Peanut Butter and Dark Chocolate, 304
Sandwiches, Peanut Butter Plus, 264
Peas
Black-Eyed Pea and Tomato Salsa, 164
Green Pea Gazpacho, Fresh, 301
Snow Peas, Garlicky-Spicy, 187
Snow Peas, Sautéed, 153
Sugar Snap Peas, Steamed, 150
Sweet Pea Relish, Seared Scallops with Lemony, 185
Pecan Mix, Orange Chipotle Spiced, 213
Peppers
Chile
Chipotle Snack Mix, Sweet, 282
Chipotle Spiced Pecan Mix, Orange, 213
Poblanos, Corn, and Clams, Paella with, 184
Grilled Peppers and Onions, Sautéed Tilapia Tacos with, 191
Muhammara with Crudites, 217
Pico de Gallo, 277
Red and Yellow Peppers, Pork Tenderloin with, 46
Red Bell Pepper, Tabbouleh with Chicken and, 302
Roasted Peppers, Onions, Feta, and Mint, Mini Farfalle with, 126
Pesto, Cilantro-Walnut, 216
Pesto, Sicilian, 276
Pickles, Easy Refrigerator, 279
Pie, Moroccan Shepherd's, 296
Pie, Rich Chocolate Pudding, 324
Pilaf
Brown Rice Pilaf, Curried Chickpea Stew with, 103
Multigrain Pilaf with Sunflower Seeds, 104
Roasted Pumpkin and Sweet Potato Pilaf, 158
Pineapple
Caramelized Pineapple, Asian, 167
Happy Hawaiian pizza topping, The, 30
Pizza
Farmers' Market Pizza, Local, 244
Roasted Vegetable and Ricotta Pizza, 245
Topping combinations
Bagel-and-Lox Treatment, The, 30
BBQ Yardbird, The, 31
Can't-Beet-This Combo, The, 30
Chicken Pesto Party, The, 30
Farmers' Market, The, 31
Greek Austerity Cure, The, 31
Happy Hawaiian, The, 30
Peppery Pig, The, 31
Pomegranate-Orange Salsa, 166
Popcorn, Maple-Chile, 283
Pork. See also Bacon.
Chops, Smoky Pan-Grilled Pork 47
Fried Rice, Almost Classic Pork, 94
Peppery Pig pizza topping, The, 31
Prosciutto, Melon Gazpacho with Frizzled, 301
Tenderloin
Red and Yellow Peppers, Pork Tenderloin with, 46
Roast Pork Tenderloin with Plum Barbecue Sauce, 321
Soup, Pork and Wild Rice, 102
Potatoes. See also Sweet Potatoes.
Baked Potato, Spinach, 323

Microwave Smashed Potatoes, 322
Bacon and Cheddar variation, 323
Roasted Garlic variation, 323
Southwest variation, 322
Roasted Potatoes with Thyme and Garlic, 148
Truffled Roasted Potatoes, 285
Twice-Baked Potatoes, Smoked Salmon and Cheese, Mini, 299
Pudding, Fontina and Parmesan Mushroom Bread, 95
Pumpkin and Sweet Potato Pilaf, Roasted, 158
Pumpkin Parfait, 134

Quinoa and Parsley, Salad, 109
Quinoa with Roasted Garlic, Tomato, and Spinach, 105

Relish, Cucumber Gazpacho with Shrimp, 258
Relish, Seared Scallops with Lemony Sweet Pea, 185
Rice
Brown Rice Pilaf, Curried Chickpea Stew with, 103
Brown Rice Risotto, Mushroom–, 101
Fried Rice, Almost Classic Pork, 94
Fried Rice, Chicken, 28
Paella with Poblanos, Corn, and Clams, 184
Wild Rice Soup, Pork and, 102
Risotto
Brown Rice Risotto, Mushroom–, 101
Farro Risotto with Mushrooms, 100
Lemon-Vegetable Risotto, Summer, 243

Salads and Salad Dressings
Avocado-Herb Dressing, 218
Chicken Salad Sandwiches, Herbed, 130
Chickpea Salad with Grilled Prawns, Crispy, 198
Edamame Salad with Crisp Steak Bits, 128
Green Goddess Dressing, Four-Herb, 259
Honey Balsamic Arugula Salad, 144
Quinoa and Parsley Salad, 109
Roasted Corn and Radish Salad with Avocado-Herb Dressing, 218
Shrimp, Avocado, and Grapefruit Salad, 145
Shrimp Cobb Salad, 129
Slaw, Cabbage, 33
Slaw, Green Apple, 166
Spinach-Strawberry Salad, 167
Tabbouleh with Chicken and Red Bell Pepper, 302
Tabbouleh with Tahini Drizzle, Chicken, 106
Three-Bean and Roasted Corn Salad, Zesty, 160
Toasted Millet and Confetti Vegetable Salad with Sesame and Soy Dressing, 108
Toppers for salads
Californian, 146
Classic Caprese, 147
Greek, 147
Nuts, Berries & Blue, 146
Perfect Pear-Up, 147
Protein-Packed, 146
Southwestern, 146
Tuna Salad, Pan-Grilled Thai, 199
Udon Noodle Salad with Broccolini and Spicy Tofu, 246
Vinaigrette
Champagne Vinaigrette, 223

Easy Herb Vinaigrette, 223
Mustard Seed-Chive Vinaigrette, 223
Sesame Vinaigrette, 223
Waldorf Salad with Steel-Cut Oats, 107
Wheat Berry Salad with Raisins and Pistachios, 107
Salmon
Burgers, Salmon, 188
Cakes with Lemon-Garlic Aioli, Cajun Salmon, 200
Hoisin Glaze, Salmon with, 187
King Salmon with Tomato-Peach Salsa, Grilled, 187
Maple-Glazed Salmon, 186
Sandwiches, Salmon, 48
Smoked Salmon and Cheese Mini Twice-Baked Potatoes, 299
Salsas
Black-Eyed Pea and Tomato Salsa, 164
Mango Salsa, Black Bean Burgers with, 236
Pomegranate-Orange Salsa, 166
Tomatillo-Lime Salsa, 277
Tomato-Peach Salsa, Grilled King Salmon with, 187
Verde, Salsa, 164
Sandwiches
Baked Falafel Sandwiches with Yogurt-Tahini Sauce, 237
Burger, Out-N-In California, 317
Burgers, Salmon, 188
Burgers with Blue Cheese Mayo and Sherry Vidalia Onions, 316
Burgers with Mango Salsa, Black Bean, 236
Chicken Salad Sandwiches, Herbed, 130
Grilled Eggplant Pita Sandwiches with Yogurt-Garlic Spread, 49
Gyros, Broiled Tilapia, 189
Open-Faced Hummus Sandwiches, 131
Open-Faced Pimiento Cheese BLTs, 49
Open-Faced Sandwiches with Ricotta, Arugula, and Fried Egg, 75
Peanut Butter Plus Sandwiches, 264
Pita Pockets, Southwestern White Bean, 303
Salmon Sandwiches, 48
Shawarma, Spicy Chicken, 35
Sloppy Lentils in Pita, 263
Tuna Sandwiches, Tuscan, 131
Sauces. See also Glaze, Pesto, Relish, Salsas, Toppings.
Barbecue Sauce, Tangy Coffee, 277
Bolognese, Eggplant, 98
Chimichurri, 25
Chimichurri, Zingy, 276
Horseradish Chive Sauce, Beef Tenderloin with, 320
Marinara, Basic, 278
Marinara, Linguine with Two-Olive, 220
Mushroom Sauce, 25
Peanut Sauce, Tempeh and Green Bean Stir-Fry with, 247
Pico de Gallo, 277
Plum Barbecue Sauce, Roast Pork Tenderloin with, 321
Puttanesca, Pasta, 193
Tomato Sauce and Clams, Pasta with Fresh, 98
Yogurt Sauce, Kibbeh Meatballs with Spiced, 34

Sauces (continued)
  Yogurt-Tahini Sauce, Baked Falafel Sandwiches
    with, 237
Scallops with Lemony Sweet Pea Relish, Seared, 185
Shrimp
  Baked Shrimp with Tomatoes, 297
  Crustacean Crunch taco filling, 33
  Linguine with Shrimp and Veggies, Creamy, 127
  Pad Thai, Shrimp, 29
  Pasta with Arugula and Shrimp, Peppery, 192
  Relish, Cucumber Gazpacho with Shrimp, 258
  Salad, Shrimp, Avocado, and Grapefruit, 145
  Salad, Shrimp Cobb, 129
Slow Cooker
  Beef Daube, Provençal, 43
  Chili, Chickpea, 42
Snacks
  Almonds, Rosemary Roasted, 213
  Almonds, Sweet Spiced, 212
  Chips, Zucchini Oven, 141
  Mix, Orange Chipotle Spiced Pecan, 213
  Mix, Sweet Chipotle Snack, 282
  Popcorn, Maple-Chile, 283
Soups. See also Chili, Stews.
  Chowder with Grilled Chicken, Avocado Corn, 219
  French Onion and Apple Soup, 300
  Gazpacho
    Cucumber Gazpacho with Shrimp Relish, 258
    Green Pea Gazpacho, Fresh, 301
    Melon Gazpacho with Frizzled Prosciutto, 301
  Pork and Wild Rice Soup, 102
  Roasted Butternut Squash Soup, 157
  Squash Soup, Indian-Spiced Roasted, 159
  Stock, Mushroom, 101
  Stock, Roasted Chicken, 279
  Tomato Soup, Double, 281
Spinach
  Chickpeas and Spinach with Smoky Paprika, 260
  Dip, Artichoke, Spinach, and White Bean, 165
  Potato, Spinach Baked, 323
  Salad, Spinach-Strawberry, 167
Spreads. See also Mayonnaise.
  Butter, Roasted Asparagus with Browned, 149
  Yogurt-Garlic Spread, Grilled Eggplant Pita
    Sandwiches with, 49
Squash. See also Zucchini.
  Acorn Squash Wedges with Maple-Harissa Glaze, 156
  Butternut
    Beef Tagine with Butternut Squash, 44
    Macaroni and Cheese, Creamy, Light, 319
    Roasted Butternut Squash Soup, 157
  Roasted Squash Soup, Indian-Spiced, 159
Stews. See also Chili, Soups, Tagine.
  Chickpea Stew, Moroccan, 239
  Chickpea Stew with Brown Rice Pilaf, Curried, 103
  Country Captain, Vegetarian, 238
  Fish Stew, Shanghai-Inspired, 195
  Fish Stew with White Beans, Saffron, 194
  Strawberry Pops, Sparkling, 305
  Strawberry Salad, Spinach-, 167
  Succotash, Edamame, 161
Sustainable Choice
  Arctic Char with Blistered Cherry Tomatoes, 182

Blackened Tilapia Baja Tacos, 190
Broiled Oysters with Garlic-Buttered
  Breadcrumbs, 183
Broiled Tilapia Gyros, 189
Chimichurri Halibut Tacos, 190
Curried Coconut Mussels, 183
Maple-Glazed Salmon, 186
Paella with Poblanos, Corn, and Clams, 184
Pan-Fried Trout with Tomato Basil Sauté, 181
Peppery Pasta with Arugula and Shrimp, 192
Saffron Fish Stew with White Beans, 194
Seared Scallops with Lemony Sweet Pea Relish, 185
Sweet Potatoes
  Roasted Pumpkin and Sweet Potato Pilaf, 158
  Shepherd's Pie, Moroccan, 296

Tabbouleh with Chicken and Red Bell Pepper, 302
Tabbouleh with Tahini Drizzle, Chicken, 106
Tacos
  Fillings
    Black Bean Fiesta, 32
    Classic, 32
    Crustacean Crunch, 33
    Fajita-Style Steak, 33
    Mahi & Mango, 32
    Maine-Mex, 33
  Halibut Tacos, Chimichurri, 190
  Tilapia Baja Tacos, Blackened, 190
  Tilapia Tacos with Grilled Peppers and Onions,
    Sautéed, 191
Tagine with Butternut Squash, Beef, 44
Tagine with Olives, Apricot, Plum, and Chicken, 221
Tempeh and Green Bean Stir-Fry with Peanut Sauce, 247
Tofu
  Lasagna, Baked Vegetable, 234
  Salad with Broccolini and Spicy Tofu, Udon
    Noodle, 246
Tomatillos
  Salsa, Tomatillo-Lime, 277
  Salsa Verde, 164
Tomatoes. See also Sauces.
  Baked Shrimp with Tomatoes, 297
  Cherry Tomatoes, Arctic Char with Blistered, 182
  Pesto, Sicilian, 276
  Pico de Gallo, 277
  Quinoa with Roasted Garlic, Tomato, and Spinach, 105
  Raita, Indian-Style, 259
  Salsa, Black-Eyed Pea and Tomato, 164
  Salsa, Grilled King Salmon with Tomato-Peach, 187
  Sauté, Pan-Fried Trout with Tomato-Basil, 181
  Soup, Double Tomato, 281
  Vinaigrette, Steamed Green Beans with Tomato-
    Garlic, 151
Toppings
  Garlic-Buttered Breadcrumbs, Broiled Oysters
    with, 183
  Lemon-Garlic Aioli, Cajun Salmon Cakes with, 200
  Ponzu, 25
  Soy-Ginger Drizzle, Steamed Baby Bok Choy with, 155
  Tomato-Basil Sauté, Pan-Fried Trout with, 181
  Tomato-Garlic Vinaigrette, Steamed Green Beans
    with, 151

Tzatziki, 25
Wasabi Cream, 25
Tuna
  Salad, Pan-Grilled Thai Tuna, 199
  Salad, Tuna and White Bean, 201
  Sandwiches, Tuscan Tuna, 131
  Sesame Albacore Tuna, 180
Turkey
  Chili, Turkey and Bean, 280
  Happy Hawaiian pizza topping, The, 30
  Tenders, Turkey, 41
Tzatziki, 25
Tzatziki, Greek-Style, 259

Vegetables. See also specific types.
  Arctic Char and Vegetables in Parchment Hearts, 197
  Farmers' Market pizza topping, The, 31
  Frittata, Summer Vegetable, 74
  Lasagna, Baked Vegetable, 234
  Linguine with Shrimp and Veggies, Creamy, 127
  Omelet, Quick Garden, 72
  Pizza, Local Farmers' Market, 244
  Pizza, Roasted Vegetable and Ricotta, 245
  Risotto, Summer Lemon-Vegetable, 243
  Salad with Sesame and Soy Dressing, Toasted Millet
    and Confetti Vegetable, 108

Walnuts
  Muhammara with Crudites, 217
  Pesto, Cilantro-Walnut, 216
  Yogurt Parfaits, Slow-Roasted Grape and, 71
Wasabi Cream, 25
Wasabi Mayonnaise, Beef Teriyaki Crisps with, 298
Wheat Berry Salad with Raisins and Pistachios, 107
Wheat Germ Muffins, Cherry-, 66
Whole-Wheat Buttermilk Pancakes, 64
Whole-Wheat Pasta with Edamame, Arugula, and
  Herbs, 97

Yogurt
  Frozen yogurt toppers
    15 calories, 307
    50 calories, 306
    70 calories, 306
    85 calories, 307
    125 calories, 306, 307
    155 calories, 307
    160 calories, 306
  Parfaits
    Blueberry-Orange Parfaits, 71
    Greek Yogurt Parfaits, 70
    Pumpkin Parfait, 134
    Slow-Roasted Grape and Yogurt Parfaits, 71
  Raita, Indian-Style, 259
  Sauce, Baked Falafel Sandwiches with
    Yogurt-Tahini, 237
  Sauce, Kibbeh Meatballs with Spiced Yogurt, 34
  Spread, Grilled Eggplant Pita Sandwiches with
    Yogurt-Garlic, 49
  Tzatziki, Greek-Style, 259

Zucchini Oven Chips, 141